Treatment and Prognosis

PAEDIATRICS

Edited by

Graham Clayden MD, FRCP

and

Richard Hawkins MBBS, FRCS

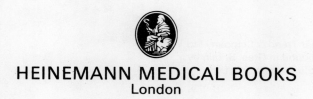

HEINEMANN MEDICAL BOOKS
London

Heinemann Medical Books,
22 Bedford Square,
London WC1B 3HH

ISBN: 0–433–06010–7

© Graham Clayden and Richard Hawkins, 1988

First published 1988

British Library Cataloguing-in-Publication Data

Paediatrics. — (Treatment and prognosis).
 1. Pediatrics   2. Prognosis
 I. Clayden, Graham S.   II. Hawkins,
 Richard, 1949–   III. Series
 618.92'075   RJ47

 ISBN 0–433–06010–7

Typeset by Latimer Trend & Company Ltd
and printed and bound in Great Britain by
Biddles Ltd, Guildford and King's Lynn

Contents

Foreword

A Breckenridge MD, MSc, FRCP
Professor of Clinical Pharmacology, University of Liverpool

For many years most medical textbooks have tended to concentrate on the pathogenesis and clinical features of disease rather than their treatment and prognosis. Yet it is in these latter areas where most progress has taken place recently. It is our intention and hope that both the young hospital doctor working for higher examinations and his more senior colleague requiring updating will be informed and helped by the *Treatment and Prognosis* series.

The main subject areas in each discipline are covered and while perforce large and important topics must be dealt with briefly, the editorial board is happy that the correct emphasis and balance has been given to the individual disease entities. Further, the distinguished panel of authors has been disciplined to adopt a reasonably uniform mode of presentation which will ease assimilation.

The *Treatment and Prognosis* series is written clearly to allow a succinct and up-to-date picture of those important aspects of modern disease management to emerge, which will be particularly appealing to the busy clinical doctor.

Preface

The successful management of sick children depends upon an up-to-date knowledge of treatment options, coupled with an understanding of the natural history of disease and how treatment options may influence it.

This book provides that information in a concise, easily accessible form geared to meet the needs of busy clinicians. For those working in hospital it maps out areas of essential treatment and provides supporting references. For those preparing for examinations it provides a base of knowledge especially valuable in 'long case' discussions on management. For general practitioners it will inform and update on procedures which a child may need in a specialist centre as well as proving a guide to treatment which can be started at home.

For ease of reference the format for each topic is identical. There is an initial account of the disease or condition containing relevant details of pathology and epidemiology. This is followed by sections on treatment, prognosis and, where appropriate, follow-up. To retain conciseness and avoid repetition it has not been possible to include for each topic the measures which should be taken to support the child and family through the unavoidable anxieties of investigation, the shock of an adverse prognosis and the rigours of treatment, but this does not mean that we underestimate the importance of these issues.

We note a healthy trend towards shared care between specialist centres, local paediatricians and general practitioners in such conditions as cystic fibrosis, asthma, epilepsy, diabetes, eczema, migraine and many others. We hope this book will go some way towards assisting and encouraging this development.

GS Clayden

RL Hawkins

List of contributors

MH Bellman MD, MRCP, DCH
Consultant Paediatrician, The Royal National Throat, Nose and Ear Hospital, London

SC Bellman MA, MB, BChir, FRCSI, DLO
Consultant Audiological Physician, The Hospital for Sick Children, London

IW Booth MSc, BSc, MBBS, MRCP, DCH, DObs, RCOG
Senior Lecturer in Paediatrics, University of Birmingham

DCA Candy MSc, MBBS, MRCP
Senior Lecturer in Paediatric Gastroenterology, University of Birmingham

GS Clayden MD, FRCP
Senior Lecturer in Paediatrics, United Medical and Dental Schools of Guy's and St. Thomas's Hospitals, London

AE Fryer BSc, MBBS, MRCP
Senior Registrar in Genetics, University Hospital of Wales, Cardiff

C Garrett MBBS, FRCP, MRCP, MRCS, LRCP
Consultant in Clinical Genetics, Royal Devon and Exeter Hospital, Wonford

JDM Gould BScEd, MB, ChB, MRCP, DObst, RCOG, DCH, RCPS
Consultant in Paediatrics, The Ipswich Hospital, Ipswich

J Graham-Pole MD
Associate Professor, University of Florida, Gainesville

GW Harley MBBS, DO, FRACO
Head of Ophthalmology Unit, Royal Children's Hospital, Melbourne

JI Harper MD, MRCP
Consultant in Paediatric Dermatology, The Hospital for Sick Children, London

JA Hulse MD, MRCP
Senior Registrar, Department of Paediatrics, St Thomas's Hospital, London

WB Knight MBBS, FRACP, MRCP
Paediatric Cardiologist, The Adelaide Children's Hospital, Adelaide

TJ Meredith MA, MRCP
Department of Medicine, Guy's Hospital, London

G du Mont
Senior Lecturer in Paediatrics, United Medical and Dental Schools of Guy's and St. Thomas's Hospitals, London

J O'Day MBBS, FRACS, FRACP, FRCS, FRACO, DO(Melb.)
Senior Ophthalmic Surgeon, St Vincent's Hospital, Melbourne

JP Osborne MBBS, MD, MRCP, DCH, DObs, RCOG
Consultant Paediatrician, Royal United Hospital, Bath

JF Price MD, FRCP
Consultant Paediatrician, King's College Hospital, London

SPA Rigden MBBS, MRCP
Senior Lecturer, United Medical and Dental Schools of Guy's and St. Thomas's Hospitals, London

D Roberts MB, ChB, MRCP
Research Registrar in Paediatrics, St. Thomas's Hospital and Guy's Hospital, London

RO Robinson FRCP
Consultant Paediatric Neurologist, Guy's Hospital, London

K Simmer MBBS, PhD, MRCP
Consultant Neonatologist, The Adelaide Children's Hospital, Adelaide

MS Tanner MSc, BSc, MBBS, MRCP, MRCS, LRCP, DCH
Senior Lecturer, Leicester Royal Infirmary, Leicester

JA Vale MD, FRCP
West Midlands Poisons Unit, Dudley Road Hospital, Birmingham, and the University of Birmingham

SN Wolkind MD, FRCPsych
Consultant Child Psychiatrist, Maudsley Hospital, London

Disease directory

13 Diseases of the ear   239

14 Diseases of the skin   249

1
Inherited and Congenital Conditions

C. Garrett

Down's Syndrome

The extra chromosome 21 in Down's syndrome gives rise to a recognisable pattern of abnormalities and is the commonest cause of severe intellectual retardation, occurring in 1 in 700 births. The mean adult height for males is 155 cm and for females is 145 cm.

TREATMENT

1. A multidisciplinary approach is needed involving both hospital and community services.
2. Congenital heart disease: surgical or medical treatment, with penicillin prophylaxis.
3. Gastrointestinal and other malformations: surgical treatment.
4. Hypothyroidism: thyroxine replacement therapy.
5. Visual and hearing defect: treatment and hearing aids.
6. Plastic surgery to alter appearance and correct macroglossia has been advocated but is not generally accepted[1].
7. Megavitamins and minerals[2], in common with other treatments such as 5-hydroxytryptamine and dimethylsulfoxide, have no beneficial effects[3].
8. Provision for special educational needs: the trend now is to integrate the children into normal schools where possible.
9. Teaching of communication skills is especially important.
10. Early intervention infant stimulation programmes may be beneficial but further studies are needed[4].
11. Difficult behaviour: guidance for parents and school.
12. Support for parents in coping with the emotional repercussions of having a handicapped child.

PROGNOSIS

- Mortality is decreasing as a result of antibiotics and cardiac surgery. 75% survive to 5 years, and 50% to middle age[5].
- Intelligence varies from dull normal to profoundly retarded, and tends to decline with age. Mean IQ at 2 years is 56, at 4 is 46 and at 11 is 37[6]. Girls score higher than boys, and those at home higher than in institutions. Birthweight and hypotonia are useful predictors. Mosaics may be less severely affected.
- Some of these children learn to read and write while others do not develop speech. Most have a happy personality and social skills exceeding those expected for their mental age.
- 13% have serious behaviour problems, e.g. hyperkinesia.
- Less than 5% develop seizures.
- Premature ageing and degenerative brain changes similar to Alzheimer's disease occur in older patients[7].
- Visual problems include strabismus 33%, myopia 33%, nystagmus 15%, keratoconus 6% and cataract 1%. Blindness occurs in 5%.
- Conductive deafness is common, and sensorineural deafness is three times more frequent than normal.
- Congenital heart disease (20–40%) is a major cause of early mortality. Main defects are atrioventricular canal, ventricular septal defect (VSD), patent ductus arteriosus (PDA) and atrial septal defect (ASD).
- Gastrointestinal malformations (5%) include duodenal atresia, atresia of jejunum, ileum or oesophagus, pyloric stenosis, mega- or microcolon, anal atresia and exomphalos.
- Respiratory infections are very common and there is a general predisposition to infection.
- Congenital hypothyroidism occurs in 1%. 17% adults are hypothyroid and 2.5% are hyperthyroid. 33% have antithyroid antibodies[8]. The incidence of other autoimmune disorders is increased.
- Acute leukaemia (1%) occurs in both children and adults: overall survival is lower than normally expected.
- Atlanto-axial instability occurs in 10–20%, but rarely causes complications. Hip dislocation is more common than normal.
- Males have cryptorchidism (14%), low libido

and sperm counts, and are probably infertile. Pregnancies have been reported in females, resulting in both Down's syndrome and normal offspring.

- Karyotypes: primary trisomy 21 (92%), mosaics (3%), translocations (5%: of which half are familial).
- The recurrence risk after a trisomy 21 child born to a young mother is 1%. After translocation it depends on the type of translocation and which parent is the carrier.
- Risk of trisomy 21 increases with maternal age, from 1 in 1500 at 25, to 1 in 350 at 35, and 1 in 100 at 40.

FOLLOW-UP

Regular assessment of the physical, educational and social needs of the child are necessary. Genetic counselling and prenatal diagnosis should be available for future pregnancies.

[1] Rozner L (1983) *Lancet*, **i,** 1320.
[2] Smith G et al. (1984) *J. Pediatr.*, **105,** 228.
[3] de la Cruz F F et al. (1981) *Trisomy 21 Research Perspectives*. Baltimore: University Park Press.
[4] Bricker D et al. (1981) *Paediatrics*, **67,** 45.
[5] Scholl T et al. (1982) *Dev. Med. Child Neurol.*, **24,** 817.
[6] Carr J (1985) In *Current Approaches to Down's Syndrome* (Lan D, Stratford B eds.) pp. 167–86. London: Holt, Rinehart & Winston.
[7] Gath A (1981) *Dev. Med. Child Neurol.*, **23,** 814.
[8] Fort P et al. (1984) *J. Pediatr.*, **104,** 545.

Klinefelter's Syndrome

Klinefelter's syndrome, with the chromosome complement 47 XXY, affects 1 in 500 males, resulting in hypogonadism, delayed puberty and infertility. Affected boys may have intellectual and behaviour problems and are relatively tall and thin with long legs.

TREATMENT

1. Speech therapy, remedial teaching and psychiatric referral if necessary.
2. Testosterone replacement therapy improves secondary sex characteristics but does not affect fertility. After the age of 12 years, small doses of testosterone (e.g. testosterone enanthate 50 mg i.m. every 3 weeks), increasing to 250 mg three weekly by the age of 15–17 years[1].
3. Cosmetic surgery for gynaecomastia.

PROGNOSIS

- Follow-up after newborn screening studies shows the effects to be milder than previously thought[2].
- Inadequate virilization to a variable degree, with small testes (less than 2.5 cm diameter in adults), small penis, delayed puberty, low testosterone and raised FSH at puberty, gynaecomastia.
- Infertility and azoospermia are features. Mosaics (20%) may be fertile.

- There is increased growth velocity, and a low upper/lower segment ratio. These individuals are tall and thin as adolescents.
- Verbal IQ is 10–15 points below siblings.
- There is language delay (50%).
- 30% have delayed emotional maturity, and learning and behaviour problems.
- There is an increased incidence of diabetes, breast cancer, and varicose veins.
- The syndrome is associated with raised maternal age, but the recurrence risk is not increased.
- The severity of retardation and number of abnormalities increases with the number of extra X chromosomes.

FOLLOW-UP

Follow-up should be yearly, and every 3–6 months during puberty.

[1] Caldwell P D et al. (1972) *J. Pediatr.*, **80,** 250.
[2] Ratcliffe S G et al. (1982) *Arch. Dis. Childh.*, **57,** 6.

Turner's Syndrome

Turner's syndrome, due to a missing or abnormal X chromosome, results in short stature, sexual infantilism and characteristic phenotypic features. One in 5000 girls is affected.

TREATMENT

1. Oestrogen replacement therapy is required from the age of 11 years until the menopause. This produces a growth spurt, but does not affect final height. Oestrogen produces breast development and menstruation and protects against osteoporosis and premature ageing. Small doses are given initially (e.g. as ethinyl oestradiol 5 μg daily continuously) and increased gradually to 20 μg daily over 1–2 years. Larger doses over a shorter time may cause nipple and areolar enlargement without adequate breast development. Progesterone (e.g. as norethisterone acetate 350 μg daily for 1 week in 4) should be given with doses of ethinyl oestradiol over 10 μg, or if breakthrough bleeding occurs. The combined pill (e.g. Loestrin 20, containing ethinyl oestradiol 20 μg and norethisterone acetate 1 mg) can then be substituted for the two separate drugs[1].
2. The effect of very small doses of oestrogen given prepubertally on final height is under investigation[2].
3. Low doses of androgens may increase final height but this is controversial[3].
4. Coarctation is treated surgically. Penicillin prophylaxis is required for congenital heart defects. Hypertension must be controlled.
5. Antibiotics and/or myringotomy for otitis media.
6. Orthodontic treatment as necessary.
7. Cosmetic surgery (e.g. for neck webbing) should be undertaken with care, because of keloid formation.
8. Attention should be paid to diet to prevent obesity.

PROGNOSIS

- Adult height is 142 ± 6 cm, and is influenced by parents' height. There is decreased growth velocity and no growth spurt[1].
- Ovaries are present in the fetus but then degenerate, becoming streaks. Amenorrhoea, absent secondary sex characteristics and high FSH levels occur at puberty. Patients are rarely fertile, and offspring are frequently abnormal[4].
- Coarctation of the aorta occurs in 20% and bicuspid aortic valve in 34%.
- Renal anomalies, especially horseshoe kidney or duplication, occur in 50%.
- Unexplained hypertension is present in 27%.
- Other features include typical facies, short web neck (50%); low posterior hair line (75%); low set prominent ears (80%); micrognathia (70%); narrow maxilla (80%); naevi (60%); and dental irregularities.
- In infants there is a tendency for redundant neck skin, lymphoedema (40%), and hypoplastic and hyperconvex finger nails (75%).
- Conductive deafness occurs in 50%.
- Telangiectasia of bowel occurs in 5%.
- There is an association with antithyroid antibodies and Crohn's disease.
- A tendency to obesity is common.
- IQ is normal but there may be difficulty with visuospatial relationships and maths.
- There may be premature ageing and osteoporosis, but life span is normal without cardiac anomalies and hypertension.
- 99% of affected fetuses abort spontaneously.
- Recurrence risk not increased after an affected child.
- 55% karyotypes are 45 X. Mosaics and structural rearrangements (45%) may be less severely affected.

FOLLOW-UP

These patients should be reviewed yearly, then 3–6 monthly during puberty. Blood pressure, height and weight should be measured.

[1] Brook C G D (1986) *Arch. Dis. Childh.*, **61**, 305.
[2] Ross J L et al. (1983) *New Eng. J. Med.*, **309**, 1104.
[3] Moore D C et al. (1977) *J. Pediatr.*, **90**, 462.
[4] Nielsen J et al. (1979) *Br. J. Obstet. Gynaecol.*, **68**, 833.

Trisomy 13 (Patau Syndrome)

The extra chromosome 13 in Patau syndrome causes a recognisable pattern of congenital malformations[1], including hare lip, polydactyly and microphthalmia, with severe developmental retardation. One in 8000 babies is affected, and few survive beyond one year.

TREATMENT

Treatment is supportive, since the prognosis is uniformly poor. The clinical picture should lead to early diagnosis, so that decisions to intervene medically or surgically can be made in full knowledge of the prognosis.

PROGNOSIS

- 50% die within one month, 80% by one year. Long-term survivors are rare, and are severely retarded[2].
- 5% are mosaics and are less severely affected.
- Characteristic defects are cleft lip and/or palate (60–80%), postaxial polydactyly (60%), microphthalmia, iris coloboma, scalp defects, capillary haemangioma, cryptorchidism and abnormal low set ears.
- 80% have congenital heart defects, often VSD or ASD.
- 60% have renal anomalies, e.g. polycystic kidneys.
- 5% have holoprosencephaly with defects of the forebrain and olfactory and optic nerves.
- Primary trisomy 13 is associated with raised maternal age. The recurrence risk is less than 1%.
- 20% are due to a translocation. The recurrence risk is 2% if a parent is a translocation carrier.

FOLLOW-UP

Genetic counselling should be offered; prenatal diagnosis by amniocentesis is available for future pregnancies.

---

[1] Hodes M E *et al.* (1978) *J. Med. Genet.*, **15,** 48.
[2] Redheendran R *et al.* (1981) *Am. J. Med. Genet.*, **8,** 167.

Trisomy 18 (Edward Syndrome)

The extra chromosome 18 in Edward syndrome causes severe developmental and growth retardation, with a characteristic pattern of congenital malformations[1]. Features include small chin, prominent occiput, low set malformed ears, clenched hands with overlapping fingers, rocker-bottom feet, short sternum and cryptorchidism. Of the 1 in 6000 babies affected, few reach the age of one year.

TREATMENT

Treatment is supportive, in view of the poor prognosis. Early diagnosis allows for the decision to consider withholding medical or surgical measures which might prolong survival.

PROGNOSIS

- 50% succumb by 2 months and 90% by 1 year[2]. 1–2% survive for 10 years or more; all are severely retarded. Long-term survivors are often mosaics[3].
- The 3:1 female preponderance of survivors reflects the increased fatality rate in males.
- Intrauterine growth retardation. Severe postnatal growth retardation with failure to thrive and feeding difficulties.
- Profound developmental delay, often with microcephaly.

- 90% have congenital heart defects, frequently VSD.
- Renal dysplasia, ureteral atresia, exomphalos and other defects occasionally occur[4].
- Primary trisomy 18 is associated with raised maternal age. The recurrence risk is less than 1%.
- It is rarely due to a sporadic or familial translocation.

FOLLOW-UP

Genetic counselling should be offered; prenatal diagnosis by amniocentesis is available for future pregnancies.

---

[1] Hodes M E et al. (1978) J. Med. Genet., **15,** 48.
[2] Weber W W (1967) Am. J. Hum. Genet., **19,** 369.
[3] Smith A et al. (1978) J. Ment. Def. Res., **22,** 277.
[4] Moerman P et al. (1982) J. Genet. Hum., **30,** 17.

2

Neonatal Disorders

K. Simmer and D. Roberts

Intrauterine Growth Retardation

Intrauterine growth retardation (IUGR) can be due to maternal factors (e.g. hypertension, undernutrition, smoking), placental factors (e.g. infarction, retroplacental clots) or fetal factors (e.g. chromosomal abnormalities). Babies suffering from IUGR are at increased risk of congenital malformations, birth asphyxia, meconium aspiration, hypoglycaemia, hypocalcaemia, hypothermia, polycythaemia, thrombocytopenia and coagulation abnormalities. However, with recent improvements in obstetric and neonatal care, these problems are uncommon.

PROGNOSIS

- After an initial phase of accelerated growth, IUGR babies continue to be smaller than controls[1-3].
- Babies with prolonged IUGR have an increased incidence of mental handicap and behavioural and learning difficulties[4,5]. Cerebral palsy occurs in approximately 1%, convulsions in 6% and minimal cerebral dysfunction, such as speech deficits, in 25%; 35–50% do poorly at school[1].
- Babies with IUGR have a higher mortality than those with birthweights appropriate for gestational age, however, within the group of very low birthweight babies (500–1500 g), the rate is lower, presumably due to intrauterine stress accelerating lung maturation[6].

FOLLOW-UP

The growth and development of these babies should be checked at 6 weeks, 3, 6, and 12 months.

[1] Fitzhardinge P M et al. (1972) Paediatrics, **49,** 50.
[2] Waltner F J et al. (1982) Acta Paediat. Scand., **71,** 651.
[3] Bhargava S K et al. (1985) Nutr. Res., **5,** 707.
[4] Fancourt R et al. (1976) Br. Med J., **2,** 1435.
[5] Low J W et al. (1978) Am. J. Obstet. Gynecol., **130,** 534.
[6] Goldenberg R L et al. (1985) Am. J. Obstet. Gynecol., **152,** 980.

Birth Asphyxia

Birth asphyxia is defined as an Apgar score of <6 at 5 minutes after delivery and regarded as 'severe' if score <3. Babies at increased risk of asphyxia include those who are: 1) preterm, 2) small for dates, (placental insufficiency), 3) 'distressed' (meconium staining of liquor, placental abruption), 4) a multiple birth, 5) anaemic, 6) experiencing a 'traumatic' delivery (forceps rotation, breech extraction). The incidence is about 1.5–6/1000 live births.

TREATMENT

1. Early, effective resuscitation, including intubation and ventilation and i.v. sodium bicarbonate (8.4%, 1 ml/kg diluted). Avoid hypoglycaemia and hypotension by giving intravenous dextrose, fresh frozen plasma or dopamine.
2. Restrict fluids by 20–30%.
3. Reduce intracranial pressure with mannitol (20%, 1 g/kg i.v.)[1].
4. Hyperventilation aiming to keep P_{CO_2} between 25 and 30 mmHg.
5. Phenobarbitone (15 mg/kg i.m. or i.v. loading, then 5 mg/kg/day i.m. or orally) may be given to prevent or to treat convulsions. If convulsions continue alternatives include: diazepam 0.2 mg/kg i.v., paraldehyde 0.1 ml/kg i.m., chlormethiazole (Heminevrin) infusion 5–20 mg/kg/hour, phenytoin 10 mg/kg i.v. stat.
6. The following investigations are usually performed when a neonate has convulsions to exclude an underlying factor that requires treatment: blood sugar, serum electrolytes including calcium, blood cultures, TORCH screen (antibody titres for toxoplasmosis, rubella and herpes, urine microscopy for inclusion bodies), lumbar puncture, and test urine for an abnormal amino acids pattern, reducing substances, pH, ketones and sugar.
7. Persistent fetal circulation or myocardial dysfunction may occur and require treatment (see p. 11).

PROGNOSIS

- Approximately 12% babies with significant asphyxia die and of those who survive, 20% are handicapped. Handicaps include cerebral palsy, visual impairment, neurosensory hearing loss, developmental delay and epilepsy.
- Babies with mild asphyxia develop normally.
- Of those with moderate asphyxia, babies with neonatal convulsions or who are abnormal neurologically on discharge have an increased risk of handicap[2].
- An abnormal EEG or an abnormal trace on the cerebral function monitor is a poor prognostic sign[3,4].
- Intensive brain-orientated treatment can reduce the mortality rate of severe asphyxia from 50 to 14% and the incidence of neurodevelopmental handicap from 50 to 18%[5].

FOLLOW-UP

Follow-up is at 6 weeks, 3, 6, and 12 months. The neurological development should be checked and an EEG performed. Head ultrasound should be carried out at 3 months.

[1] Levene M I et al. (1985) Arch. Dis. Childh., **60,** 12.
[2] Robertson C et al. (1985) Dev. Med. Child. Neurol., **27,** 473.
[3] Rose A L et al. (1970) Paediatrics, **45,** 404.
[4] Archbald F et al. (1984) Dev. Med. Child. Neurol., **26,** 162.
[5] Svenningsen N W et al. (1982) Arch. Dis. Childh., **57,** 176.

Respiratory Distress in the Newborn

Respiratory distress syndrome

Respiratory distress syndrome (RDS) is the commonest cause of death in preterm babies. The lungs are immature and the surfactant abnormal in quantity, composition and physical properties. The incidence is proportional to gestational age, and is increased in boys, twins, infants of diabetic mothers (IDM), birth asphyxiated infants and after caesarian section. The signs of tachypnoea, recession, grunting and cyanosis develop within four hours of birth and usually improve after a few days. The chest x-ray has a fine granular appearance with an air bronchogram. Classically the disease improves after a few days.

TREATMENT

1. Prevention

    a) If preterm delivery is anticipated, the ratio of lecithin to syringomyelin in amniotic fluid will indicate lung maturity (< 2.0 indicates immature lungs); analysing the surfactant lipids improves the sensitivity of this test (a low level of phosphatidyl-inositol, without phosphatidylglycerol indicating lung immaturity).

    b) Antenatal glucocorticoïd therapy reduces the incidence of RDS; the greatest effect is seen in the group with gestational age 30–34 weeks, delivered 24 hours to 7 days after initiation of maternal treatment[1].

    c) Birth asphyxia, hypothermia, hypoxia and hypercarbia increase the severity of RDS and should be avoided. Early, effective resuscitation is beneficial to lung function.

2. Administer humidified headbox O_2. If > 60% O_2 required, commence continuous positive airways pressure (CPAP) (nasal prongs or endotracheal tube) or intermittent positive pressure ventilation (IPPV) (oral or nasal endotracheal tube) early. Aim to keep arterial oxygen between 45–70 mmHg. Monitor blood gases via an intravascular O_2 electrode or transcutaneous Po_2 monitor, and intermittent arterial blood samples.

Ventilator settings:

    a) Commence at pressures of 25/5 cmH$_2$O, rate of 30/minute and inspiratory:expiratory time (I:E) ratios of 1:1, and if Pao_2 low increase I:E ratio to 2:1 and if necessary, the peak pressure to 28–30 cmH$_2$O^2.

    b) Alternatively, increase the rate up to 100/minute in ventilated infants who are making spontaneous efforts[3]. Active expiration against ventilator inflation is believed to be associated with the development of pneumothoraces[4] and can be abolished either by the use of a faster ventilator rate and a more normal I:E ratio (1:1) or by paralysis with pancuronium (30–100 µg/kg 2 hourly).

    c) High frequency ventilation has been used as an experimental treatment for RDS. Gas exchange is maintained by the use of small tidal volumes at frequencies of 60–1800 breaths/minute (1–30 Hz). There are three techniques: high frequency positive pressure ventilation, high frequency jet ventilation and high frequency oscillation[5].

3. Frusemide may be beneficial when a spontaneous diuresis does not occur.

4. Antibiotics are usually given as it is difficult to differentiate initially RDS from group B streptococcal pneumonia (see p. 265).

5. Treacheal instillation of surfactant may lessen the severity of RDS. Enhorning et al. (1985) used lung lavage fluid from newly slaughtered calves and demonstrated an increased arterial: alveolar Po_2 ratio and the need for less respiratory support[6]. Morley et al. (1981) used an artificial dry powder (dipalmitolylphosphatidyl-choline:phosphatidylglycerol 7:3 w/w) and demonstrated a small but significant improvement in the treated babies[7].

6. Pneumothoraces are drained with a size 10 or

12 thoracentesis tube into the pleural space, usually in the second or third intercostal space anteriorly or on the sixth intercostal space laterally; the chest drain is connected to 5–15 cmH$_2$O negative suction. The drain is removed when the lung has re-expanded and drainage ceased for 24 hours. When cardiac tamponade results from a pneumopericardium, air is aspirated from a substernal approach.

7. Persistent fetal circulation may develop due to hypoxia. Tolazoline 1 mg/kg may be effective at improving oxygenation, rarely an infusion at 1 mg/hour is required. Systemic hypotension can be expected after tolazoline and treated with fresh frozen plasma 10 mg/kg i.v. or dopamine 5–10 µg/kg/minute i.v.

PROGNOSIS

- The survival rate is 88%[8].
- Of those who are ventilated, approximately 20% die, 29% develop intraventricular haemorrhages, 33% develop pneumothoraces and 17% chronic lung disease.
- Approximately 20% infants ventilated for RDS develop pulmonary interstitial emphysema (PIE) which is associated with malposition of the endotracheal tube and the use of high peak pressures[9]. 40% neonates with birthweights less than 1 kg develop pulmonary air leaks (35% PIE, 20% pneumothorax, 3% pneumomediastinum and 2% pneumopericardium)[10].
- Extremely low birthweight babies with pulmonary air leaks have a poor prognosis; survival is 30% with air leak and 71% without[10].
- Neurological handicap occurs in 10–20% survivors of RDS; the incidence depending on the gestational age, however, long-term studies are difficult to evaluate as neonatal intensive care changes rapidly[11].
- The re-admission rate to hospital due to chest infections is high.
- Subglottic stenosis occurs in 1.8% intubated neonates (2.6% survivors). Tracheostomy is required in 84% cases of subglottic stenosis and of these 60% will later require surgical reconstruction of the larynx. 5–14% infants who required a tracheostomy die[12].

Chronic lung disease

Chronic lung disease is diagnosed when O$_2$ is required for more than 28 days and the chest x-ray shows irregular linear strands of dense opacities alternating with areas of emphysematous cysts that eventually coalesce causing marked overinflation. Bronchopulmonary dysplasia (BPD) occurs in babies who have been ventilated for RDS; there is massive damage to the bronchi with necrosis, peribronchial fibrosis and squamous metaplasia. Wilson Mikity syndrome (WMS) (pulmonary insufficiency of prematurity) occurs in infants who have not had RDS but who develop respiratory distress in the first three weeks of life (the incidence is decreasing with the early initiation of ventilation).

TREATMENT

1. Oral diuretics have been reported to improve lung function in infants with chronic lung disease (chlorothiazide 40 µg/kg/day and spironolactone 3 mg/kg/day or frusemide 1–4 mg/kg/day). Potassium and phosphorus depletion are potential complications[13], as is nephrocalcinosis.
2. Rapid weaning from the ventilator of infants with chronic lung disease may be achieved by using dexamethasone at 2–6 weeks of age (0.5 mg/kg/day i.v. for three days, 0.3 mg/kg for three days, then decrease the dose by 10% every three days until 0.1 mg/kg/day, then alternate days for one week)[14].
3. Vitamin A deficiency, which results in necrotising tracheobronchitis and squamous metaplasia, is common in very low birthweight (VLBW) infants and recent studies of vitamin A supplementation suggest that such treatment may well decrease the incidence of BPD[15].

PROGNOSIS

- Morbidity and mortality for those with severe BPD is high during the first two years of life, however, most survivors show a gradual improvement in lung function and can eventually be weaned from respiratory support[16].
- Similarly children who have had WMS have an increased incidence of chest infections for a few years, abnormal chest x-rays for 2–6 years and persistent small airways damage at 8–10 years[17].

FOLLOW-UP

Follow-up should be at 6 weeks and 3, 6 and 12 months. Vision, bearing and development should be checked. If chronic lung disease exists, pulmonary hypertension should be excluded.

Transient tachypnoea of the newborn

Transient tachypnoea of the newborn occurs in 5–10% babies. The chest x-ray shows hyperinflation and oedema of the interlobar septa and fluid in the fissures.

TREATMENT AND PROGNOSIS

Up to 40% O_2 is required for 2–3 days before there is a complete recovery.

Meconium aspiration

Meconium aspiration occurs in up to 3% term or post-term babies. Chest x-ray shows focal or generalised infiltrates and hyperinflation. Pulmonary air leaks and persistent fetal circulation occur.

TREATMENT AND PROGNOSIS

1. *Prognosis*

   a) The prognosis is good unless there is severe birth asphyxia and respiratory failure.

   b) Patients who require ventilation have a 40% incidence of barotrauma and mortality may exceed 60%[18].

2. Vigorous nasopharyngeal and endotracheal suction is essential during and immediately after delivery.

3. Ventilation is difficult and should be commenced at rates of 30–40 and I:E ratios of 1:2 (increasing the rate is preferable to increasing the pressures).

4. Sedation and paralysis are often required.

[1] Liggins G C et al. (1972) Paediatrics, 50, 515.
[2] Herman S et al. (1973) Arch. Dis. Childh., 48, 612.
[3] Field D et al. (1984) Arch. Dis. Childh., 59, 1151.
[4] Greenough A et al. (1983) J. Pediatr., 103, 769.
[5] Special Conference Report (1983) Paediatrics, 71, 280.
[6] Enhorning G et al. (1985) Paediatrics, 76, 145.
[7] Morley C J et al. (1981) Lancet, i, 64.
[8] Greenough A et al. (1985) Br. Med. J., 290, 597.
[9] Greenough A et al. (1984) Arch. Dis. Childh., 59, 1046.
[10] Yu V Y H et al. (1986) Arch. Dis. Childh., 61, 239.
[11] Alberman E et al. (1985) Arch. Dis. Childh., 60, 913.
[12] Quiney R E et al. (1986) Arch. Dis. Childh., 61, 689.
[13] Kao L C et al. (1984) Paediatrics, 74, 37.
[14] Avery G B et al. (1985) Paediatrics, 75, 106.
[15] Shenai J P et al. (1985) Pediatr. Res., 19, 185.
[16] Morray J P et al. (1982) Pediatr. Res., 16, 290.
[17] Coates A L et al. (1978) J. Pediatr., 92, 247.
[18] Vidyasagar D et al. (1975) Paediatrics, 56, 208.

Apnoea

Recurrent apnoea occur in 1% babies and usually commence in the first two days of life. The incidence is 75% at 25–29 weeks falling to 7% at 34–35 weeks. Immaturity of the brainstem centres is an important underlying factor[1], but conditions such as hypoxia, metabolic disturbances, infection, anaemia, convulsions, heart failure and even the introduction of oral feeds predispose the newborn to apnoea. Apnoea may be central or obstructive in type. Bradycardia occurs in 24% cases apnoea, as a response to falling oxygen saturation probably through a peripheral chemoreceptor reflex that is manifest when breathing efforts are absent or ineffective[2].

TREATMENT

1. Monitor with alarms set at 10–20 s using either an apnoea mattress, pressure-sensor pad or capsule that is attached to the abdominal wall.
2. Correct underlying predisposing factors.
3. Gentle stimulation.
4. Nurse in slightly higher O_2 concentrations and cooler ambient temperatures.
5. Theophylline-3 mg/kg 8–12-hourly orally (therapeutic blood levels 5–15 µg/l); 4 mg/day i.v. after a loading dose of 8 mg/kg; 10 mg/kg/day rectally.
6. CPAP (3–5 cmH$_2$O) or IPPV.

PROGNOSIS

- Up to one-third of preterm infants (<32 weeks) suffering from recurrent apnoea and other preterm complications (such as sepsis or necrotising enterocolitis) die and, of survivors, 20% are handicapped[3].
- Provided the apnoea are not prolonged, respond to treatment and there are no other complications, the risk of neurological handicap is no greater than in infants of similar gestational age.
- Recurrent apnoea decrease in frequency and eventually cease at term[4].

[1] Henderson-Smart D J et al. (1983) New Eng. J. Med., **308,** 353.
[2] Henderson-Smart D J et al. (1986) Arch. Dis. Childh., **61,** 227.
[3] Jones R A K et al. (1982) Arch. Dis. Childh., **57,** 766.
[4] Henderson-Smart D J (1981) Aust. Paediatr. J., **17,** 273.

Jaundice

Physiological jaundice appears after 48 hours and is due to an increased bilirubin load and delayed maturation of the excretory pathway. Bilirubin levels are related to gestational age and race (higher in normal Chinese, Japanese and American Indian babies). 50% term and 80% preterm infants develop jaundice which is considered abnormal if it appears within 24 hours of life or persists for more than 10 days in term or 14 days in preterm infants.

Unconjugated hyperbilirubinaemia

TREATMENT

1. Exchange transfusion

   a) In UK exchange transfusion is mandatory if the level of bilirubin (μmmol/l) $> 10 \times$ gestational age in weeks. In USA, exchange transfusion is recommended if bilirubin $> 340\,\mu mol/l$ in term infants, $> 250\,\mu mol/l$ in infants with birthweight 1500 g, and $> 170\,\mu mol/l$ in those with birthweight of 1000 g. The clinical situation and the postnatal age are also considered with a lower threshold for low birthweight, hypoxic, septic or hypoalbuminaemic infants. Indications in isoimmune haemolytic disease are a cord haemoglobin $< 12\,g/dl$, cord bilirubin $> 89\,\mu mol/l$ or a postnatal bilirubin rise of $> 17\,\mu mol/l/hour$.

   b) Twice the blood volume (160 ml/kg) is exchanged over 1.5–2.0 hours via an umbilical arterial or venous catheter. This replaces 90% circulating plasma and erythrocytes. Aliquot size is dependent on weight and tolerance of infant and ranges from 5 ml in 1000 g infants to 20 ml in 4000 g infants. Smaller aliquots and slower rate of exchange produce better equilibration of bilirubin from the extravascular space and the rebound rise after the exchange is less marked. Donor blood must be warm and fresh; blood older than a few days has a high potassium load and the erythrocytes have a shorter life span.

   c) Complications occur in 4.2% infants and include emboli, sepsis and electrolyte imbalance.

   d) Mortality is 0.5%[1].

2. Phototherapy

   a) Phototherapy facilitates biliary excretion of unconjugated bilirubin as the photoproduct is a water soluble isomer which is excreted without conjugation. The increased amount of unconjugated bilirubin in the bowel stimulates peristalsis resulting in decreased transit time and therefore decreased enterohepatic circulation.

   b) Phototherapy significantly reduces the incidence of exchange transfusion in low birthweight infants and has maximal effect in the first 24–48 hours of therapy[2].

   c) Effective reduction in bilirubin requires blue light of wavelength 450–460 nm at minimum irradiance flux of $4\,\mu W/m^2/nm$ which is provided by standard phototherapy units with $8 \times 20\,W$ fluorescent lamps and the infant positioned 45 cm below.

   d) Guidelines for phototherapy take account of birthweight, gestational age and serum bilirubin. Phototherapy should be commenced when bilirubin is $> 170\,\mu mol/l$ in babies with birthweights 1500–2000 g, $> 200\,\mu mol/l$ in those with birthweights 2000–2500 g and $> 255\,\mu mol/l$ in those with birthweights $> 2500\,g$.

   e) Normograms are available that define levels for obligatory phototherapy and exchange and have a zone between the two where exchange may be required because of factors other than bilirubin levels[3].

   f) Eyes should be shielded during phototherapy to prevent retinal damage.

   g) Fluids should be increased by 30 ml/kg/day to account for increased insensible water loss.

h) Side-effects include a transient rash, loose stools and lethargy.

3. Enzyme induction

   a) Induction of UDP-glucuronyl transferase can be achieved by pre- or postnatal exposure to agents with a similar route of metabolism.
   b) Prenatal administration of phenobarbitone, phenytoin or ethanol is associated with lower serum bilirubin levels in the newborn[4,5]. To enhance bilirubin clearance in neonates, phenobarbitone (12 mg/kg/day)[6] has to be given in doses that unfortunately affect behaviour.

4. Early feeding: Approximately 200 mg of bilirubin is present in the newborn gut[7], some of which is available for uptake by the enterohepatic circulation. Peristalsis, established by early feeding, promotes excretion of retained unconjugated bilirubin and bile flow. Increased transit time and bulk reduces the amount available for enterohepatic circulation. In addition, bacterial colonisation further degrades bilirubin to less absorbable pigments[7].

PROGNOSIS

- Severe, uncontrolled, unconjugated hyperbilirubinaemia may lead to the development of kernicterus (lethargy, opisthotonus, seizures, high-pitched cry and abnormal Moro reflex). Kernicterus has a 50% mortality rate and survivors have high frequency hearing loss, choreoathetoid palsy and mental retardation. Before effective treatment of isoimmune haemolytic disease was possible, kernicterus was a common finding in infants dying from jaundice. Kernicterus is now rare in term infants but bilirubin staining the basal ganglion is found at post-mortem in 3–10% low birthweight babies without documented toxic bilirubin levels.
- Impaired early motor performance is associated with moderate elevations of bilirubin (170–240 µmol/l)[8], however, the majority of infants are functioning normally in later childhood[9].
- Sensorineural deafness occurs in 36% very low

birthweight infants with bilirubin levels > 240 µmol/l[10].

- Prolonged jaundice develops in 1–2% normal breast-fed infants. It may persist for several weeks but, if breastfeeding is discontinued for 24–48 hours, the bilirubin level falls; kernicterus has never been documented. Prognosis is excellent.

Conjugated hyperbilirubinaemia

Conjugated hyperbilirubinaemia is characterised by a raised conjugated bilirubin and evidence of hepatocellular injury. It occurs in 1% jaundiced infants and in 8% those with prolonged jaundice[11]. Bile duct obstruction should be distinguished from intrahepatic disease by ultrasound, percutaneous liver biopsy (bile duct proliferation in extrahepatic biliary atresia) and ^{131}I-rose bengal faecal excretion test (there is cholestasis if < 10% injected dose is excreted in the stool in 72 hours).

TREATMENT

1. General treatment is supportive.
2. If bleeding time is prolonged, vitamin K (0.3 mg/kg) or fresh frozen plasma (10 ml/kg) may be required.
3. Nutrition can be improved by additional medium chain triglycerides, carbohydrate and fat soluble vitamins.

PROGNOSIS

- Prognosis depends on the aetiology and it is therefore important to identify potentially remedial causes (septicaemia, toxoplasmosis, syphilis, galactosaemia, fructosaemia, cystic fibrosis, choledochal cysts).
- Biliary atresia (incidence 1/15 000 births) has a poor prognosis without surgical intervention. Death occurs in the second year from progressive hepatic fibrosis. Biliary-intestinal anastomosis achieves biliary drainage in up to 90% patients if the procedure is carried out before two months of age, beyond this the prognosis is poor. The three-year survival rate is 66%[2].
- Intrahepatic cholestasis has been reported in over 20% infants receiving total parenteral

nutrition. The incidence is higher in very low birthweight babies[13]. Prognosis is good with liver function tests returning to normal over several months after cessation of TPN.

FOLLOW-UP

Follow-up should be at 6 weeks, 3, 6 and 12 months. Check for anaemia in those with rhesus disease as there may be a need for a top-up transfusion. Auditory evoked responses should be checked in at-risk infants prior to discharge. In those with conjugated hyperbilirubinaemia, monitor liver function tests at each visit to ensure resolution.

[1] Keenan W J et al. (1985) Paediatrics (Suppl.), **75**, 417.
[2] Brown N A K et al. (1985) Paediatrics (Suppl.), **75**, 393.
[3] Cockington R A (1979) J. Pediatr., **95**, 281.
[4] Stern L et al. (1970) Am. J. Dis. Child., **120**, 26.
[5] Waltman R et al. (1969) Lancet, **ii**, 108.
[6] Wallin A et al. (1984) Acta Paediatr. Scand., **73**, 488.
[7] Cashore W J et al. (1984) Clin. Perinatol., **11**, 339.
[8] Boggs T R et al. (1967) J. Pediatr., **71**, 553.
[9] Rubin R A et al. (1979) J. Pediatr., **94**, 601.
[10] DeVries L S et al. (1985) Paediatrics, **76**, 351.
[11] Matthew P M et al. (1981) Arch. Dis. Childh., **56**, 949.
[12] Barkin R M et al. (1980) J. Pediatr., **96**, 1015.
[13] Beale E F et al. (1979) Paediatrics, **64**, 342.

Necrotising Enterocolitis

Necrotising enterocolitis (NEC) is an acquired gastrointestinal disorder characterised by ischaemic necrosis of bowel, which affects 1–5% admissions to a neonatal unit. The incidence in very low birthweight babies is 10–31%[1]. Factors implicated in the aetiology include gut ischaemia, colonisation by pathogenic enteric bacteria and excess protein intake[2]. The clinical course is variable but can progress rapidly to gangrene, perforation and shock. The diagnosis is confirmed by the presence of pneumatosis intestinalis on the abdominal x-ray.

TREATMENT

1. Bowel decompression, nasogastric suction and total parenteral nutrition for 10–14 days. Enteral feeds are then reintroduced with progressive increase in volume and concentration of feeds to full calories by mouth by 7–14 days. A lactose-free formula may be necessary if carbohydrate intolerance occurs.
2. Intravenous antibiotics against enteric microflora are used for 10–14 days; penicillin (50 mg/kg b.d.), gentamicin (2.5 mg/kg 12–24 hourly depending on gestational age) and metronidazole (7.5 mg/kg b.d.) is a suitable regimen. Alternatively gentamicin and clindamycin (15–40 mg/kg/day) can be used. Oral aminoglycosides do not prevent perforation or alter the course of the disease[3].
3. Fluids: Up to 200 ml/kg/day above maintenance requirements in the form of plasma; whole blood may be required to maintain blood pressure, urine output and tissue perfusion in the presence of endotoxic shock and peritonitis.
4. Infusion of bicarbonate may be necessary to correct metabolic acidosis.
5. Inotropes may be indicated to improve cardiac output (dopamine or dobutamine 5–10 µg/kg/minute).
6. Ventilation is frequently necessary for apnoea or hypoxia secondary to abdominal distension.
7. Analgesia with morphine (0.1 mg/kg 8-hourly or 0.02 mg/kg/hour i.v.) for painful distension and peritonitis may be necessary.
8. Infectious disease control measures should be implemented if an outbreak develops.
9. Surgical treatment

   a) 20% infants with NEC undergo surgery[4] which is indicated for: perforation, right lower quadrant mass, persisting dilated loop of bowel, and failure to respond to medical treatment.

b) Abdominal x-rays are performed every 6–8 hours in the acute stage to detect intestinal perforation.

c) It may be possible to select patients with gangrenous bowel prior to perforation by paracentesis – brown peritoneal fluid or the presence of bacteria on microscopy is indicative of gangrene[5].

d) The diseased bowel is resected with proximal diversion and mucus fistula construction. Bowel continuity is restored after 2–6 months.

e) Infants with ileostomies are at risk of fluid and electrolyte losses therefore early anastomosis is advised[6].

f) If the extent of bowel involved is limited, a primary anastomosis may be possible.

g) If the neonate's condition is unstable or the whole bowel gangrenous, local drainage of the peritoneum only is performed.

PROGNOSIS

- Mortality is approximately 40%. (For a more detailed breakdown see p. 77.)
- Recurrence rate is 4%[1].
- Strictures, secondary to cicatricial scarring, occur in 10% and usually present 2–8 weeks after the initial illness with abdominal obstruction and/or bleeding[7]; 70% strictures occur between the transverse and sigmoid colon. Surgically treated patients have a higher incidence of two or more strictures.
- Removal of more than 70% the bowel results in serious nutritional disturbances with malabsorption of fats, vitamin B_{12} and bile salts.
- Long-term development is comparable to that of babies born at a similar gestational age[8].

FOLLOW-UP

Follow-up should be at 6 weeks and 3, 6 and 12 months. Malabsorptive diarrhoea should be excluded. If there has been a terminal ileum resection or ileostomy, check vitamin B_{12} levels. If the infant is constipated, consider Hirschsprung's disease or stricture. Stricture may also present as subacute obstruction.

[1] Kliegman R M et al. (1981) Am. J. Dis. Child., **135,** 603.
[2] Kosloske A M (1984) Paediatrics, **74,** 1086.
[3] Hansen T N et al. (1980) J. Pediatr., **97,** 836.
[4] Bell M J et al. (1978) Ann. Surg., **187,** 1.
[5] Kosloske A M et al. (1982) Arch. Surg., **117,** 571.
[6] Rothstein F C et al. (1982) Paediatrics, **70,** 249.
[7] Costin B S et al. (1978) Radiology, **128,** 435.
[8] Bohane T D et al. (1979) J. Pediatr., **94,** 552.

Intraventricular Haemorrhage

Intraventricular haemorrhage (IVH) usually occurs within 72 hours of birth. The incidence is 40% in infants with birthweight less than 1.5 kg or gestational age under 35 weeks[1]. Ultrasound is the diagnostic method of choice; clinical criteria predict only 50%[2]. Associated factors are prematurity, hypoxia, hypercapnia, mechanical ventilation and pneumothorax. The aetiology is thought to be a combination of physiological mechanisms of the preterm infant (diving reflex, pressure passive cerebral flow) and therapeutic measures (volume expanders, pressor agents). Haemorrhage is initially into the subependymal germinal matrix overlying the caudate nucleus, which is prominent at 24–32 weeks' gestation and the source of glial precursors. It may spread to the ventricles, basal cisterns, subarachnoid space or cerebral parenchyma. The condition is usually graded according to severity: 1 subependymal haemorrhage; 2 IVH without dilatation; 3 IVH with dilatation; and 4 parenchymal extension[3].

TREATMENT

1. Prevention of preterm deliveries.
2. No other preventative therapy is universally recommended although a beneficial effect has been reported with fresh frozen plasma 10 ml/kg at birth and repeated at 24 hours[4]; ethamsylate 12.5 mg/kg 6-hourly from birth for 16 doses[5]; vitamin E 20 mg/kg at birth and on three consecutive days[6].
3. Close surveillance of ventricular size is indicated for post-haemorrhagic hydrocephalus; of these, spontaneous arrest or resolution occurs in 50%[7]. Serial lumbar punctures (20 ml CSF) have been reported to arrest progression in 73%[8]. Ventricular taps are used to provide immediate relief of rapidly increasing intracranial pressure, but ventriculoperitoneal[9] or atrial shunt is the definitive treatment. Shunt insertion is usually delayed until the CSF is free of blood. Shunt related problems include infection and blockage. The system requires revision in 46%. Isosorbide (8 g/kg/day) may be useful in controlling intracerebral pressure until a shunt can be inserted, although hypernatraemia and diarrhoea may limit the dose used[10]. High dose acetazolamide (100 mg/kg/day) with frusemide (1 mg/kg/day) may also be useful[11].

PROGNOSIS

- Small haemorrhages do not affect survival. Mortality is 10% with moderate haemorrhage and 50–60% with large haemorrhage[3,12].

- Progressive post-haemorrhagic ventricular dilatation occurs in 20% infants with moderate IVH and in 65–100% those with severe IVH. Dilatation occurs at the time of initial haemorrhage but usually does not become progressive for a further 1–3 weeks, after which the clinical signs of hydrocephalus develop[7].
- Porencephalic cysts may follow parenchymal haemorrhage.
- Neurodevelopmental outcome at two years for infants with grade 1–2 IVH is comparable to that of infants of similar gestational age without IVH: 10% have major handicap. Infants with grade 3–4 IVH have delayed development[13] and 58% have major handicap (cerebral palsy, blindness, deafness or fits)[14]. The presence of hydrocephalus does not further influence neurodevelopmental outcome[12].
- The presence of periventricular leucomalacia in addition indicates a poor prognosis. Severe cerebral palsy, blindness and mental retardation occur in most survivors[15].

FOLLOW-UP

Development is checked at 6 weeks, 3, 6 and 12 months. Cerebral ultrasound should be performed at 6 weeks and 6 months (more frequently if rapidly increasing head size).

[1] Levene M I et al. (1981) Arch. Dis. Childh., 36, 416.
[2] Lazzara A et al. (1980) Paediatrics, 65, 30.
[3] Papile L et al. (1978) J. Pediatr., 92, 529.

Contd.

[4] Beverley D W et al. (1985) Arch. Dis. Childh., **60,** 710.
[5] Cooke R W I et al. (1984) Arch. Dis. Childh., **59,** 82.
[6] Chiswick M L et al. (1983) Br. Med. J., **287,** 81.
[7] Hill A et al. (1981) Paediatrics,**68,** 623
[8] Papile L et al. (1980) J. Pediatr., **97,** 273.
[9] Bada H S et al. (1979) Child's Brain, **5,** 109.

[10] Lorber J et al. (1983) Dev. Med. Child Neurol., **25,** 502.
[11] Bergman E et al. (1978) Ann. Neurol., **4,** 189.
[12] Krishnamoorthy K S et al. (1979) Paediatrics, **64,** 233.
[13] Catto-Smith A G et al. (1985) Arch. Dis. Childh., **60,** 8.
[14] Papile L et al. (1983) J. Pediatr., **103,** 273.
[15] DeVries L S et al. (1985) Lancet, **i,** 137.

Retinopathy of Prematurity

Retinopathy of prematurity (ROP, previously called retrolental fibroplasia) is a condition affecting developing vessels at the junction of the vascularised and non-vascularised retina. The incidence is 20% in survivors with birthweights < 2.5 kg, but 68% in those with birthweights < 1 kg[1]. The median postnatal age at which acute ROP is first seen is 51 and 40 days for those < 28 and > 28 weeks' gestational age respectively, the first signs usually being seen between 32.5 and 38.5 weeks postmenstrual age[2]. The condition is the commonest cause of acquired blindness in the neonatal period, causing total blindness in 8% infants with birthweights < 1 kg and 0.5% of those with birthweights 1–1.5 kg[3]. Children with ROP have an IQ distribution similar to or slightly lower than controls. They may also be at increased risk of emotional problems, largely as a function of early maladaptive interaction patterns[4].

TREATMENT AND PREVENTION

1. Prevention.

   a) Although the role of hyperoxaemia in the aetiology has not been clearly defined, the use of oxygen in the management of pre-term babies must be carefully controlled.
   b) The protective role of vitamin E is still controversial[5].

2. The eyes of all preterm babies should be examined between 32 and 38 weeks' postmenstrual age; the pupils are dilated with 0.5% cyclopentolate and examined by indirect ophthalmoscopy.
3. Clinical trials are in progress to determine whether ablative cryotherapy has a role to play but it may halt progression of advanced disease[1].

PROGNOSIS

- The international classification is based on the location of the disease in the retina and the extent of the developing retinal vessels involved in the pathological process[6]. The more posterior the disease and the greater the amount of involved retinal tissue, the more likely it is that permanent scarring will occur.
- 80–90% early disease resolves completely without visual sequelae.

FOLLOW-UP

Follow-up at 6 weeks, 3, 6, and 12 months, with an ophthalmologist.

[1] Reisner S H et al. (1985) Arch. Dis. Childh., **60,** 698.
[2] Fielder A R et al. (1986) Arch. Dis. Childh., **61,** 774.
[3] Phelps D L (1981) Lancet, **i,** 606.
[4] Teplin S W (1983) Paediatrics, **71,** 6.
[5] Schaffer D B et al. (1985) Ophthalmology, **92,** 1005.
[6] International Classification of Retinopathy of Prematurity (1984) Paediatrics, **74,** 127.

Ophthalmia Neonatorum

Ophthalmia neonatorum (ON) is a purulent discharge from the eyes of an infant within 28 days of delivery. It occurs in 10% neonates. The infection is commonly contracted during delivery. A bacterial pathogen is isolated in 60%.

Gonococcal ON

The prevalence varies from 0.4/1000 deliveries (USA) to 10/1000 deliveries (parts of Africa).

TREATMENT AND PREVENTION

1. Prevention

   a) Antenatal treatment of maternal infection.
   b) Neonatal prophylaxis: the eyelids are cleaned and either 1% silver nitrate or 1% tetracycline eyedrops instilled at delivery. Prophylaxis reduces the incidence in babies at risk from 28% to 2%[1]. Silver nitrate itself produces a chemical conjunctivitis which resolves in 48 hours.

2. Admit to hospital and isolate.
3. Administer i.v. penicillin 50 000 units/kg/day in divided doses for seven days[2]. Topical treatment alone has a 20% failure rate and the risk of haematogenous spread remains.
4. Irrigate eyes with saline while discharge persists.
5. In areas where penicillin-resistant gonococcal prevalence is greater than 1%, use single dose kanamycin 25 mg/kg or cefotaxime 100 mg/kg i.m. with 1% tetracycline or 0.5% erythromycin eye ointment for 10 days[3].
6. Notify patient to local health authorities.
7. Treat the parents.

PROGNOSIS

- Before the advent of antibiotics, gonococcal ON was the commonest form of blindness in early childhood. Rapid invasion of the eye and corneal ulceration result in visual handicap[3].
- 16% affected infants have extraocular gonococcal infection: rhinitis, arthritis and meningitis[3].

Chlamydia

Chlamydial ON accounts for 28% ON[1]. The prevalence is 1.1–3.7/1000 deliveries[4]. 40% babies born to infected mothers develop chlamydial ON[5].

TREATMENT

1. Erythromycin (50 mg/kg/day orally in divided doses) for 2 weeks with 1% tetracycline eye ointment q.d.s.
2. Topical treatment alone is inadequate as 50% have concurrent nasopharyngeal colonisation[6].
3. Treat parents with erythromycin or tetracycline for 2 weeks.

PROGNOSIS

- Chlamydial ON is less destructive than gonococcal ON, but severe inflammation with conjunctival scarring and persistence of infection for years can occur.
- Sight is rarely impaired[6].

Herpes simplex type II

Primary or recurrent herpetic genital infections occur in 1% pregnant women. The risk of infection for their infant is 40–60%[7] and 20% infected infants have eye involvement.

TREATMENT

1. Topical antiviral agents (1% acyclovir or adenosine arabinoside) 3-hourly until resolution[8].
2. Consider systemic therapy with acyclovir as disseminated infection may follow, or precede, eye involvement.

PROGNOSIS

- Keratitis, choroidoretinitis and cataracts develop secondary to conjunctivitis[9].

- Recurrence of keratitis can occur and affected infants need re-evaluation throughout childhood as amblyopia and irreversible visual loss can occur.

Other organisms

Other organisms, including coagulase-positive staphylococcus, *Streptococcus pneumoniae*, *Klebsiella* spp. and *Haemophilus* spp. are responsible for 30% ON.

TREATMENT

The majority respond to topical 0.5% chloramphenicol or 1% tetracycline, and all (except streptococci) to topical neomycin or gentamicin.

PROGNOSIS

- These organisms do not produce destructive eye disease.

FOLLOW-UP

Follow-up at 2 weeks and again if infections persist, for example due to a blocked tear duct.

[1] Armstrong J H *et al.* (1976) *Paediatrics*, **57**, 884.
[2] American Academy of Paediatrics (1980) *Paediatrics*, **65**, 1047.
[3] Fransen L *et al.* (1984) *Lancet*, **ii**, 1234.
[4] Pierce J M *et al.* (1982) *Br. J. Ophthal.*, **66**, 728.
[5] Harrison H R (1985) *Am. J. Dis. Child.*, **139**, 550.
[6] Rees E *et al.* (1981) *Arch. Dis. Childh.*, **56**, 193.
[7] Kibrick S (1980) *J. Am. Med. Assoc.*, **243**, 157.
[8] Whitley R J *et al.* (1980) *Paediatrics*, **66**, 495.
[9] Friendly D S (1983) *Pediatr. Clin. North. Am.*, **30**, 1033.

Fluid and Electrolyte Balance

Sodium and water

Fluid and electrolyte balance in neonates is difficult because of their limited renal homeostatic function and large insensible water losses. Glomerular filtration rate (GFR) is low at birth but increases in the first month; the rise is slower in preterm infants[1,2]. The kidney's ability to regulate sodium excretion is a function of gestational and postnatal age[2]. Sodium balance is negative in 100% babies born at <30 weeks' gestation, 70% at 30–32 weeks' and 46% at 33–35 weeks'. Hyponatraemia may also be due to water retention with inappropriate increases in urinary arginine vasopressin excretion and osmolality[3]. Conversely both a limited ability to concentrate urine and high insensible water loss (IWL) predisposes the newborn to hypernatraemia. The maximum osmolality of urine tends to increase exponentially with age.

TREATMENT

1. Fluid requirements are approximately 60 ml/kg for day 1, 90 ml/kg for days 2–3, 120 ml/kg for days 3–4, 150 ml/kg for days 5–7. Preterm babies often need 180–200 ml/kg/day in the second week of life. Babies weighing less than 1 kg or who are receiving phototherapy require more fluid, while babies with a persistent ductus arteriosus (PDA) require less. Efficient warming and humidification of inspired gas in an infant receiving headbox O_2 continuous positive airways pressure (CPAP) or intermittent positive pressure ventilation (IPPV) and nursing the baby under a plastic sheet, decrease IWL.

2. Daily measurements of body weight and plasma sodium are the two most reliable indicators of changes in water balance. Total body water usually decreases in the first few days of

life; weight loss from this cause usually does not exceed 10%.

3. Urine output should be >1 ml/kg/hour and the urine specific gravity <1012 (280–400 mosmol/kgH$_2$O). Caution is needed when interpreting urine specific gravity because a rise may indicate dehydration or inappropriate arginine vasopressin secretion for which the treatment is a reduction in water intake. Inappropriate antidiuretic hormone (ADH) secretion is suspected in the presence of hyponatraemia and a plasma osmolality of <270 mosmol/kgH$_2$O in the presence of hyperosmolar urine and continuing sodium losses (renal and adrenal diseases excluded), and is managed by fluid restriction.

4. Sodium requirement at term is 3 mmol/kg. Sodium supplementation to 4–5 mmol/kg in preterm infants appears to improve growth without undesirable side-effects[4].

Neonatal hypocalcaemia

Neonatal hypocalcaemia is diagnosed when the total serum calcium <1.75 mmol/l (ionised calcium 0.6 mmol/l). 30–50% calcium in blood is protein bound mostly to albumin, therefore, total serum calcium should be corrected for albumin levels by ± 0.1 mmol/l for each 4 g/l albumin above or below the mean albumin for age. Preterm, small-for-gestational-age, polycythaemic and asphyxiated infants and infants of diabetic mothers (IDM) are particularly at risk of hypocalcaemia. Hypocalcaemia can also result from maternal vitamin D deficiency and maternal or neonatal hypoparathyroidism. Symptoms include jitteriness, hypertonicity, vomiting, apnoea, convulsions and laryngospasm. There may be increased Q-T intervals on the ECG.

TREATMENT

1. Oral supplements of calcium 2 mmol/kg/day.
2. If symptomatic, i.v. correction – 0.4 mmol/kg i.v. slowly, followed by 1 mmol/kg/day i.v.
3. Check plasma magnesium level. If <0.6 mmol/l treat with magnesium sulphate i.m. in 50% solution, 0.075 ml/kg single dose i.m.
4. In older infants, exclude high phosphate feeds (e.g. cow's milk) and neonatal rickets.

Neonatal hypercalcaemia

Neonatal hypercalcaemia is diagnosed when the total serum calcium is 2.75 mmol/l or higher. Hypercalcaemia occurs in hyperparathyroidism, vitamin A and D intoxication, phosphate depletion and Williams syndrome (idiopathic hypercalcaemia of infancy). Symptoms include hypotonia, weakness, irritability, weight loss, constipation, vomiting, polydipsia and polyuria.

TREATMENT

1. Increase fluid intake.
2. Frusemide (1 mg/kg).
3. Steroids (hydrocortisone 1 mg/kg 6-hourly).
4. Correct underlying cause.

PROGNOSIS

● Untreated hypercalcaemia can result in nephrocalcinosis, with hypertension and renal failure.

Neonatal hypoglycaemia

Neonatal hypoglycaemia is diagnosed when the blood glucose <1.7 mmol/l in term, and <1.1 mmol/l in preterm infants. (Note: collecting tube must contain fluoride to inhibit *in vitro* glycogenolysis; venous blood glucose concentration is 10% below that of capillary or arterial blood.) Glucose is the most important substrate for brain metabolism and a continuous supply is essential for normal neurological function. Preterm and small-for-gestational-age (SGA) infants and infants of diabetic mothers (IDM) are particularly at risk as are infants with respiratory distress syndrome, septicaemia, hypothermia, birth asphyxia, severe rhesus (Rh) disease, congenital heart disease, hypopituitarism, congenital adrenal hyperplasia and inborn metabolic errors such as galactosaemia. Infants of diabetic mothers and those with Rh disease have hyperinsulinism; SGA infants have reduced hepatic glycogen stores and a high ratio of brain:liver weight with an increased rate of oxygen consumption. Preterm infants have metabolic needs that are increased out of proportion to substrate stores and calorie supply. The symptoms of jitteriness, apnoea, lethargy, hypotonia, pallor, irritability and convulsions are nonspecific. The frequency of significant hypoglycaemia is 2–3/1000 live births, excluding IDM. The prevalence in IDM is 50% (of whom 10–20% are symptomatic), in infants of gestational diabetics it is 20% (25% symptomatic) and in low birthweight infants 6% (80–90% symptomatic)[5].

TREATMENT

1. Monitor at-risk babies. If dextrostix is low (<2.2 mmol):

    a) Measure blood sugar and feed with milk hourly.
    b) Measure plasma insulin (to exclude islet cell disorders).
    c) Add 50% dextrose to feeds (1 ml/kg).

2. Give an i.v. bolus of 50% dextrose (1 ml/kg diluted 1:1 with N. saline), followed by a glucose infusion (10 mg/kg/minute = 6 ml/kg/ hour 10% dextrose or 3 ml/kg/hour 20% dextrose). Infusions should not be discontinued abruptly as reactive hypoglycaemia can occur.
3. Steroids (cortisone 5 mg/kg 12-hourly or prednisolone 1 mg/kg/day) are occasionally used, and diazoxide is indicated if there is hyperinsulinism.

Neonatal hyperglycaemia

Neonatal hyperglycaemia is particularly common in low birthweight infants as a result of parenteral glucose administration and drugs (e.g. aminophylline). Transient diabetes mellitus, which is occasionally seen in SGA infants, is a rare cause.

TREATMENT

1. Maintain fluid requirements but reduce the amount of glucose infused.
2. Give insulin (0.5–1 unit/kg subcutaneously stat or 0.1 unit/kg/hour i.v.).
3. Monitor blood glucose levels regularly.

PROGNOSIS

● Hyperglycaemia will result in excess water loss secondary to an osmotic diuresis and may result in brainstem dehydration, capillary dilatation and intracranial haemorrhage.

Potassium

Hyperkalaemia (see *Renal failure*, p.128). Neonatal hyperkalaemia (serum $K^+ > 7$ mmol/l) should be treated with calcium resonium (1 g/day pr) and if necessary glucose and insulin infusion (1 unit soluble insulin/4 g glucose). Peritoneal dialysis should be used if the neurological outlook is favourable. Cardiac monitoring is essential.

Neonatal acidosis

Neonatal acidosis is defined as when pH falls to 7.2 or less, or when base deficit rises above 10 mmol/l. Metabolic acidosis often occurs with birth asphyxia, congenital heart disease, infection, necrotising enterocolitis, renal failure and disorders of amino and organic acids.

TREATMENT

1. Respiratory acidosis

    a) Improve alveolar ventilation and reduce P_{CO_2} by increasing the ventilator rate or pressure.
    b) Occasionally prolonged hypoxia or hypotension will lead to metabolic acidosis which will need correction with alkali.

2. Metabolic acidosis. The underlying cause must be treated while the acidosis is corrected with sodium bicarbonate (mmol = base deficit × birth weight (kg) × 0.3).

PROGNOSIS

● Depends on underlying condition.
● Severe acidosis (pH 6.9) is fatal.

FOLLOW-UP

The development of children who have had fits due to hypoglycaemia or hypocalcaemia should be monitored closely.

[1] Aperia A et al. (1981) *Acta Paediatr. Scand.*, **70**, 183.
[2] Al-Dahhan J et al. (1983) *Arch. Dis. Childh.*, **58**, 335.
[3] Rees L et al. (1984) *Arch. Dis. Childh.*, **59**, 429.
[4] Al-Dahhan J et al. (1984) *Arch. Dis. Childh.*, **59**, 945.
[5] Beard A et al. (1971) *J. Pediatr.*, **79**, 314.
[6] Griffiths A D et al. (1971) *Arch. Dis. Childh.*, **46**, 819.

3

Diseases of the Respiratory System

J. F. Price

Tonsillitis and Adenoiditis

The commonest causes of pharyngotonsillitis are viral infections particularly with adeno-, coxsackie-, influenza, parainfluenza, respiratory syncytial viruses and infectious mononucleosis. The β-haemolytic streptococcus is the most important bacterial cause but accounts for only 10–15% throat infections. Bacterial infection is suggested if it is localised to the tonsils, pus is present, the onset is sudden with systemic symptoms and there is tender cervical lymphadenopathy, but none of these features is diagnostic.

TREATMENT

1. Acute infections

   a) Viral infection requires symptomatic treatment only.
   b) If streptococcal infection is suspected a throat swab should be taken and penicillin administration started. Oral penicillin must be given for 10 days to eradicate streptococci from the throat. When there is doubt about patient compliance a single injection of benzathine penicillin 600 000–1 200 000 units (dose related to the size of the child) is the alternative. Erythromycin 20–40 mg/kg/day is an acceptable substitute for children who are penicillin allergic. Since failure to eliminate streptococci may be due to the presence of β-lactamase producing organisms in the tonsils[1], the addition of flucloxacillin may prove effective.

2. Surgery

   a) Indications for adenotonsillectomy include:
      i) Obstructive sleep apnoea
      ii) Frequent severe attacks of pharyngotonsillitis which have not responded to adequate antibiotic therapy and are resulting in failure to thrive. Undocumented histories of recurrent throat infections are not a basis for tonsillectomy[2].
      iii) Peritonsillar abscess; controversial – see below.
      iv) Tonsillar hypertrophy alone is not an indication.
      v) Recurrent otitis media with effusion and deafness may be an indication for adenoidectomy but not tonsillectomy.
   b) Complications from adenotonsillectomy, although uncommon include haemorrhage, pneumonia, lung abscess, septicaemia and death.

PROGNOSIS

- With viral infections complications are unusual.
- Streptococcal infections may be accompanied by erythema multiforme, erythema nodosum and, uncommonly, scarlet fever. Infection may spread locally and cause peritonsillar or retropharyngeal abscess, sinusitis and otitis media. Acute glomerulonephritis and rarely rheumatic fever are late complications. Protection from the former is not guaranteed by penicillin therapy.
- Chronic infection of tonsils and adenoids can result in:

   a) Failure to thrive, loss of appetite, poor weight gain and frequent acute upper respiratory infections.
   b) Severe upper airway obstruction, obstructive sleep apnoea, and chest deformity with a depression at the site of insertion of the diaphragms.
   c) Deafness, due to otitis media with effusion, which can lead to speech delay and withdrawn behaviour.

- The frequency and severity of pharyngotonsillitis decreases with age and there is a corresponding reduction in the size of the tonsils and adenoids.

FOLLOW-UP

Obstructive sleep apnoea and failure to thrive due to adenotonsillar hypertrophy usually respond dramatically to surgery. Hearing and speech development need regular review after treatment.

[1] Brook I *et al.* (1981) *Ann. Otol. Rhinol. Laryngol.*, **90**, 261.
[2] Paradise J L *et al.* (1978) *New Eng. J. Med.*, **298**, 409.

Peritonsillar Abscess

Infection arises either by local extension from the tonsil or via lymphatics. Symptoms are progressive dysphagia, drooling, a muffled voice and, in severe cases, trismus. It occurs mainly in adolescents, is rare in young children and is most often caused by β-haemolytic streptococci.

TREATMENT

1. Admit the child to hospital and give high dose intravenous antibiotics – initially benzylpenicillin.
2. Peritonsillar cellulitis may respond to antibiotics alone but it is often difficult to distinguish cellulitis from abscess. If in doubt the tonsil should be incised and drained; pus should be cultured and the antibiotic changed if necessary.
3. It has been suggested that immediate tonsillectomy speeds recovery and reduces the risk of recurrence[1]; recent work suggests recurrence is infrequent anyway and there should be additional evidence of chronic disease of the tonsils before removing them.

PROGNOSIS

- Rare complications include extension of infection into the neck, jugular vein thrombosis and mediastinitis.
- Rupture of the abscess may result in inhalation pneumonia.
- Recurrence is uncommon.

FOLLOW-UP

GP follow-up after discharge to check for recurrence.

[1] McCurdy J A (1977) *Arch. Otolaryngol.*, **103**, 414.

Retropharyngeal Abscess

The presentation is stridor, drooling, dysphagia and fever mainly in children under 6 years. Infection extends from the naso- or oropharynx or results from trauma due to a foreign body, fingernails or endoscopy. Causative organisms are streptococci, anaerobes and staphylococci. The posterior pharynx is difficult to examine in an ill small child. A lateral neck radiograph may show a mass in the posterior pharynx; interpretation of such radiographs requires special care; for example the prevertebral space is wider than in adults[1].

TREATMENT

1. Admit the child to hospital and treat with intravenous antibiotics; initially penicillin and gentamicin.
2. Although early retropharyngeal infection has been successfully treated with antibiotics alone[2], it is best to evaluate the condition under general anaesthesia. The child should be intubated and, with the airway protected, the abscess incised, drained and pus cultured. The tracheal tube can then be removed.

PROGNOSIS

- The mass may completely occlude the upper airway endangering life.
- Spontaneous rupture anteriorly may be followed by aspiration pneumonia or sudden death.
- The infection may spread to cause mediastinitis, spinal osteomyelitis, thrombosis of the jugular vein and septicaemia.
- With appropriate management complete resolution takes place in a few days.

FOLLOW–UP

Recurrence is rare.

[1] Seid A B et al. (1979) Laryngoscope, **89**, 1717.
[2] Schloseberg D et al. (1981) Laryngoscope, **91**, 1738.

Upper Respiratory Tract Infection

An average pre-school child has 6–8 respiratory infections per year; 90% are caused by viruses. Most are mild with symptoms mainly of nasal obstruction and discharge. Rhinoviruses are the commonest cause. There may also be pharyngitis, and infection can spread to the paranasal sinuses and middle ear. A cough indicates inflammation of the larynx, trachea or bronchi.

TREATMENT

1. Careful management of fluid intake in infants is important.
2. Give paracetamol for fever.
3. Cleaning the nose before feeds, and local decongestants (ephedrine, xylometazoline) may be helpful in young infants. Vasoconstrictor drops should not be used for more than one week.
4. Pseudo–ephedrine has been shown to reduce sneezing and nasal blockage[1].
5. Antihistamines are widely used but their efficacy is not proven.
6. There is no evidence that antibiotics reduce the duration of symptoms, or limit the risk of secondary bacterial infection[2].

PROGNOSIS

- Symptoms typically last 1–3 days. Cough may persist for up to two weeks in a child whose symptoms were initially upper respiratory[3].
- There is usually complete recovery without antibiotic treatment.
- Nasal obstruction interferes with feeding in infants under three months of age who are obligate nose breathers.

FOLLOW-UP

If symptoms persist for more than a week the child should be re-examined for evidence of secondary bacterial infection.

[1] Bye C E et al. (1980) Br. Med. J., **1,** 189.
[2] Taylor B et al. (1977) Br. Med. J., **2,** 552.
[3] Scott N C H (1979) Br. Med. J., **1,** 29.

Acute Epiglottitis

Acute epiglottitis is an uncommon serious illness nearly always caused by *Haemophilus influenzae* type B. Inflammatory oedema of the epiglottis and aryepiglottic folds leads to severe airway obstruction. The peak age of onset is 2–3 years. The child becomes pyrexial and toxic with an acutely painful throat, low pitched stridor and drooling but little cough, over 3–6 hours. Diagnosis is made on history and general examination. Inspection of the throat, manipulation for a lateral neck radiograph, or lying the child supine can precipitate acute airway occlusion.

TREATMENT

1. Chloramphenicol i.v. 50 mg/kg then 25 mg/kg 6 hourly. Amoxycillin may be substituted if blood cultures show the *Haemophilus* to be sensitive to it.
2. An artificial airway should be established as soon as the diagnosis is made. Nasotracheal intubation is preferable, extubation is usually possible after 6–18 hours[1]. Tracheostomy is the alternative.

PROGNOSIS

- This condition should be taken seriously because death from laryngeal occlusion may occur before the child reaches hospital.

- Once antibiotics are started and an airway established, improvement is rapid and the outcome excellent.
- There may be associated *Haemophilus* pneumonia, otitis media, osteomyelitis or meningitis[2].
- Pulmonary oedema develops occasionally probably due to severe hypoxia.

FOLLOW-UP

If there is associated otitis media or pneumonia, the ears should be examined, hearing checked and a chest radiography done one month after discharge. Recurrence of epiglottitis is rare.

---

[1] Phelan P D *et al.* (1980) *Anaes. Intensive Care*, **8,** 402.
[2] Molteni R A (1976) *Paediatrics*, **58,** 526.

Acute Laryngotracheitis (Croup)

Croup is a viral infection caused most often by the parainfluenza viruses. The peak age incidence is 1–2 years. It is the commonest cause of acute laryngeal obstruction in children. Symptoms are coryza, then a barking cough, hoarseness and inspiratory stridor. Sternal recession during inspiration indicates severe airway obstruction.

TREATMENT

1. Minimal upset and reassurance help to prevent hyperventilation which itself increases airway obstruction and oxygen requirement. Careful monitoring of pulse, colour and chest recession is important. Fluids should be given orally if possible.
2. Warm moist air seems to bring relief in 30–60 minutes, the mechanism is unknown. At home the child can be taken to the bathroom and the hot taps turned on. In hospital mist therapy is not needed provided the ward is warm and has reasonable relative humidity. There is no evidence of benefit from cold water mists via 'croupettes'[1].
3. Oxygen administration may upset the child and may mask signs of worsening laryngeal obstruction; it should not be given routinely.
4. Drugs. Antibiotics are not necessary. Claims of benefit from steroids are unsubstantiated[2]. Nebulised racemic adrenaline transiently improves obstruction and is occasionally useful as a temporary measure, e.g. when arranging intubation.
5. The decision to establish a mechanical airway is made on the clinical state not the blood gases. Nasotracheal intubation is preferable to tracheostomy but the choice will depend on the facilities available. An intubated child should be managed in an intensive care unit. Duration of intubation is 1–10 days (mean 3).

PROGNOSIS

- Stridor usually disappears in 1–3 days, a dry cough may persist for 1–2 weeks.
- 1–2% of hospitalised children develop severe laryngeal obstruction and need intubation. Usually they recover completely – subglottic stenosis is rare.
- Secondary bacterial infection is rare but may be caused by *Staphylococcus aureus*: a mucopurulent membrane forms on the larynx and subglottis and the child develops symptoms similar to acute epiglottitis.
- Some children have recurrent episodes of 'croup'. There is a familial tendency, many have allergic features and hyper-reactivity of the airways[3].

FOLLOW-UP

GP follow up for recurrence, and for the very rare development of sub-glottic stenosis after intubation.

[1] Henry R (1983) *Arch. Dis. Childh.*, **58,** 577.
[2] Tunnessen W W *et al.* (1980) *J. Pediatr.*, **96,** 751.
[3] Zach M *et al.* (1981) *Arch. Dis. Childh.*, **56,** 336.

Bronchitis

Viral infection is the commonest cause of acute bronchitis. The main symptom is cough and after a few days coarse crackles are heard over the large airways. Bronchitis is a feature of measles and whooping cough and occurs sometimes with mycoplasma infection. Primary acute bacterial bronchitis is rare. Recurrent or 'chronic' bronchitis may indicate serious underlying disease; it is also associated with inhalation of food, gastric contents or air pollutants notably cigarette smoke.

TREATMENT

1. There is no effective treatment for uncomplicated acute bronchitis. Expectorants are of no value and cough suppressants are contraindicated in a child with a productive cough.
2. Purulent-looking sputum does not necessarily mean bacterial infection, but a cough persisting without improvement for 10–14 days is an indication for administration of an antibiotic effective against common secondary invaders such as *Streptococcus pneumoniae* and *Haemophilus influenzae*.
3. A chest radiograph should be performed if there is no response to the antibiotic, to exclude segmental collapse, foreign body or serious underlying chest pathology.
4. Recurrent episodes of cough with wheezing should be treated with bronchodilators not antibiotics.

PROGNOSIS

- Acute bronchitis usually resolves without treatment in 1–2 weeks.

- Recurrent cough and wheezing with viral respiratory infection (wheezy bronchitis) is almost always due to asthma.
- Recurrent or chronic bronchitis occurs in cystic fibrosis, the immotile cilia syndrome and immune deficiency.
- Bronchitis in early childhood is associated with chronic cough and abnormal lung function by young adulthood[1,2]. The decline in lung function is accelerated by cigarette smoking[3].

FOLLOW-UP

Uncomplicated acute bronchitis needs no follow-up. Recurrent episodes or persistent symptoms of bronchitis require investigation for the underlying cause.

[1] Colley J R T *et al.* (1973) *Br. Med. J.*, **3**, 195.
[2] Woolcock A J *et al.* (1979) *Am. Rev. Respir. Dis.*, **120**, 5.
[3] Burrows B *et al.* (1977) *Am. Rev. Respir. Dis.*, **115**, 751.

Acute Viral Bronchiolitis

Acute viral bronchiolitis is the most common serious lower respiratory tract infection of infancy. About 1% infants are admitted to hospital, mainly in the winter months, with acute bronchiolitis. In 85% cases respiratory syncytial virus is the cause. The peak age incidence is 2–4 months. Coryzal symptoms are followed by cough, wheezing, dyspnoea and difficulty in feeding. The lungs become overinflated and fine crackles and wheezing can be heard.

TREATMENT

1. Hospital admission is indicated if there is respiratory distress or difficulty with feeding.
2. Good nursing care with minimal handling and careful monitoring is very important.
3. Humidified oxygen should be given via a headbox or clear plastic oxygen cot. An initial concentration of 30–40% can be increased if necessary without fear of making CO_2 retention worse. Small particle water vapour mist is of no value.
4. Fluids need to be given by intragastric tube or intravenously if the baby is too breathless to take oral feeds.
5. Bronchodilators (salbutamol or ipratropium bromide), and corticosteroids have no beneficial effect.
6. Antibiotics are not generally needed. Occasional secondary infection may be due to *Haemophilus influenzae* or *Staphylococcus aureus*.
7. Ribavirin aerosol, given 18 hours per day for three days, reduces the severity of bronchiolitis. This antiviral agent may prove useful in severe cases, or in infants with underlying abnormalities[1].

PROGNOSIS

- Respiratory distress increases for 2–4 days. Respiratory failure develops in 1–2% hospitalised infants. Malnourished infants or those with congenital heart disease, immune deficiency or bronchopulmonary dysplasia may be severely affected.
- Recovery is usually in 7–10 days.
- Mortality is less than 1–2% and can be reduced further by mechanical ventilation for respiratory failure.
- At least 50% have subsequent episodes of wheezing and increased bronchial reactivity, but allergic features are no greater than in the general population[2].
- 60% children have evidence of lung overinflation two years after acute bronchiolitis[3].
- The frequency of lower respiratory symptoms decreases as the children grow older and most stop wheezing by school age.

FOLLOW-UP

Regular review because many children have subsequent episodes of cough and wheezing and persisting abnormalities of lung function.

[1] Barry W *et al.* (1986) *Arch. Dis. Childh.*, **61,** 593.
[2] Pullen C R *et al.* (1982) *Br. Med. J.*, **284,** 1665.
[3] Henry R L *et al.* (1983) *Arch. Dis. Childh.*, **58,** 713.

Bacterial Pneumonia

In neonates the likeliest causes are group B streptococci and gram-negative rods. Pneumococcus and *Haemophilus influenzae* predominate in older infants and young children, *Staphylococcus aureus* is now uncommon. In adolescents *Mycoplasma* and pneumococcus are the most common causes. Haemolytic streptococci and *Klebsiella* are infrequent causes.

TREATMENT

1. General measures

   a) Maintain fluid intake, reduce pyrexia and give oxygen according to PaO_2 if there is respiratory distress.
   b) Clearance of nasal secretions helps.
   c) There is little place for physiotherapy in the acute management but it may be of value if resolution is slow.

2. Antibiotics

   a) Blood cultures are positive in 30–40% cases pneumococcal, 70–80% *H. influenzae* and *Staph. aureus* pneumonia. If present pleural fluid should be tapped diagnostically before starting antibiotics. Throat swabs are of little value, and sputum is difficult to obtain in young children. A chest radiograph will show the distribution of pneumonia and pleural fluid.
   b) Antibiotics covering the most likely organisms (according to age) should be started while awaiting results of cultures.

      i) Pneumococcus – benzylpenicillin 50 000–150 000 units/kg/day or amoxycillin for 10–14 days.
      ii) *H. influenzae* – amoxycillin 50–100 mg/kg/day for 10–14 days. If resistant use a cephalosporin or chloramphenicol.
      iii) *Staph. aureus* – flucloxacillin 50–100 mg/kg/day for 4–6 weeks.

3. Pleural fluid: small effusions will resolve spontaneously; large serosanguineous effusions require tapping; purulent fluid needs continuous drainage (see *Empyema*).

PROGNOSIS

- Pneumococcus causes lobar or segmental pneumonia in older children, and bronchopneumonia in infants. Pleurisy is common, empyema rare. With chemotherapy there is rapid and complete resolution, mortality is less than 5%, and residual lung damage is rare.
- *Haemophilus influenzae* causes lobar or bronchopneumonia. In one series 75% developed a pleural effusion, 50% otitis media, 6% meningitis, and 5% pericarditis[1]. Pneumatocoeles and empyema both occur. Bronchiectasis is uncommon.
- *Staphylococcus aureus* causes severe infection lasting for up to 6 weeks in infants, or in children with underlying disease and immunodeficiency. Complications are pleural effusion/empyema (55%), pneumothorax (21%), and abscess or pneumatocoeles (13%)[2]; pyopneumothorax may cause sudden lung collapse. Focal sepsis elsewhere in the body arises in 10–15% cases.
- With good management resolution is nearly always complete, without bronchiectasis; pneumatocoeles and pleural thickening can take 6–12 months to clear.
- Mortality is less than 10%, higher in preterm infants.

FOLLOW-UP

Pneumococcus and *H.influenza*—chest radiograph after 10–14 days. If resolution is incomplete give regular physiotherapy and repeat chest radiograph in one month; if normal and the child is asymptomatic no further follow-up. *Staphylococcus aureus*—resolution is much slower, regular review with chest radiograph until resolution is complete. Post-pneumonia bronchiectasis (rare) requires postural drainage, antibiotics for acute exacerbations and regular review throughout childhood. Improvement frequently occurs during adolescence.

[1] Ginsburg C M *et al.* (1979) *Paediatrics*, **64,** 283.
[2] Rebhan A W *et al.* (1969) *Can. Med. Assoc. J.*, **82,** 513.

Viral/Mycoplasmal Pneumonia

Viral pneumonia occurs most often in infants and pre-school children. Important causes are respiratory syncytial virus (RSV), parainfluenza virus 3, adenovirus types 3, 7, 14, 21 and influenza viruses A and B. Mycoplasmal pneumonia is frequent in children aged 5–15 years.

TREATMENT

1. Rapid immunofluorescent techniques on naso-pharyngeal washings are valuable to diagnose RSV, parainfluenza and influenza viruses but less so for adenovirus pneumonia.
2. General supportive measures are important, the course of viral pneumonia is not influenced by antibiotics.
3. *Mycoplasma pneumoniae* is sensitive to erythromycin *in vitro* and this drug may shorten the duration of the illness.

PROGNOSIS

● Viral pneumonia

a) Full recovery in 2–3 weeks without long-term sequelae is usual.
b) Up to 20% develop transient pleural effusions.
c) Mortality is low but occurs in preterm or malnourished infants or those with congenital malformations.
d) Bronchiolitis obliterans, bronchiectasis and pulmonary fibrosis follow about 40% cases of severe adenovirus pneumonia[1], particularly when contracted soon after measles[2].

Adenoviral infection is one cause of the small hyperlucent lung (Macleod's syndrome).
e) Rarely influenza A infection can result in permanent lung damage.

● Mycoplasmal pneumonia

a) A non-productive paroxysmal cough may persist for 3 weeks.
b) There is evidence of long-term lung function abnormalities in symptom-free children[3]. Macleod's syndrome is a rare complication.

FOLLOW-UP

A chest radiograph should be done just before discharge from hospital and repeated a month later if the pneumonia has not completely resolved. Children with adenovirus pneumonia need long-term follow-up because of the risk of permanent lung damage.

[1] James A G *et al.* (1979) *J. Pediatr.*, **9,** 530.
[2] Warner J O *et al.* (1976) *Br. J. Dis. Chest*, **70,** 89.
[3] Mok J Y Q *et al.* (1979) *Arch. Dis. Childh.*, **54,** 506.

Chlamydial Pneumonia

Chlamydia trachomatis is an important cause of neonatal conjunctivitis; 10–20% infected infants develop pneumonia typically before three months of age. Symptoms are dyspnoea and staccato cough, there is no pyrexia and systemic effects are minimal[1].

TREATMENT

1. Diagnosis is made on the basis of an afebrile pneumonia, hyperexpansion and symmetrical interstitial infiltrates on chest radiograph, identification of *C. trachomatis* in nasopharyngeal secretions by immunofluorescent staining or culture and rising serum antibody titres.
2. Hospitalisation is necessary because PaO_2 is often reduced to 50–60 mmHg and coughing spasms interfere with feeding.
3. Supplemental oxygen via a headbox; parenteral fluids are often indicated.
4. Erythromycin is given for 14 days. Clinical improvement begins 3–5 days after starting treatment.
5. Ventilatory support is rarely needed.

PROGNOSIS

- Fever suggests secondary bacterial infection – this is uncommon.
- Recovery occurs after 5–7 weeks. No late sequelae of chlamydial pneumonia have been recognised.

FOLLOW-UP

The infant should be followed-up until symptoms have resolved and the chest radiograph returned to normal.

[1] Tipple M A *et al.* (1979) *Paediatrics*, **63**, 192.

Interstitial Pneumonia

Interstitial pneumonia comprises a group of diseases, mainly of unknown aetiology, with a similar presentation of gradual onset of dyspnoea, cough and weight loss, hypoxia, fine crackles at the lung bases and diffuse infiltrates on chest radiograph. A lung biopsy should be carried out to determine the histology.

TREATMENT

1. Prednisolone 2 mg/kg/day starting dose, may need to be continued for many months. Relapse may follow withdrawal.
2. Immunosuppressive drugs – azathioprine and cyclophosphamide have been used in adults, their value is not established in children.

PROGNOSIS

- Classical (fibrosing alveolitis): onset in infancy. Complications include haemoptysis and pneumothorax. Pulmonary hypertension and right heart failure occur late. The course is usually progressive; most die in respiratory failure before the age of two years[1].
- Desquamative: rare, about 20 reported cases in childhood. The earliest onset is at $2\frac{1}{2}$ weeks[2]. Most respond initially to steroids, some remit spontaneously. Alveolitis with minimal alveolar-capillary damage is a good prognostic sign.

- Bronchiolitis obliterans: follows adenovirus infection. Without treatment most patients die. It may respond to steroids.
- Lymphoid: extremely rare in childhood. The earliest onset is at 15 months. It is associated with dysproteinaemia and Sjögren's syndrome. The course is usually progressive.

FOLLOW-UP

Specialist supervision with serial chest radiographs, lung function tests (measurement of lung volumes, gas diffusion and PaO_2), ECGs and assessment of growth. Response to steroids should be apparent within 6–8 weeks. Steroid withdrawal should be gradual and may take 1–2 years.

---

[1] Hewitt C J et al. (1977) Arch. Dis. Childh., **52,** 22.
[2] Howatt W F et al. (1973) Am. J. Dis. Child., **126,** 346.

Inhalation Pneumonia

Inhalation (most often of food, occasionally irritating chemicals) results from dysphagia (very frequent), oesophageal dysfunction with regurgitation (frequent) or an abnormal connection between the airways and gut (rare).

TREATMENT

1. Massive milk inhalation (preterm infants are particularly at risk) requires oxygen, vigorous physiotherapy and suction, and early intervention with positive pressure ventilation.
2. Bacterial infection is uncommon after hydrocarbon inhalation; steroids are not effective[1].
3. Recurrent inhalation requires careful observation of feeding, neurological assessment, barium studies of swallowing and reflux, and an oesophagogram (prone) to look for a tracheo-oesophageal fistula.
4. Infants with reflux should be nursed upright and feeds thickened.
5. Indications for surgery (fundoplication) include recurrent pneumonia, apnoeic episodes, failure to grow despite medical management, oesophagitis, and a large hiatus hernia.

PROGNOSIS

- The prognosis is determined by the nature and quantity of inhaled material and the underlying cause.
- Recurrent inhalation can cause obliterative bronchiolitis, interstitial pneumonitis and pulmonary fibrosis. Symptoms are cough, wheezing, dyspnoea, recurrent fever and failure to grow.
- Occasionally secondary bacterial infection results in bronchiectasis or even lung abscess.
- Acute pneumonia following kerosene inhalation resolves rapidly, but chronic lung damage can occur after inhalation of hydrocarbons and of nut oils.

FOLLOW-UP

Children who have had recurrent or massive inhalation before receiving appropriate treatment should be followed-up because they are at risk of developing chronic lung damage.

[1] Marks M I et al. (1972) J. Pediatr., **81,** 3666.

Foreign Body in Larynx/Trachea

In England and Wales over 200 deaths per year result from foreign body inhalation. The highest rate is in children under the age of four years. Nearly all deaths are due to acute upper airway obstruction. Sharp foreign bodies such as pieces of bone or plastic, egg shells or pins impact in the larynx. Large seeds or nuts may become stuck in the trachea.

TREATMENT

Several techniques have been described to dislodge a foreign body in the larynx. The American Academy of Pediatrics recommends blows on the back as the most effective method[1]. Alternatives are abdominal thrusts (Heimlich manoeuvre[2]) or chest thrusts. If these relatively simple procedures fail direct laryngoscopy/tracheoscopy should be carried out immediately to remove the foreign body, or if this is impossible cricothyroidotomy or tracheostomy[3].

PROGNOSIS

- Partial laryngeal obstruction causes sudden explosive coughing, loud stridor or aphonia.
- Complete laryngeal obstruction leads to rapid loss of consciousness and death.

FOLLOW-UP

Once the foreign body has been removed there is rapid recovery. Developmental assessment should be done if there was severe hypoxia.

[1] Greensher J et al. (1982) Paediatrics, **70**, 110.
[2] Heimlich H J (1982) Paediatrics, **70**, 120.
[3] Gass D S (1980) J. Am. Med. Assoc., **243**, 1141.

Foreign Body in Lung

Edible nuts make up over half of intrabronchial foreign bodies. Two-thirds are diagnosed within one week but others may go unrecognised for many months. Most lodge in a main or stem bronchus, the right side more than the left. Chest radiography in inspiration and expiration usually show obstructive hyperinflation or lobar/segmental collapse.

TREATMENT

1. If the clinical and radiological pattern of illness is suggestive bronchoscopy should be carried out even without a history of inhalation.
2. Removal via a ventilating bronchoscope under general anaesthesia is usually successful[1]. Uncommon complications include glottic oedema and pneumothorax. Occasionally a peanut may break up and make removal extremely difficult.
3. Physiotherapy and bronchodilators are neither an effective nor safe alternative.
4. If diagnosis has been late, infection is likely distal to the bronchial obstruction. Antibiotics and physiotherapy should be given postoperatively.
5. Failure of bronchoscopy on two occasions is an indication for thoracotomy and resection; necessary in <5% cases.

PROGNOSIS

- Asphyxia is uncommon and death rare.

- There are five main patterns of illness resulting from delayed diagnosis; recurrent wheezing, persistent chest infection, chronic cough with haemoptysis, chronic cough and lung collapse and acute respiratory failure[2].
- Long-term pulmonary abnormalities have been demonstrated particularly when removal of the foreign body has been delayed.

FOLLOW-UP

A child should be followed-up if the diagnosis is delayed by more than one week. A ventilation perfusion lung scan is a more sensitive index of lung damage following foreign body inhalation than a chest radiograph. If the ventilation perfusion scan is normal long-term lung damage is very unlikely.

[1] Hight E W et al. (1981) J. Pediatr. Surg., **16**, 694.
[2] Williams H E et al. (1969) Med. J. Aust., **1**, 625.

Cystic Fibrosis

Cystic fibrosis, a recessively inherited disorder, is the commonest cause of chronic suppurative lung disease in white children. The diagnosis is based on chronic pulmonary disease, pancreatic insufficiency and elevated sweat sodium and chloride concentrations. Lung changes include bronchiolar obstruction and air trapping, bronchitis, bronchiectasis, pneumonia and abscess formation. Important infecting organisms are *Staphylococcus aureus* and *Pseudomonas aeruginosa*.

TREATMENT OF LUNG DISEASE

1. The principles are clearance of mucopurulent secretions and prevention or treatment of pulmonary infection.
2. Physiotherapy: chest percussion and postural drainage for 10–15 minutes one to three times per day according to need. Drainage of dependent lobes is important and special attention should be given to localised disease. In older children self treatment with forced expiration and vigorous coughing and increased physical activity may be an effective substitute[1].
3. Antibiotics

   a) Antistaphylococcal antibiotics are sometimes given throughout infancy although benefit is unproven.
   b) Exacerbations of cough in children with lung disease should be treated with oral antibiotics (e.g. flucloxacillin and amoxycillin) for 3–6 weeks. They may be poorly absorbed and penicillins are rapidly excreted so high doses are needed.
   c) Acute severe exacerbations or failure to respond to oral antibiotics at home are indications for hospital admission and intravenous treatment usually with two antibiotics (e.g gentamicin or tobramycin plus azlocillin or ceftazidime).
   d) Regular aerosol antibiotics given at home have been shown to be beneficial in patients with *Pseudomonas* lung infection. Gentamicin is used most frequently.
   e) Some antibiotics used in cystic fibrosis include:

Drug	Dose (mg/kg/day)	Route
Flucloxacillin	50–100	i.v./oral
Amoxycillin	50–100	i.v./oral
Gentamicin	3–9	i.v.
Tobramycin	3–9	i.v.
Azlocillin	200–300	i.v.
Ceftazidime	100–150	i.v.
Co-trimoxazole	80/400– 320/1600 daily	oral

4. Mucolytics: agents such as acetylcysteine and 2-mercaptoethane have only a small therapeutic effect but may be useful when combined with azlocillin in patients with *Pseudomonas* infection[2].
5. Bronchodilators: the response to bronchodilators is unpredictable and should be tested before they are used regularly. A nebulised β-agonist before physiotherapy may help some children.
6. If a large pneumothorax exists insert an intercostal drain; failure to resolve in 7–10 days or recurrence are indications for pleurodesis, or thoracotomy and pleurectomy[3].
7. Nutrition

   (a) The diet should be high protein, high energy with normal or low fat content (Medium Chain Triglycerides can be used as a partial substitute for fat).
   b) Pancreatic enzyme replacement (e.g. Pancrex V. Forte 0.5–8 g before meals depending on age; other popular preparations include Creon, Nutrizyme and Pancrease). Dosage is a compromise between persistence of offensive stools if too low and anal irritation if too high.
   c) Vitamin supplementation (including vitamin E) supplied usually as Ketovite liquid and tablets.

8. Gastrointestinal problems:

   a) Neonatal meconium ileus—obstruction may be relieved by the detergent effect of the diagnostic Gastrografin enema (unless evidence of perforation or dehydration present). Acetyl cysteine orally and rectally may help but sur-

gery is required if medical treatment fails.
b) Meconium ileus equivalent—treatment is similar to the neonate.
9. Sodium supplementation in hot weather to combat excessive loss in sweat.

PROGNOSIS

- The survival to young adulthood in large cystic fibrosis centres is 70–80%[4].
- There appears to be genetic variation which affects disease severity.
- Early diagnosis is desirable but there is no proof it improves outlook. Infants with meconium ileus who survive the neonatal period and infants diagnosed soon after birth because of family history have the same prognosis as unselected patients.
- There is evidence that early referral to specialist centres improves prognosis.
- Children presenting with mainly respiratory symptoms do worse than those presenting with predominantly gastrointestinal symptoms.

- *Pseudomonas* infection is associated with severe lung disease and adversely affects prognosis.
- Haemoptysis (60%) and pneumothorax (19%) are complications seen particularly in adolescents and adults.

FOLLOW-UP

Specialist supervision is needed, with 2–3 monthly clinical assessment, review of antibiotics, physiotherapy, diet and pancreatic supplements, weight, height, spirometry and sputum culture. Chest radiographs and more complex lung function tests should be done six monthly. It is important to monitor for complications such as nasal polyps, liver disease, diabetes, arthropathy etc. Follow-up will be throughout life and adolescence is a particularly important period.

[1] Blomquist M et al. (1986) Arch. Dis. Childh., **61**, 362.
[2] Heaf D P et al. (1983) Arch. Dis. Childh., **58**, 824.
[3] Penketh A R L et al. (1982) Thorax, **37**, 850.
[4] Wilmott R W et al. (1983) Arch. Dis. Childh., **58**, 835.

Empyema

An empyema is a thick purulent exudate resulting from pleural bacterial infection. The most common cause is *Staphylococcus aureus*; others include aerobic bacteria causing pneumonia (see p. 34), and anaerobes particularly after inhalation in children with dental sepsis. Tuberculous empyema is rare.

TREATMENT

1. General supportive measures, antipyretics, analgesia, and maintenance of fluid balance are important.
2. Intravenous antibiotics (see *Bacterial pneumonia* p. 34). There is no evidence that intrapleural antibiotics are beneficial.
3. An intercostal drain should be inserted attached to an underwater seal.
4. If the exudate is thick or loculated, a thoracotomy is indicated. Adhesions should be broken down, pus and fibrin removed and a large drain inserted, if necessary with rib resection.
5. At least three weeks' drainage may be necessary for empyema due to anaerobes and late diagnosis of staphylococcal infection.

PROGNOSIS

- With prompt treatment mortality is virtually nil, most fatalities are due to delay in achieving adequate drainage.
- The prognosis is worst in children under two years of age, or if there is underlying malignant disease or immunodeficiency.
- Complications include tension pyopneumothorax, and bronchopleural fistula.
- Unlike adults pleural thickening usually resolves, with no effect on future lung growth or function.

FOLLOW-UP

After discharge from hospital this should be until the chest radiograph has returned to normal.

Asthma

Symptoms include recurrent cough, wheezing and breathlessness provoked by variable obstruction of the intrathoracic airways. The prevalence is 7–10%; 80% start wheezing before five years of age and boys are affected twice as often as girls. The basic abnormality is bronchial hyper-responsiveness and most asthmatic children are atopic. Important triggers are viral upper respiratory infection, exercise, climatic changes, cold air and smoke, allergic reactions and emotional upset.

TREATMENT

1. General

   a) Explanation and education about therapy is vital.
   b) Sport should be encouraged and exercise-induced wheezing prevented by pre-treatment with an inhaled β-agonist.
   c) Inhaled bronchodilators are preferable to oral therapy because the effective dose is smaller and there is less risk of side-effects. The method of administration depends on the child's age:

Under 4 years	Nebuhaler/nebuliser
4–8 years: as above plus	Rotahaler/tube spacer
Over 8 years: as above plus	Unmodified metered aerosol.

2. Drugs

   a) In infancy bronchodilator and prophylactic therapy is relatively ineffective, although babies with eczema and an atopic family are more likely to respond. Oral presentations are less effective than nebulised bronchodilators. Steroid therapy may enhance the effect of β-agonists. Hospital admission is indicated if acute wheezing is severe enough to cause feeding difficulty or hypoxia[1].
   b) Mild episodic cases should receive intermittent treatment with β-agonists (salbutamol/terbutaline); particularly when they have viral respiratory infections and before exercise.
   c) For patients with frequent attacks prophylaxis is needed. Sodium cromoglycate and slow-release theophyllines are equally effective; the choice depends on patient compliance. Theophylline metabolism varies widely; optimum blood levels are 5–20 mg/l. Inhaled steroids (beclomethazone, budesonide) are more potent prophylactic agents than cromoglycate or theophylline and can be given twice daily. Children taking prophylaxis should always have available a fast-acting bronchodilator to treat attacks. A long-acting theophylline given at bedtime (10–14 mg/kg) may improve nocturnal wheezing[2].
   d) Chronic persistent cases: all need inhaled steroids, and β-adrenergic bronchodilators. Adding regular slow-release theophylline may improve control. If continuous oral prednisolone is used it should be given as a single dose on alternate days to reduce side-effects.

3. Immunotherapy: housedust mite eradication measures incompletely or transiently remove the mites so they are of limited value in reducing night-time symptoms. Immunotherapy with mite extract gives moderate benefit in selected patients. The injections are painful, potentially dangerous, and at present have little place in treatment[3].

4. Acute severe asthma

   a) Indications for hospital referral include:
      i) Dyspnoea causing difficulty speaking.
      ii) Cyanosis.
      iii) Peak flow less than 25% expected.
      iv) No response to two additional doses of bronchodilator.
      v) Known pattern of severe attacks.
   b) Assessment
      i) Record peak flow on admission, then four hourly.

ii) Pulsus paradox greater than 25 mmHg indicates severe airways obstruction.

iii) Chest radiography will show pulmonary air leaks or collapse but does not define severity of an acute attack.

iv) Blood gases should be estimated if the child is very young, there is cyanosis or there is deterioration despite initial treatment.

c) Management

i) Oxygen and nebulised salbutamol 2.5–5 mg or terbutaline 2.5–5 mg, 2–4 hourly.

ii) If there is no rapid improvement, i.v. aminophylline 6 mg/kg bolus (omit if on oral theophylline) then 1 mg/kg/hour plus i.v. hydrocortisone 4 mg/kg bolus then 4 hourly.

iii) Correct dehydration. Note that ADH secretion may be increased and over-hydration could cause pulmonary oedema.

iv) If there is decreasing respiratory effort and rising P_{CO_2} despite vigorous treatment, ventilation should be considered.

v) Antibiotics are rarely needed, sedatives should never be used.

PROGNOSIS

- Mild episodic: this type involves about 75% childhood asthmatics. It is mainly precipitated by viral respiratory infection. Lung function is normal between attacks. 50% stop wheezing by the age of 14 years, many of the others improve, 15% have troublesome asthma as adults.

- Frequent: about 20% childhood asthmatics. There are multiple trigger factors. 40% have airways obstruction between attacks, but chest deformity is uncommon. 20% become asymptomatic in adolescence; 20% more improve; 25% have severe adult asthma.

- Chronic persistent: 2–5% of childhood asthmatics. All have abnormal lung function between attacks, many have chest deformity. 5% become wheeze free before adulthood, over 50% have continuing severe symptoms[4].

- Mortality: there are 40–45 cases per year in England and Wales. The highest number is in the 10–14 year age group.

FOLLOW-UP

Out-patient treatment should always be reassessed after a hospital admission. Children require increased medication for several weeks after an acute asthma attack. Patients with frequent or chronic persistent asthma need regular assessment with a review of symptom frequency, chest deformity, pulmonary function, and medication including compliance, dosage and route of administration. Inhaler technique should be checked frequently. A diary card record of symptoms and twice daily peak flow rate at home is useful particularly in unstable asthma and when treatment is being altered.

[1] Silverman M (1984) *Arch. Dis. Childh.*, **59**, 84.
[2] Pedersen S (1985) *Clin. Allergy*, **15**, 79.
[3] Price J F et al. (1984) *Clin. Allergy*, **14**, 209.
[4] Martin A J et al. (1980) *Br. Med. J.*, **280**, 1397.

Allergic Rhinitis

Seasonal symptoms are provoked by windborne pollens of grasses, weeds and trees. Antigens in household dust, particularly *Dermatophagoides pteronyssinus* are probably responsible for perennial rhinitis. Some children become sensitised to feathers and the epithelia of pets. Symptoms include sneezing, rhinorrhoea, nasal obstruction and itching of the nose and pharynx. Many also have conjunctivitis.

TREATMENT

1. Inhaled steroids: beclomethasone and budesonide are very effective given twice daily. The side-effects of crusting and bleeding of the nasal mucosa affect 5%. Nasal infection is not increased, *Candida* infection is rare and therapeutic doses do not cause adrenal suppression in children[1].

2. Antihistamines

   a) Selective histamine antagonists (astemizole, terfenadine) control sneezing, rhinorrhoea and nasal obstruction as effectively as topical steroids (without causing drowsiness), and may control conjunctivitis better[2].

   b) Histamine antagonists and topical steroids used concurrently are particularly effective in severe cases.

3. Sodium cromoglycate: nasal cromoglycate is useful prophylaxis for summer hayfever if started before the onset of the pollen season. It is less effective than topical steroids.

4. Vasoconstrictors: local decongestants (oxymetazoline, xylometazoline) are useful when starting a topical steroid, but if used for more than one week can themselves cause severe nasal congestion. Oral sympathomimetic agents are less effective than topical preparations.

5. Systemic steroids give rapid relief but symptoms recur when they are stopped. They should only be used in short courses for 'emergencies' such as examinations, or to achieve initial control of very severe symptoms.

6. Immunotherapy has some beneficial effect in seasonal but not in perennial rhinitis. The injections are unpleasant and potentially hazardous. Oral and sublingual immunotherapy seems safe but there is considerable doubt about its efficacy[3].

PROGNOSIS

- Seasonal rhinitis affects 5–9% children and is uncommon before the age of five years. Children with nasal symptoms only often have hyper-reactive bronchi but few develop asthma – 1–3% after the age of four years.

- About 10% of the population have perennial rhinitis. Over 30% of them develop symptoms before the age of 10 years.

- 90% children with allergic rhinitis still have symptoms after 5 years, and 80% after 20 years.

FOLLOW-UP

Children with seasonal symptoms should be seen and treatment started before the expected time of onset of symptoms each year. Those with perennial rhinitis and particularly those receiving topical steroids, need a regular review and examination of the upper airway.

[1] Mygind N (1982) *Clin. Otolaryngol.*, **7**, 343.
[2] Wood S F (1986) *Clin. Allergy*, **16**, 195.
[3] Cooper P J *et al.* (1984) *Clin. Allergy*, **14**, 541.

4

Diseases of the Cardiovascular System

W. B. Knight

Heart Failure[1,2]

Heart failure in children occurs most commonly in the first six months of life. In many cases it is precipitated by the postnatal fall in pulmonary vascular resistance in patients with left to right shunts, or spontaneous closure of the ductus arteriosus in patients with coarctation. It is important to distinguish heart failure from oedema of non-cardiac origin (e.g. nephrotic syndrome) and from circulatory insufficiency due to dehydration or hypovolaemia (e.g. diarrhoea, burns) or anaemia. The prognosis and treatment depend on the underlying pathophysiological and anatomical causes.

CAUSES OF HEART FAILURE

1. Left to right shunt, e.g. ventricular septal defect, patent ductus arteriosus, truncus arteriosus, total anomalous pulmonary venous drainage, aortopulmonary window.
2. Obstructive lesions, e.g. coarctation, critical aortic or pulmonary stenosis, hypoplastic left heart syndrome.
3. Regurgitant lesions, e.g. Ebstein's anomaly, rheumatic mitral regurgitation.
4. Depressed ventricular contractility, e.g. congestive cardiomyopathy, severe birth asphyxia, anomalous origin of the left coronary artery.
5. Abnormalities of cardiac rhythm, e.g. complete heart block with inadequate ventricular rate, prolonged neonatal supraventricular tachycardia.
6. Large systemic arteriovenous malformations (most frequently intracerebral).
7. Cardiac tamponade, e.g. purulent pericarditis, post-pericardiotomy syndrome.

DRUG DOSES IN THE TREATMENT OF HEART FAILURE

1. Diuretics

   a) Frusemide 1–2 mg/kg/dose orally, i.v. or i.m. 2–3 times daily in combination with
   b) Spironolactone 1–2 mg/kg/dose orally 12 hourly.
   c) Alternatively, hydrochlorothiazide 1–2 mg/kg/dose orally 12 hourly.

2. Digoxin

   a) In term babies and infants: 10 µg/kg/day in two divided doses for maintenance therapy (may be monitored by serum levels), and 50 µg/kg/24 hours orally or 35 µg/kg/24 hours i.v. as digitalising dose (as $\frac{1}{2} + \frac{1}{4} + \frac{1}{4}$ of total dose every 8 hours).
   b) In preterm babies and older children, maintenance dose is 8 µg/kg/day in two divided doses, and oral digitalising dose is 40 µg/kg/24 hours. Intravenous digitalising dose is 30 (preterm) and 40 (children) µg/kg/24 hours.

3. Afterloading reducing agents

   a) Hydralazine 0.5–2 mg/kg/dose orally 8 hourly.
   b) Captopril 0.5–1 mg/kg/dose orally 12 hourly (less for neonates and infants).
   c) Prazosin 5–25 µg/kg/dose orally 6 hourly (first dose 5 µg/kg).
   d) Nitroprusside 0.5–10 µg/kg/minute i.v.

4. Intravenous inotropic agents

   a) Dopamine 2–10 µg/kg/minute i.v.
   b) Dobutamine 2–10 µg/kg/minute i.v.
   c) Isoprenaline (isoproterenol) 0.05–0.5 µg/kg/minute i.v.
   d) Adrenaline (epinephrine) 0.05–0.5 µg/kg/minute i.v.
   e) Noradrenaline (norepinephrine) 0.05–0.5 µg/kg/minute i.v.

5. Prostaglandins

   a) Prostaglandin E_2 0.005–0.02 µg/kg/minute i.v. (starting dose 0.005 µg/kg/minute).
   b) Prostaglandin E_1 0.005–0.05 µg/kg/minute i.v. (starting dose 0.005 µg/kg/minute).

Contd.

c) Prostaglandin E$_2$ 20–25 µg/kg/hour orally, decreasing dose frequency after first week.

[1] Friedman W F et al. (1984) Pediatr. Clin. North Am., **31**, 1197.
[2] Silove E D et al. (1985) Arch. Dis. Childh., **60**, 1025.

Ventricular Septal Defect

Ventricular septal defect (VSD) occurs in 1.5–2.5/1000 live births and is the second most common form of congenital heart anomaly after bicuspid aortic valve. By itself and in combination with other defects it occurs in 25–30% all cases of congenital heart disease. Anatomical variations of isolated VSD result from variations in their number, size and site (perimembranous, muscular, subarterial). Clinical manifestations and prognosis without treatment depend on overall functional size, site, associated lesions and the reaction of the small pulmonary arteries to excessive pulmonary blood flow and/or pressure.

TREATMENT OF ISOLATED VSD

1. Children with a small VSD are asymptomatic and require no treatment apart from antibiotic prophylaxis against infective endocarditis.
2. Medical treatment is indicated in all infants with heart failure: digoxin, diuretics, blood transfusion if anaemic and caloric supplements if fluid restriction is necessary (see p. 46).
3. Patch closure (with Dacron or pericardium) is indicated for

   a) Intractable heart failure, failure to thrive due to a large left to right shunt, or a progressive rise in pulmonary vascular resistance (PVR) (but is inoperable >8 units.m^2). In these patients with moderate to large size defects, surgery will usually be required before the age of two years.
   b) A large shunt persisting beyond infancy (with risk of development of pulmonary vascular disease (PVD) later in adult life, as in atrial septal defect (ASD)), after more than one episode of infective endocarditis (debatable), and after development of significant right ventricular outflow tract or mid-cavity obstruction.

4. Hospital mortality for primary VSD closure is <10% in infancy[1]. It is <2% beyond 2 years of age when PVR is normal.
5. For multiple muscular (Swiss cheese) VSD, pulmonary artery banding is carried out in infancy, followed by debanding and closure of residual defects usually beyond 2–3 years of age.

PROGNOSIS

- Most defects become smaller or close completely, usually within the first 2 years of life. Spontaneous closure may even occur after the age of 30 years. Life span should be normal in these subjects provided they do not develop infective endocarditis.
- Without surgery, the left to right shunt in symptomatic infants with large VSD may remain large (with death from heart failure in about 15%) or may become smaller due to:

   a) Spontaneous reduction in size or complete closure of the defect.
   b) Increasing PVR (with eventual irreversible PVD in some).
   c) Acquired right ventricular outflow tract or, less commonly, mid-cavity obstruction[2].

- Provided there are no chronic postoperative problems, e.g. residual VSD, aortic regurgitation or heart block, life span following surgical closure may be normal.
- Slowly progressive aortic regurgitation develops after infancy in about 5% patients with VSD. When severe, there is a significant mortality rate without surgery[3].

- Those with PVD (PVR > 8 units/m^2) are inoperable and most will become cyanosed at a variable age, due to increasing right to left shunt, and die in the second to fourth decade, the commonest terminal events being haemoptysis, heart failure and sudden (presumed arrhythmic) death[4]. In rare cases PVD develops despite surgical closure of VSD.

FOLLOW-UP

Infants with a VSD should be seen by a cardiologist at least every 3 months until the natural history of the defect in each individual is clear. Doubts about the pulmonary artery pressure and PVR must be resolved (by cardiac catheterisation) before 12–18 months of age. Patients with small defects need only be seen every 1–3 years beyond infancy. Doppler echocardiography may be helpful in following spontaneous closure or localising a defect which is unlikely to close. Following successful closure of VSD, patients need only be followed up by a cardiologist every 2–3 years with ECG and chest x-ray and Doppler echocardiography to check for the development of arrhythmias, pulmonary hypertension, aortic regurgitation and subaortic stenosis.

[1] Yeager S B et al. (1984) J. Am. Coll. Cardiol., 3, 1269.
[2] Collins G et al. (1972) Am. Heart J., 84, 695.
[3] Keane J F et al. (1977) Circulation, 56 (Suppl. I), I-72.
[4] Wood P. (1958) Br. Med. J., 2, 755.

Atrial Septal Defect

Atrial septal defect (ASD) occurs in 0.6/1000 live births and is twice as common in girls. In most cases the ASD involves the fossa ovalis (secundum ASD). There may be associated anomalies of pulmonary venous drainage. Less common is the so-called ostium primum ASD in which the left atrioventricular (AV) valve is frequently regurgitant. Rarer forms of ASD are sinus venosus defects associated with anomalous drainage of one or both right pulmonary veins, coronary sinus defects and posterior defects.

TREATMENT

1. Heart failure in infancy

   a) Medical treatment initially with diuretics and digoxin (see p. 46).
   b) If intractable (rarely with isolated secundum ASD, more commonly with primum ASD with moderate to severe left AV valve regurgitation) surgical closure with patch and left AV valve repair is required. Current hospital mortality should be $< 10\%$.

2. Asymptomatic or minimally symptomatic children: surgical closure either by direct suture or by patch at two years of age (or soon after diagnosis if this is not made until after the age of two) because there are occasional reports of spontaneous closure before this age. Long-term right ventricular dysfunction is less likely with operation at a younger age. Anomalies of pulmonary venous drainage and left mitral valve regurgitation are dealt with at the same time with very little extra risk. Hospital mortality is $< 2\%$.

3. By way of comparison, patients > 45 years of age with pulmonary hypertension or congestive heart failure or both, have operative mortality rates of 15–20%[1].

PROGNOSIS

- Those who have a small ASD (Qp:Qs < 1.5) will in general have no symptoms related to it apart from the small possibility of paradoxical embolism and do not require surgical treatment.
- Without treatment, the long-term survival rate

in moderate to large secundum ASD is high until the third decade when it begins to decline steadily, death being mainly due to pulmonary vascular disease and heart failure, the latter frequently being precipitated by atrial arrhythmias. Only rarely does heart failure occur in infancy[2] or childhood.

- The natural history of ostium primum ASD with mild or no left AV valve regurgitation is probably similar to that of patients with a large secundum ASD. With moderate to severe left AV valve regurgitation the prognosis is much worse, with death from heart failure a definite risk in early childhood.
- Late survival following closure of isolated secundum ASD in asymptomatic children will probably be the same as that for the normal population.
- Late survival after operation in ostium primum

ASD is closely related to the severity of left AV valve regurgitation preoperatively[3].

FOLLOW-UP

Follow-up with ECG is required every 2–5 years following successful closure of ASD to detect the onset of atrial arrhythmias which may occur many years after operation. When AV valve regurgitation or stenosis is suspected after repair of ostium primum ASD, at least yearly cardiological follow-up with chest x-ray and ECG and/or Doppler echocardiography is necessary.

[1] Rahimtoola S H et al. (1968) Circulation, **37** (suppl. V), V-2.
[2] Hunt C E et al. (1973) Circulation, **47**, 1042.
[3] Kirklin J W, Barratt-Boyes BG (1985) Cardiac Surgery, p. 584. New York: John Wiley & Sons.

Pulmonary Stenosis

Pulmonary valve stenosis (PVS) with intact ventricular septum comprises 8–10% all congenital heart disease. There is a wide variation in the clinico-pathological spectrum, from duct-dependent critical stenosis with hypoplasia of the right ventricle and pulmonary arteries resulting in cyanosis and heart failure in the newborn period to minimal commissural fusion causing no symptoms.

TREATMENT

1. Neonates with critical PVS and cyanosis

   a) Prostaglandin E infusion (until after operation) and diuretics followed by
   b) Pulmonary valvotomy usually with systemic-pulmonary artery shunt[1]. Current hospital mortality should be <30%.
   c) Further operations will be necessary in >50% cases and may include transannular patching of the right ventricular outflow tract, repeat valvotomy, ASD and shunt closure[1].

2. Moderate to severe PVS (pressure gradient >50 mmHg) beyond the neonatal period

   a) Balloon pulmonary valvuloplasty[2] or, if this fails
   b) Open pulmonary valvotomy. Occasionally infundibular resection and, especially with dysplastic valves, a transannular patch are required. Hospital mortality is <5%. If heart failure has occurred preoperatively, hospital mortality is higher.

PROGNOSIS

- Without surgery, virtually all neonates with cyanosis and heart failure due to critical PVS die within the first month of life. .
- Without surgery, infants and children with severe PVS who were not symptomatic in the first month, increasingly develop symptoms as

they grow older[3]. The pressure gradient across the valve frequently increases in early childhood (often due to secondary infundibular narrowing) and the right ventricle becomes fibrotic.

- Mild PVS (pressure gradient <40 mmHg) carries an excellent prognosis without any treatment[3]. The obstruction rarely increases with age.
- Following surgery, long-term prognosis is excellent for those without heart failure and for those who do not require operation until after the first month. Symptomatic neonates with critical PVS have a worse outcome, >50% survivors requiring further operations within 10 years of the initial operation[1].
- The long-term results of balloon pulmonary valvuloplasty are unknown.

FOLLOW-UP

For those who have had successful pulmonary valvotomy/valvuloplasty and those with mild PVS, cardiological follow-up is required every 1–3 years. Chest x-ray, ECG and Doppler echocardiography may be required. The same tests are performed more frequently for more severe unoperated PVS and for those who have undergone surgery for critical PVS.

[1] Coles J G et al. (1984) Ann. Thorac. Surg., **38**, 458.
[2] Walls J T et al. (1984) J. Thorac. Cardiovasc. Surg., **88**, 352.
[3] Nugent E W et al. (1977) Circulation, **56** (suppl. I), I-38.

Aortic Stenosis

Aortic stenosis occurs less commonly than pulmonary stenosis. Obstruction to left ventricular emptying results in left ventricular hypertrophy and varying degrees of subendocardial ischaemia. Congenital aortic valve stenosis (AVS) frequently presents in infancy as opposed to discrete subaortic stenosis (SAS) which rarely becomes severe before the age of three years. Supravalvar aortic stenosis is rarer and is frequently associated with peripheral pulmonary artery stenoses, elfin facies, mental retardation and infantile hypercalcaemia (William's syndrome).

TREATMENT

1. Critical AVS with heart failure in infancy

   a) Palliation before surgery with prostaglandin E infusion in the neonatal period[1], digoxin and diuretics, followed by
   b) Aortic valvotomy. Hospital mortality is disappointingly high (30–50%)[2].

2. Beyond infancy aortic valvotomy carries a hospital mortality <2%. A second valvotomy and/or aortic valve replacement may, with time, become necessary in all survivors. For this reason aortic valvotomy should only be performed when the stenosis is severe (pressure gradient across the valve >60–90 mmHg)[3]. In

the meantime, competitive sport should be avoided.

3. Balloon aortic valvuloplasty may be indicated in certain cases but long-term results are unknown (see Pulmonary stenosis p. 49).

4. Because operation for SAS is more likely to be curative and because progression of obstruction is faster, surgery to resect the obstruction is generally performed at lower levels of outflow tract gradient. Hospital mortality is <5%[4]. Reoperation for residual or recurrent SAS may be required.

PROGNOSIS

- Without surgery, most patients with critical

AVS presenting with heart failure in infancy will die. Those with less severe AVS who are only diagnosed following detection of a murmur do not usually develop heart failure in childhood, but have a significant incidence of sudden death, especially during strenuous exertion. Mild and moderate AVS predisposes to infective endocarditis and may progress slowly to severe stenosis.

- Subaortic stenosis causes progressive left ventricular outflow tract obstruction from childhood to early adulthood. The lesion rarely progresses after that time. Untreated, sudden death or death from heart failure may occur.
- Without surgery patients with William's syndrome have a significant incidence of sudden death especially when there are associated diffuse peripheral pulmonary artery stenoses.
- Postoperatively, most patients with AVS will require repeat aortic valvotomy or aortic valve replacement, frequently within 20 years of the first operation. More than 90% hospital survivors are alive 15 years postoperatively and

functional state is very good in the majority.
- Late survival and functional status are similar following surgery for SAS. Although recurrent stenosis does occur, reoperation is required less frequently than for AVS.
- Postoperative late survival for isolated localised supravalvar stenosis is good.

FOLLOW-UP

Yearly or more frequent follow-up with ECG, chest x-ray, serial Doppler echocardiography and/or exercise ECG is required to evaluate the need for surgery. Postoperatively the same investigations may be required every 1–2 years for cardiological follow-up visits.

[1] Artman M et al. (1983) Am. J. Dis. Child., 137, 339.
[2] Dobell A R C et al. (1981) J. Thorac. Cardiovasc. Surg., 81, 916.
[3] Hossack K F et al. (1980) Br. Heart J., 43, 561.
[4] Wright G B et al. (1983) Am. J. Cardiol., 52, 830.

Coarctation of the Aorta

Coarctation of the aorta (CoAo) accounts for 7.5% symptomatic cardiovascular disease in infants. It consists of a discrete narrowing of the aortic isthmus sometimes associated with tubular hypoplasia of the aortic arch. In severe CoAo, heart failure and lower body hypoperfusion with oliguria and metabolic acidosis follow constriction of the ductus arteriosus. Less severe CoAo is often not diagnosed until adolescence or later. 40–50% patients with CoAo also have a bicuspid aortic valve which is usually haemodynamically insignificant in childhood. Very rarely CoAo may occur at other sites in the thoracic or abdominal aorta.

TREATMENT

1. Infants with heart failure

   a) Resuscitation with correction of acidosis, prostaglandin E infusion, i.v. frusemide and/or ventilation followed by
   b) Surgical repair of CoAo, most commonly subclavian flap aortoplasty. Hospital mortality since the advent of prostaglandin E is <5% for isolated CoAo. Hospital mor-

tality is 25% when there are major associated cardiac anomalies[1].

2. Asymptomatic infants and children require surgical repair (subclavian flap or end-to-end anastomosis) soon after diagnosis. Hospital mortality is <1%.

3. Late post-surgical problems include recoarctation (more frequent with repair at younger age) and persistent hypertension (less frequent with repair at younger age)[1] which, depending

51

on severity, may require surgical or medical treatment respectively. Balloon dilatation is often effective in cases of recoarctation but long-term results are not known.

PROGNOSIS

- Symptomatic infants: the majority also have associated cardiac lesions, especially VSD[2].

    a) 60% with isolated CoAo die without surgical treatment.
    b) Almost all patients with associated major cardiac lesions will die without surgical treatment.
    c) In those with associated major lesions, prognosis following successful CoAo repair depends on the severity of the associated lesion.

- Those without heart failure in infancy have a significant incidence of subarachnoid haemorrhage, endocarditis (especially on bicuspid aortic valve) and endarteritis. Death from heart failure occurs with increasing frequency from age 20 years, especially in patients with bicuspid aortic valve who develop calcific aortic stenosis.

- 15-year survival following surgical repair of isolated coarctation in infancy or childhood is >90%[3].

FOLLOW-UP

Cardiological follow-up every 1–3 years with blood pressure measurements, ECG, chest x-ray and/or Doppler echocardiography is necessary to detect persistent postoperative hypertension, recoarctation and aortic or subaortic stenosis.

[1] Williams W G et al. (1980) J. Thorac. Cardiovasc. Surg., **79,** 603.
[2] Sinha S N et al. (1969) Circulation, **40,** 385.
[3] Kirklin J W, Barratt-Boyes BG (1985) Cardiac Surgery, p. 1059. New York: John Wiley & Sons.

Patent Ductus Arteriosus

The prevalence of isolated patent ductus arteriosus (PDA) beyond 14 days of age is 0.6/1000 live term babies. In preterm infants prolonged ductal patency is much more frequent, becoming almost universal at less than 30 weeks' gestation[1]. In this group, however, spontaneous ductal closure will occur in almost all babies, often at 32–34 weeks after conception.

TREATMENT

1. Infants in heart failure require initial diuretic therapy and fluid restriction followed by duct ligation or division, which is curative. Hospital mortality is <1%.
2. All other infants and children with isolated PDA should have duct ligation or division at six months of age or non-urgently after the diagnosis is made (if beyond six months of age). The operation is curative. Hospital mortality is <1%.
3. Preterm babies who are in heart failure, or ventilator-dependent with signs of a ductal shunt require fluid restriction and diuretics. If necessary this is followed within 48 hours by intravenous indomethacin, a prostaglandin-synthetase inhibitor, 0.2 mg/kg every 8–12 hours for three doses unless medically contraindicated (renal impairment, disorders of clotting, recent intraventricular haemorrhage and necrotising enterocolitis). A second course may be given 48 hours or more later[2]. If medical therapy fails (20–30% cases), surgical ligation should be performed. Operative mortality is 1%, but because of associated medical problems hospital mortality in this group is 20–25%[3].
4. Children and adults with dominant right to left

shunt (Eisenmenger syndrome) are inoperable.

PROGNOSIS

- Untreated, large ducts may result in severe heart failure and death in infancy. The incidence and outcome of pulmonary vascular disease are comparable to that in VSD.
- Moderate and even small ducts may lead to heart failure early or late in adult life[4].
- The smallest ducts may result in no symptoms at all, although there is a small but definite risk of infective endarteritis.

- Late survival after surgical duct closure in childhood is probably the same as that for the normal population.

FOLLOW-UP

In general no regular cardiological follow-up is required beyond one year after PDA ligation.

[1] Rigby M L et al. (1984) Arch. Dis. Childh., **59**, 341.
[2] Gersony W M et al. (1983) J. Pediatr., **102**, 895.
[3] Wagner H R et al. (1984) J. Thorac. Cardiovasc. Surg., **87**, 870.
[4] Marquis R M et al. (1982) Br. Heart J., **48**, 469.

Complete Transposition of the Great Arteries

Hearts with concordant atrioventricular and discordant ventriculo-arterial connections (TGA) occur in 0.2–0.3/1000 live births. This anatomical arrangement results in two separate uncrossed circulations with life only possible while there is adequate mixing between the two; the site of mixing may be the atria (patent foramen ovale or ASD), ventricles (VSD) or great arteries (PDA). The clinical features, treatment and prognosis depend upon the presence or absence of associated lesions (ASD, VSD, PDA, left ventricular outflow tract obstruction (LVOTO), coarctation).

TREATMENT

1. Initial treatment

   a) Prostaglandin E infusion for severe hypoxia in order to increase intercirculatory mixing.

   b) Balloon atrial septostomy (BAS). Surgical septectomy is sometimes required.

   c) Diuretics and digoxin for heart failure (e.g. in patients with TGA and VSD).

2. Definitive surgical treatment

   a) Either anatomical correction (arterial switch operation)[1]:
      i) For simple TGA in the first 2 weeks of life current hospital mortality is <10%.
      ii) For TGA and large VSD (or PDA),

within the first 3 months current hospital mortality is <20%.

   b) Or intra-atrial redirection operations (Senning or Mustard), when 2(a) not possible:
      i) For simple TGA: from three to six months of age or earlier if inadequate improvement after BAS. Hospital mortality is 5–10%[2].
      ii) For TGA and VSD: VSD closure in addition to intra-atrial redirection operation. Hospital mortality is 15–30%[3].
      iii) Palliative procedure for TGA with pulmonary vascular disease. Hospital mortality is <5%.

   c) Or Rastelli operation for TGA and VSD and LVOTO: closure of VSD by a patch directing LV blood into aorta, closure of pulmonary valve, external valve conduit from RV to pulmonary trunk and closure of ASD. This is often performed after a preliminary systemic to pulmonary artery shunt, but not before 4–5 years of age. Hospital mortality is 10–20%.

PROGNOSIS

- Untreated, 30% die in the first week and 90% die in the first year.
- Overall mortality from the time of balloon atrial septostomy to definitive intra-atrial redirection operation is 10–20%. Five-year survival for hospital survivors of this type of operation is 90–95% for simple TGA[2] but less when VSD closure was part of the repair.
- Long-term disability after intra-atrial redirection operations may result from right ventricular dysfunction, venous obstruction, tricuspid regurgitation and atrial arrhythmias[4]. Pulmonary vascular disease may develop even after successful early operation.

- Long-term results of anatomical correction are not known. Mid-term results are encouraging[1].

FOLLOW-UP

Yearly follow-up by a paediatric cardiologist with ECG, chest x-ray and/or Doppler echocardiography is required after atrial or arterial surgery to detect arrhythmias, venous obstruction, right ventricular dysfunction, pulmonary hypertension, neo-aortic regurgitation or stenosis and right ventricular outflow tract obstruction.

[1] Quaegebur J M et al. (1987) J. Thorac. Cardiovasc. Surg., **92**, 361.
[2] Marx G R et al. (1983) J. Am. Coll. Cardiol., **1**, 476.
[3] Penkoske P A et al. (1983) Ann. Thorac. Surg., **36**, 281.
[4] Zuberbuhler J R (ed.) (1983) Am. J. Cardiol., **51**, 1513.

Total Anomalous Pulmonary Venous Connection

Total anomalous pulmonary venous connection (TAPVC) accounts for 1–2% congenital heart disease. In TAPVC there is no communication between the confluence of pulmonary veins behind the heart and the left atrium. This results in an obligatory right to left shunt and heart failure in infancy due to excessive pulmonary blood flow and/or pulmonary venous hypertension secondary to obstructed drainage. The commonest form is supracardiac drainage to the innominate vein via a vertical vein. Infradiaphragmatic forms are inevitably obstructive while cardiac forms (to right atrium and coronary sinus) are rarely so.

TREATMENT

1. Diuretics and digoxin and/or positive pressure ventilation while preparing for surgery.
2. Surgical correction in infancy. Surgery is urgent for obstructive but less so for non-obstructive forms. Surgery comprises creation of a wide communication between the pulmonary veins and left atrium with closure of the anomalously draining vein and the interatrial communication. Overall hospital mortality is 15–30%.

PROGNOSIS

- Without operation, 80% die within the first year. Survival with obstructive is significantly less than with non-obstructive forms[1].
- Rarely an untreated patient with non-obstructive TAPVC and large atrial communication survives into adult life but develops pulmonary vascular disease.
- Following successful surgical correction in infancy the prognosis is excellent in most cases. Late deaths (10–15%) are mostly due to pulmonary venous obstruction[2].

Cardiological follow-up with ECG and chest x-ray every 1–2 years is essential to detect the development of pulmonary hypertension due to pulmonary venous obstruction, and atrial arrhythmias.

[1] Gathman G E et al. (1970) Circulation, **42**, 143.
[2] Dickinson D F et al. (1982) Br. Heart J., **48**, 249.

Tetralogy of Fallot

Tetralogy of Fallot comprises 5–10% all congenital heart disease. The anatomical features of large VSD with overriding aorta and subpulmonary and pulmonary valve stenosis and often pulmonary artery stenosis result in right ventricular hypertrophy and a right to left shunt with diminished pulmonary blood flow. Wide variations in the anatomy of the right ventricular outflow tract (RVOT) and pulmonary arteries account for the variable clinical presentation, surgical treatment and prognosis. Severe degrees of RVOT obstruction lead to severe cyanosis in early infancy, while lesser degrees result in later presentation, and 'acyanotic' forms.

TREATMENT

1. Initial medical

   a) Treatment of spells: knee–chest position, oxygen, i.v. propranolol (0.1–0.2 mg/kg) and $NaHCO_3$ (1–2 mmol/kg) or subcutaneous morphine (0.1–0.2 mg/kg).
   b) Suppression of spells: propranolol 1 mg/kg q.d.s. orally while awaiting operation.
   c) Avoidance of anaemia and adequate intake of iron.
   d) Avoidance of dehydration (predisposing to stroke or, later, shunt thrombosis).

2. Surgical

   a) Infants with early severe cyanosis and older infants and children who have pulmonary artery anatomy unsuitable for complete repair require a subclavian to pulmonary artery shunt (prosthetic or classical Blalock) to stimulate growth of the pulmonary arteries and annulus[1]. Hospital mortality is <3%.
   b) When the pulmonary arteries are of adequate size, infants >3–6 months and children require complete repair preferably before the age of three years. Operation includes relief of RVOT obstruction with or without transannular patch and relief of pulmonary artery stenosis, patch closure of VSD, and ligation of any previous shunt. Hospital mortality is <10%.

PROGNOSIS

- Without surgery the prognosis depends on severity of obstruction to pulmonary blood flow; one-third die in the first year, one-half by 3 years, and three-quarters by 10 years[2]. Death is usually due to hypoxia, stroke, brain abscess or arrhythmia.
- With surgery the 8-year survival for hospital survivors of complete correction is >95%[3]. The great majority are asymptomatic.
- Risk factors for late postoperative death include[3]

   a) High right ventricular pressure after repair.
   b) Older age at operation.
   c) Early postoperative complete heart block and use of transannular patch may also increase the risk.

- Causes of late postoperative death include ventricular arrhythmias[4], complete heart block and re-operation (e.g. for residual VSD, unrelieved right ventricular outflow tract obstruction).

FOLLOW-UP

Preoperatively, infants should be seen by a cardiologist every 1–2 months to assess the need for surgical intervention. After shunt surgery 3–6 monthly visits are required to plan timing of catheterisation and definitive surgery. After correction, follow-up every 1–2 years with ECG and chest x-ray and/or Doppler echocardiography is necessary to detect arrhythmias, unrelieved right ventricular outflow tract obstruction, right ventricular dysfunction and tricuspid regurgitation.

[1] Gale A W et al. (1979) J. Thorac. Cardiovasc. Surg., 77, 459.
[2] Bertranou E G et al. (1978) Am. J. Cardiol., 42, 458.
[3] Katz N M et al. (1982) Circulation, 65, 403.
[4] Garson A et al. (1985) J. Am. Coll. Cardiol., 6, 211.

Rheumatic Fever

Acute rheumatic fever (RF) is a systemic disease which is related to preceding streptococcal group A pharyngitis or tonsillitis in susceptible individuals. The pathogenesis is presumed to be immunological. Although the incidence of RF began to fall dramatically in affluent countries even before the availability of antibiotics, in developing countries it is still common and rheumatic heart disease (RHD) is the most common form of heart disease in children.

TREATMENT

1. Primary prophylaxis (to prevent a first attack)[1]: treatment of group A streptococcal pharyngitis or tonsillitis. Either

   a) Penicillin V 125–250 mg q.d.s. for 10 days, or
   b) Benzathine penicillin G 1 200 000 units (916 mg) i.m.

2. Secondary prophylaxis (to prevent recurrence of streptococcal throat infection and, therefore, RF) should be continued until 20 years of age or 5 years after the last attack of RF, and possibly to age 40 in patients with RHD[1]. Either:

   a) Benzathine penicillin G 1 200 000 units (916 mg) i.m. every 3 weeks, or
   b) Penicillin V 125–250 mg b.d., or
   c) Sulphadiazine orally 0.5–1 g once a day, or
   d) For patients allergic to both penicillin and sulphonamides, erythromycin orally 250 mg b.d.

3. Treatment of acute RF

   a) Eradication of group A streptococci from the throat (as in (1) above).

   b) Bed rest while fever and acute manifestations persist.
   c) Aspirin 100 mg/kg/day in 4 doses for 2 weeks followed by 75 mg/kg/day for 4–6 weeks.
   d) Steroids do not reduce the incidence or severity of RHD but they may reduce the incidence of death in an acute attack[2].
   e) Treatment of heart failure with diuretics and/or afterload reducing agents.

4. Treatment of symptomatic chronic rheumatic heart disease

   a) Medical treatment: diuretics and digoxin and/or afterload reducing agents and/or anticoagulants.
   b) Rarely, surgical mitral valvotomy may be required in childhood for severe mitral stenosis.
   c) Mitral and aortic valve replacement are almost never required in childhood but may be necessary later in life.

5. Antibiotic prophylaxis against infective endocarditis for those with underlying RHD.

Contd.

PROGNOSIS

- Of all the manifestations of RF, only carditis causes death in the acute phase (rare) or results in significant chronic sequelae (RHD).
- One-third of all patients with an initial attack of RF will go on to develop RHD. Recurrences of RF are more common in those who have developed RHD after the initial attack and the incidence and severity of RHD is much higher among those who have had multiple attacks of RF[3].
- Fatality of RF and RHD in childhood is 2–3%[2].
- In the absence of recurrences of RF, new valve lesions do not appear even in those who had carditis with their first attack of RF, but old lesions may evolve.
- 70% patients with acute mitral regurgitation will lose their murmur from 4 days to 8.5 years after it was first heard. In contrast, in only 27% of patients with acute aortic regurgitation does the murmur disappear[4].

- The commonest long-term valvular sequelae are pure mitral stenosis, mitral regurgitation and mitral stenosis, and aortic regurgitation. Although it is uncommon for symptomatic RHD to occur within 10 years of the first attack of RF, in the tropics severe mitral stenosis may develop even in childhood.

FOLLOW-UP

The details of follow-up depend on the severity of the acquired valvular lesion or nature of the operation performed. Regular chest x-ray, ECG and Doppler echocardiography may be required and, when indicated, 24 hour ECG, exercise and radionuclide studies.

[1] Shulman S T et al. (1984) Circulation, **70,** 1118A.
[2] United Kingdom and United States Joint Report (1960) Circulation, **22,** 503.
[3] DiSciascio G et al. (1980) Am. Heart J., **99,** 635.
[4] Tompkins D G et al. (1972) Circulation, **45,** 543.

Infective Endocarditis

Infective endocarditis (IE) is an inflammatory process resulting from bacterial or fungal infection of cardiac valves or endocardium. Infective endarteritis is a similar process involving arterial endothelium particularly in cases of PDA and CoAo. Because of lack of suspicion the diagnosis of IE is frequently missed or made difficult by indiscriminate use of antibiotics without prior blood cultures in children at risk. Partly because of the longer survival of children at risk, the occurrence of IE appears to be increasing. Infective endocarditis may rarely occur in a previously normal heart.

TREATMENT

1. *Prophylaxis*

   a) Good dental hygiene is very important for all those at risk of IE.
   b) Antibiotics[1]
      i) For whom? Children with prosthetic heart valves or tube grafts, congenital heart disease including bicuspid aortic valve (exceptions: isolated secundum ASD, >6 months after suture closure of secundum ASD or ligation and division of PDA), rheumatic heart disease, other acquired valve dysfunction, hypertrophic cardiomyopathy, arterio-venous fistulae (systemic or pulmonary), past history of infective endocarditis, mitral valve prolapse with regurgitation.
      ii) For which procedures? All dental procedures likely to induce gum bleeding, tonsillectomy or adenoidectomy, upper and lower respiratory tract surgery,

rigid bronchoscopy, incision and drainage of infected tissue, genitourinary procedures. Only patients with prosthetic valves routinely require prophylaxis for obstetric, gynaecological or gastrointestinal procedures[2].

c) Dental, oral or respiratory tract procedures[2]

  i) Amoxycillin 3 g orally 1 hour before the procedure; children aged <10 and <5, one-half and one-quarter of this dose respectively. If prophylaxis is required twice in one month, amoxycillin should be given on both occasions. For those allergic to penicillin or on regular penicillin prophylaxis or who have recently had a course of penicillin, erythromycin stearate 1.5 g orally 1–2 hours before the procedure and 0.5 g 6 hours later; children aged <10 and <5 years, one-half and one-quarter of these doses respectively.

  ii) For those having a general anaesthetic (GA) amoxycillin 1 g i.m. in 2.5 ml of 1% lignocaine hydrochloride before induction and 0.5 g orally six hours later; one-half and one-quarter of these doses for children aged <10 and <5 years respectively. Alternatively[3], amoxycillin 3 g orally 4 hours before GA and 3 g orally as soon as possible after the procedure (same reductions in dosage for younger children).

  iii) For those on regular penicillin prophylaxis and those who have recently had a course of penicillin who require GA, or those who have a prosthetic valve or a history of endocarditis, amoxycillin 1 g i.m. in 2.5 ml of 1% lignocaine hydrochloride and gentamicin 120 mg i.m. immediately before induction of GA, or, if no GA, 15 minutes before the procedure and amoxycillin in 0.5 g orally 6 hours later. Children aged <10 and <5 years, one-half and one-quarter the dose of amoxycillin, and gentamicin 2 mg/kg.

  iv) For those who are allergic to penicillin and who require GA, or who have a prosthetic valve, or who have had a past history of IE, vancomycin 1 g i.v. over 1 hour followed by gentamicin 120 mg i.v. before induction of GA or, if no GA, 15 minutes before the procedure; for children aged <10 years, vancomycin 20 mg/kg and gentamicin 2 mg/kg.

d) For genitourinary procedures (and obstetric, gynaecological or gastrointestinal procedures in patients with prosthetic valves)

  i) For those with sterile urine who are not allergic to penicillin, antibiotics as in (iii) above.

  ii) For those with sterile urine who are allergic to penicillin, antibiotics as in (iv) above.

  iii) For those with known urine infections give antibiotics based on culture and sensitivity.

  iv) Antibiotics are not routinely required before urethral catheterisation for those with sterile urine.

2. For most organisms, a combination of two or even three bactericidal antibiotics of different classes (usually a penicillin for 4–6 weeks and an aminoglycoside for 2–6 weeks) given intravenously is mandatory. The antibiotics and their doses are governed by the *in vitro* sensitivities of the organism(s) grown from the blood and minimal bactericidal concentrations of the antibiotics for the organism, the serum bactericidal activity (back-titrations) and blood levels of antibiotics. A bacteriologist should be part of the decision-making team[4].

3. Absolute indications for surgery are progressive heart failure and recurrent emboli. Surgical options include valve replacement, drainage of paravalvular and myocardial abscesses and clearance of large, potentially embolic vegetations detected by echocardiography.

4. Dental consultation and, if indicated, treatment within 48 hours of commencing antibiotics.

PROGNOSIS

- Untreated, infective endocarditis is fatal[5].
- Despite treatment, overall mortality is approximately 20% in the young[4] and is higher in those who develop heart failure and (adults) in whom vegetations are detected by cross-sectional echocardiography[6].

[1] Shulman S T et al. (1984) Circulation, **70,** 1123A
[2] Working Party of the British Society for Antimicrobial Chemotherapy (1982) Lancet, **ii,** 1323.
[3] Working Party of the British Society for Antimicrobial Chemotherapy (1986) Lancet, **i,** 1267.
[4] Kaplan E L et al. (1983) Endocarditis. In Heart Disease in Infants, Children, and Adolescents, 3rd edn. (Adams F H, Emmanouilides G C eds). Baltimore: Williams & Wilkins.
[5] Johnson D H et al. (1975) Circulation, **51,** 581.
[6] Stafford W J et al. (1985) Br. Heart J., **53,** 310.

FOLLOW-UP

Early follow-up with home temperature chart, ECG, chest x-ray and/or Doppler echocardiography is mandatory to ensure that infection is eradicated. If there is any doubt blood cultures and counts and C-reactive protein/ESR should be repeated. Long-term follow-up is the same as that for the underlying lesion or for the surgery performed (e.g. valve replacement).

Myocarditis

Myocarditis is an inflammatory condition of the heart (and often the pericardium) which occasionally results in severe heart failure. Most cases of myocarditis probably go undiagnosed, disguised by symptoms affecting other systems. It is most frequently of viral aetiology, e.g. coxsackie, ECHO, influenza and mumps viruses. It can occur at any age, and may be present at birth following a maternal viral infection (especially coxsackie virus B).

TREATMENT

1. Bed rest with or without oxygen, diuretics and digoxin, with or without afterload reducing agents. Occasionally even positive pressure ventilation is required.
2. ECG monitoring and prompt treatment of arrhythmias or heart block in the acute phase.
3. Prednisolone ($50 \ mg/m^2$/day) and azathioprine ($50 \ mg/m^2$/day) are thought to improve prognosis, especially where there is histological evidence of inflammatory infiltrate in endomyocardial biopsy samples. Duration of treatment is usually 3–6 months, guided by further biopsies[1].
4. Digoxin and avoidance of strenuous exercise should be continued until the ECG and cardiac examination have returned to normal.

PROGNOSIS

- The majority (probably >80%) recover completely from acute viral myocarditis[2] while a small number die of rapidly progressive heart failure or arrhythmia.
- Neonatal coxsackie virus B myocarditis carries a high mortality rate (70–75%)[3].
- In a few, diffuse or focal abnormalities of left ventricular function persist for many years, while in others there is progressive deterioration. This group probably comprises a significant proportion of patients with congestive cardiomyopathy.

FOLLOW-UP

Cardiological follow-up with ECG, chest x-ray, echocardiography with or without 24 hour ECG, is required at least every 3 months in the early stages after symptomatic myocarditis. Serial radionuclide angiography and myocardial biopsy may be helpful.

[1] Mason J W et al. (1980) Am. J. Cardiol., **45,** 1037.
[2] Editorial (1972) Br. Med. J., **iii,** 783.
[3] Kilbrick S (1961) In Perspectives in Virology, p. 140. Minneapolis: Burgess.

Cardiomyopathies

Cardiomyopathies (CM) are disorders of ventricular myocardium. Congestive (or dilated) cardiomyopathy is frequently idiopathic, although some cases are sequelae of acute myocarditis. Some idiopathic cases are familial. The left ventricle is dilated and systolic function is diminished. Dilatation of the mitral valve ring may result in significant regurgitation. Hypertrophic CM is either familial or sporadic, or associated with Friedreich's ataxia, and rarely other conditions. It may occur in infants of diabetic mothers. Most commonly it is the ventricular septum which is inappropriately thickened but right and left ventricular free walls may also be involved. Left and right ventricular outflow tract obstruction may be present. The ventricular cavities are not dilated and diastolic rather than systolic function is abnormal.

TREATMENT

1. Congestive

   a) Diuretics and digoxin with or without afterload reducing agents with or without antiarrhythmic agents with or without anticoagulants.
   b) Heart transplantation is indicated in older patients with severe heart failure.

2. Hypertrophic

   a) Avoidance of competitive sport.
   b) Propranolol or verapamil appear to improve symptoms by reducing outflow tract obstruction or increasing ventricular compliance but may not protect against sudden death. Digoxin is contraindicated.
   c) Surgery (septal myotomy-myomectomy or resection of right ventricular outflow tract muscle) is only performed in patients who have severe left or right ventricular outflow tract obstruction and who are symptomatic despite medical treatment. Hospital mortality is 5–10%.

PROGNOSIS

- Some patients with congestive cardiomyopathy improve, often only transiently, while the majority die mostly from intractable heart failure within 5 years of diagnosis despite medical treatment[1].
- Of infants and children with idiopathic hypertrophic CM, about one-third die suddenly over a follow-up period of 7–9 years, possibly due to ventricular arrhythmias, while most of the remainder are asymptomatic or stable in childhood. Death from heart failure is common in symptomatic infants[2,3].
- Respiratory distress and heart failure occur in 10–50% infants of diabetic mothers who have hypertrophic CM. In survivors (the great majority), the hypertrophy resolves by 6 months of age[4].

FOLLOW-UP

Symptomatic children with congestive cardiomyopathy should be seen at frequent intervals in order to optimise drug therapy and, when appropriate to refer for heart transplantation. Chest x-ray, ECG, serial echocardiography (or radionuclide angiography) and/or 24 hour ECG are required. The same are required for children with hypertrophic cardiomyopathy who should be seen by a cardiologist at least yearly.

[1] Taliercio C P et al. (1985) J. Am. Coll. Cardiol., 6, 1126.
[2] Maron B J et al. (1982) Circulation, 65, 7.
[3] McKenna W J et al. (1984) Arch. Dis. Childh., 59, 971.
[4] Gutgesell H P et al. (1980) Circulation, 61, 441.

5

Diseases of the Alimentary Tract

D. C. A. Candy and I. W. Booth

Gastro-oesophageal Reflux

Some reflux, manifest by frequent, small regurgitation is common in infancy. More serious reflux may lead to failure to thrive, oesophagitis with bleeding, oesophageal stricture, or recurrent aspiration singly or in combination. A sliding hiatus hernia occurs in some infants but is not an invariable accompaniment of severe reflux, and many infants with a hiatus hernia are asymptomatic.

TREATMENT[1]

1. Mild reflux responds well to thickened feeds (0.5–1.5% Nestargel or Carobel added to milk).
2. Positioning after feeds is important: 30 degrees head-up prone reduces reflux and improves lower oesophageal acid clearance.
3. More severe reflux, particularly if associated with complications, may require nasogastric feeding by continuous infusion for 2–3 weeks, or until the ideal weight for length is achieved.
4. Drugs which enhance gastric emptying and/or increase lower oesophageal sphincter pressure may be added (e.g. domperidone, 0.2–0.4 mg/kg orally, at 4–8 hourly intervals). Bethanechol has too low a therapeutic index to be recommended.
5. Fundoplication is reserved for those patients with complications failing to respond to intensive medical treatment; oesophageal stricture and severe aspiration are absolute indications[2].

PROGNOSIS

- 95% infants with uncomplicated reflux are better by 12 months of age following maturation of the lower oesophageal sphincter, more solids in diet, and adoption of an upright posture; most require no treatment[3].
- Reflux associated with failure to thrive, oesophagitis or recurrent aspiration is associated with an excellent prognosis; only a small minority who fail to respond will require surgery[3].
- Prognosis in children allowed to develop peptic oesophageal stricture is more guarded.

FOLLOW-UP

Three monthly; monitor growth and look out for evidence of aspiration, and iron deficiency from oesophagitis.

[1] Balistreri W F et al. (1983) New Eng. J. Med., **309**, 790.
[2] Euler A R et al. (1977) Gastroenterology, **72**, 260.
[3] Friedland G W et al. (1975) J. Pediatr. **87**, 71.

Peptic Ulceration

In the neonate, peptic ulcers, usually gastric, tend to present with gastric perforation. With increasing age, duodenal ulcers become more common than gastric, and primary much more common than secondary ulcers[1,2]. Nocturnal pain and a family history of peptic ulceration are important pointers towards the diagnosis in childhood.

TREATMENT

1. Antacids given in high dosage (aluminium hydroxide and magnesium hydroxide mixture 30 ml/1.73 m^2, given 1 and 3 hours after meals and at bed-time) are effective in healing ulcers[3].
2. Compliance is likely to be poor with antacids, therefore H$_2$-receptor antagonists are preferred. Side-effects more likely with cimetidine than ranitidine[4]. De-Nol or sucralfate may be tried for H$_2$-blockade resistant ulcers.
3. The chances of a further relapse for patients who have relapsed after their first course of ranitidine/cimetidine may be lessened by 12 months maintenance therapy. However, 10–25% still relapse.
4. Surgical management is reserved for complications: pain resistant to H$_2$-receptor blockade, repeated relapses, haemorrhage, perforation and obstruction. Highly selective vagotomy and pyloroplasty is the operation of choice in children and adolescents. The need for surgery is likely to fall with the availability of H$_2$-receptor blockers.

PROGNOSIS

- Prognosis is poor in the neonate with acute gastric perforation.
- Under six years of age, about 25% relapse within four years, rising to a 60–70% relapse rate in older children and adolescents. The advent of H$_2$-receptor blockers may improve the prognosis.
- Vagotomy and pyloroplasty is usually successful, with a very low relapse rate (6%).

FOLLOW-UP

Follow-up is likely to be long term and should be continued at least until any possible surgical intervention.

[1] Nord K S et al. (1980) Am. J. Gastroenterol., **73,** 75.
[2] Tudor R B (1972) Gastroenterology, **62,** 823.
[3] Peterson W L et al. (1977) New Eng. J. Med., **297,** 341.
[4] Zeldis J B et al. (1983) New Eng. J. Med., **309,** 1368.
[5] Murphy M S et al. (1987) J. Pediatr. Gastroenterol. Nutr., **6,** 721.

Recurrent Abdominal Pain

Abdominal pain, severe enough to interfere with normal activities, and lasting longer than three months, occurs in 10% children. In only about 5% children is there an underlying organic cause. Of the remainder, only a few cases are likely to be psychogenic.

TREATMENT

1. Organic pain is treated as appropriate to the underlying disorder.
2. In the non-organic group treatment begins with the first consultation; attempted explanation and reassurance are meaningless unless preceded by a thorough history and full examination.
3. Explanation begins with pointing out the relationships between emotions and abdominal symptoms ('butterflies' in the tummy, sick with fear, diarrhoea and anxiety).
4. Many parents and children can understand: 'his/her intestines seem to get so sensitive from time to time, that he/she can almost feel the food going round the bends', and find this explanation helpful.
5. Occasional children with overt psychosocial problems may benefit from psychiatric referral, although psychosocial disturbances are not more common in children with non-organic pain than in pain-free controls[1].

PROGNOSIS[2,3]

- The prognosis in the organic group is that of the underlying disorder.
- In the non-organic group, pain in about one-third of the children resolves spontaneously, one-third continue to have other symptoms (e.g. migraine, dysmenorrhoea), and the remainder continue to experience both abdominal pain and other symptoms.
- Onset of pain under the age of five years, a family history of recurrent abdominal pain, and a history of more than six months before consultation may be associated with a poorer prognosis.

FOLLOW-UP

The need for hospital follow-up must be carefully considered; prolonged, organically-orientated follow-up is likely to foster the entrenchment of somatic symptoms.

[1] McGrath P J et al. (1983) Arch. Dis. Childh., **58,** 888.
[2] Apley J et al. (1973) Br. Med. J., **3,** 7.
[3] Christensen J F et al. (1975) Arch. Dis. Childh., **50,** 110.

Coeliac Disease

Coeliac disease is a gluten-induced enteropathy, probably life long, of uncertain aetiology; the gliadin fraction of gluten probably starts a harmful immune response in the small bowel mucosa.

TREATMENT

1. A gluten free diet is instituted following the finding of flat mucosa on jejunal biopsy. The expert advice of a dietitian is essential[1]. Monitor carefully for clinical response, as failure to respond may indicate continuing gluten intake or incorrect diagnosis.
2. Removal of disaccharides from the diet may be necessary if clinical intolerance persists, but this is rare.

PROGNOSIS

- The prognosis is excellent on a gluten free diet.
- The incidence of small bowel malignancy is increased[2], and it is not clear that this becomes normal on treatment with a gluten free diet.

FOLLOW-UP

Follow-up should be continued and a gluten challenge[3] carried out after 2–4 years in order to confirm the diagnosis (preferably before the child begins school). A pre-challenge jejunal biopsy will confirm that the mucosa is in remission. A gluten-containing diet is then begun (minimum 10 g wheat protein/day as, for example four slices of bread per day or alternatively as gluten powder if preferred, for 3–4 months). The jejunal biopsy is then repeated (post-challenge biopsy); mucosal relapse confirms diagnosis. The post-challenge biopsy should be performed earlier if a confirmed clinical relapse occurs before 3–4 months have passed. If the post-challenge biopsy is normal, maintain the patient on a normal diet and re-biopsy after two years, or sooner if symptoms recur. If gluten challenge confirms diagnosis, continue on gluten free diet for life.

[1] Francis D E M (1986) *Diets for Sick Children*, 4th edn. Oxford: Blackwell.
[2] Isaacson P *et al.* (1978) *Lancet*, **i,** 67.
[3] McNeish A S *et al.* (1979) *Arch. Dis. Childh.*, **54,** 783.

Intestinal Atresia

Intestinal obstruction may occur by extrinsic compression (Ladd's bands in malrotation, volvulus), or intrinsic abnormality (atresia, stenosis, internal diaphragm, bolus obstruction). Duodenal atresia occurs in 1 in 5000 live births, jejunal and ileal atresia in 1 in 6000, while colonic atresia is only one-twentieth as common as small intestinal atresia[1].

TREATMENT

1. Duodenal atresia

   a) Aspirate stomach with adequate bore naso-gastric tube and leave on free drainage with hourly aspiration.
   b) Correct fluid and electrolyte deficits if necessary.
   c) At surgery, carefully inspect the rest of the gastrointestinal tract for associated abnormalities.
   d) A fine bore transanastomotic silicon feeding tube, placed at surgery, will assist early postoperative enteral nutrition.
   e) Recovery of gastric emptying is often delayed postoperatively.

2. Jejunal and ileal atresias

   a) Treat as for duodenal atresia, except that transanastomotic tube is impractical in distal atresias.
   b) Record length and type of remaining small intestine.
   c) If resection is massive, see *Protracted diarrhoea* (p. 73).

3. Colon atresia: manage as for small intestinal atresia.

PROGNOSIS

● Duodenal atresia

   a) One-third of patients with duodenal atresia have Down's syndrome[2].
   b) Survival is over 80%[1].

● Jejunal atresia

   a) Survival is over 90%[1].
   b) Mortality is high if
      i) Multiple atresias are present.
      ii) Massive resection has been carried out.
      iii) There are associated abnormalities.

● Colonic atresia: survival is over 90%[1].

FOLLOW-UP

If terminal ileum is resected, monitor the plasma B_{12} status 6 monthly. If B_{12} levels falls (may take several years) assess terminal ileal function with a Schilling test. If some residual absorptive function is present try large oral doses (25–50 mg) B_{12}, otherwise 1000 μg B_{12} 6 weekly i.m. For remaining follow-up see *Short bowel syndrome (p. 76)*.

[1] Dickson J A S (1977) In *Essentials of Paediatric Gastroenterology*, p. 63. Edinburgh: Churchill Livingstone.
[2] Young D G et al. (1968) *Surgery*, **63**, 832.

Transient Dietary Protein Intolerances

Transient dietary protein intolerances usually manifest themselves as protracted diarrhoea and/or vomiting with failure to thrive, acute colitis or anaphylaxis. Cow's milk protein is the most commonly incriminated antigen. Also described are soya, wheat, fish, egg, chicken and rice protein intolerance. Intolerances occur more commonly in those infants with a strong family history of atopy, or IgA deficiency.

TREATMENT

1. Elimination of the offending antigen results in rapid resolution of symptoms. In the uncommon case of severe protracted diarrhoea, more intensive nutritional support, sometimes parenteral, may be needed.
2. The advice of an experienced dietitian is essential in the supervision of all exclusion diets in infancy and childhood[1].
3. In the case of cow's milk protein intolerance, a casein hydrolysate-based formula (e.g. Nutramigen, Pregistimil) is preferred to a soya-based feed, as 20–30% infants will also be, or become, intolerant to soya.
4. Occasionally older infants and toddlers will refuse a milk substitute, and it is then important to add a calcium supplement (e.g. Sandocal one or more tablets daily).
5. Most patients have grown out of their intolerance by the age of two years, which is therefore a reasonable time to conduct a challenge. Anaphylaxis occurs infrequently, nevertheless it is important to monitor carefully the start of the challenge in hospital. Begin with a skin test, followed by application of antigen to lips, and ingestion of increasing amounts (e.g. 1 ml cow's milk initially). Do not abandon the challenge until there is unequivocal evidence of intolerance; intercurrent infections may make interpretation of response difficult.

PROGNOSIS

- Dietary protein intolerances are usually outgrown by 2–3 years of age.
- Thereafter the prognosis is excellent, although some children will go on to develop other atopic disorders, such as asthma.
- Death from anaphylaxis is rare, and from protracted diarrhoea very uncommon. The latter has a small morbidity.

FOLLOW-UP

Three to six monthly, until dietary challenges are performed at two to three years of age.

---

[1] Francis D E M (1986) *Diets for Sick Children*, 4th edn. Oxford: Blackwell.

Congenital Chloridorrhoea

In this rare, autosomally recessive inherited disorder of electrolyte transport, exchange of Cl^- (inward) and HCO_3^- across the intestinal brush border is defective. Watery diarrhoea, due to unabsorbed Cl^- begins antenatally, causing hydramnios. The diagnosis is made by demonstrating that the stool Cl^- concentration exceeds the sum of stool Na^+ and K^+ concentrations.

TREATMENT

Replacement of electrolyte losses of both NaCl and KCl[1], initially i.v. then orally.

PROGNOSIS

- Normal growth and development if treated early. Nutrient absorption is normal.
- Frequent brain damage due to late diagnosis and treatment.
- Renal impairment may occur due to chronic dehydration.
- Diarrhoea uninfluenced by treatment.

FOLLOW-UP

Follow-up should be at specialist centres where satisfactory growth and development will be checked.

[1] Milla P J (1982) *Clin. Gastroenterol.*, **11**, 31.

Sucrose Intolerance

Secondary sucrose intolerance is less common than secondary lactose intolerance, as the enzyme appears more robust than lactase (see *Secondary lactase deficiency* p. 69). Primary sucrose intolerance occurs as part of the rare autosomal recessive disorder, sucrase isomaltase deficiency[1].

TREATMENT

1. Avoidance of sucrose-containing foods and added sucrose. Starch may need to be excluded in early life.
2. Vitamin C supplements may be required because of avoidance of fruit and potatoes.

PROGNOSIS

- The affected infant is well until weaning, when sucrose- and starch-containing foods are introduced. Starch intolerance occurs because of the associated low small intestinal mucosal isomaltase activity, and because 60% maltase activity is due to sucrase.
- There is a broad spectrum of susceptibility to sucrose and starch; thus symptoms may vary from life-threatening watery diarrhoea to irritable bowel syndrome[2].
- Adults with this condition may tolerate a normal diet.

FOLLOW-UP

Regular weight centile checks and dietary advice should be given.

[1] Harries J T (1982) *Clin. Gastroenterol.*, **11**, 17.
[2] Ament M E et al. (1973) *J. Pediatr.*, **83**, 721.

Lactose Intolerance

Low small intestinal lactase activity is usual in non-Caucasian individuals over the age of 5 years. Lactase deficiency may complicate any small intestinal disorder (e.g. coeliac disease in relapse gastrointestinal surgery, post-gastroenteritis). Congenital lactase deficiency may also occur as a rare autosomal disorder[1].

TREATMENT

A diet free of cow's milk (including whey, dry milk solids and curds), using soy formula or Pregestimil as a substitute.

PROGNOSIS

- Non-caucasian lactase deficiency

a) The amount of lactose which individuals with non-caucasian lactase deficiency can tolerate is highly variable.
b) In parts of Africa, and around the Mediterranean where this is the norm, little milk is consumed by adults, except as hard cheese and yoghurt in which lactose has been largely converted to lactic acid.
c) In areas such as northern Europe, where milk farming has been carried out for at least 12 000 years, persistence of production of lactase into adult life is the norm; this ability is inherited as an autosomal dominant condition[2].

- Secondary lactase deficiency: the prognosis depends on the underlying disorder.
- Congenital lactase deficiency[1]: this may be fatal in the neonatal period if not diagnosed and treated, due to dehydration from the osmotic diarrhoea.

FOLLOW-UP

Weight centiles should be checked and dietary advice given. With *secondary* lactose intolerance following acute gastroenteritis a careful trial of diluted lactose-containing milk can be started 3 months after the lactose withdrawal.

[1] Hadorn B *et al.* (1981) *Clin. Gastroenterol.*, **10**, 671.
[2] Harries J T (1982) *Clin. Gastroenterol.*, **11**, 17.

Glucose Galactose Malabsorption

This rare inborn error of monosaccharide transport due to an absent or defective brush border carrier, presents with severe watery diarrhoea from birth. Diagnosis is confirmed by rapid resolution on a lactose/glucose free diet with diarrhoea following rechallenge with glucose[1].

TREATMENT

1. A lactose, sucrose and glucose free diet is required.
2. Fructose is well tolerated and can be used as a source of carbohydrate (e.g. Galactomin 19).

PROGNOSIS

- Delay in diagnosis may result in death due to dehydration. Diarrhoea begins within a few days of birth due to the osmotic effect of monosaccharide malabsorption.
- The overall prognosis is good if the inborn error is diagnosed early because tolerance for glucose and galactose improves with age.

FOLLOW-UP

Weight centiles should be checked and dietary advice given. With *secondary* glucose galactose intolerance following acute gastroenteritis, a careful trial of diluted baby milk can be started 3 months after glucose galactose withdrawal.

[1] Harries J T (1982) *Clin. Gastroenterol.*, **11**, 17.

Abetalipoproteinaemia

Abetalipoproteinaemia is an inborn error of metabolism which presents with steatorrhoea and failure to thrive. The absence of betalipoproteins means the affected infant is unable to form chylomicrons to transport cholesterol in plasma. Small intestinal enterocytes therefore become laden with dietary fat as seen on jejunal biopsy. Plasma cholesterol levels are very low, and associated red cell membrane abnormalities result in the appearance of acanthocytes in the peripheral blood[1].

TREATMENT

1. Low fat diet. Medium chain triglycerides are useful as a supplementary source of calories because they do not need lipoprotein for transport.
2. Vitamin E (water soluble) 100 mg/kg/day.
3. Vitamin A (5000 IU/day), vitamin D (500 IU/day) and vitamin K supplements.

PROGNOSIS

- Untreated, the associated vitamin E malabsorption results in ataxia, neuropathy and pigmentary retinopathy.
- Other fat soluble vitamin deficiencies may occur.

FOLLOW-UP

Growth must be monitored since a low fat diet may have inadequate calories. Plasma vitamin E levels are undetectable because of the absence of chylomicra, hence vitamin E activity is monitored six monthly by red cell peroxide haemolysis and maintained in the normal range by adjusting the dose of the supplement. Plasma vitamin A, alkaline phosphatase and prothrombin should also be monitored because fat soluble vitamins are poorly absorbed.

[1] Muller D P R (1982) *Clin. Gastroenterol.*, **11**, 119.

Acrodermatitis Enteropathica

Acrodermatitis enteropathica is an inborn error of zinc absorption. The disorder presents in infancy after cessation of breast feeding with failure to thrive, symmetrical eczematous perioral and perianal rash, paronychia, diarrhoea, baldness, depression, and immunodeficiency[1].

TREATMENT

1. Zinc sulphate 2 mg/kg/day.
2. Monitor plasma zinc and copper.

PROGNOSIS

- All manifestations resolve on high dose zinc supplements.
- As an autosomal recessive condition, the risk in subsequent siblings is one in four.

FOLLOW-UP

Weight measurements and weight centiles should be performed regularly and zinc and copper levels checked.

[1] Hambridge K M *et al.* (1982) *Clin. Gastroenterol.*, **11**, 87.

Acute Infectious Diarrhoea

Infectious diarrhoea remains a significant cause of morbidity in industrialised societies. In developing countries it is the leading cause of childhood mortality. The commonest viral causes are rotavirus and adenovirus, and the commonest bacterial causes are *Campylobacter jejuni*, shigellae, enterotoxigenic *Escherichia coli* (developing countries) and enteropathogenic *E. coli* (developed countries).

TREATMENT

1. Treatment is based on a clinical assessment of the degree of dehydration[1].
2. If the child is shocked (peripheral cyanosis, weak rapid pulse, hypotension) i.v. 0.9% saline or plasma (20 ml/kg) is given rapidly until the peripheral circulation is restored, followed by 70 ml/kg 0.9% saline with added K^+ over three hours. Rehydration can generally be continued by the oral route.
3. If there are clinical signs of dehydration (dry mouth, sunken eyes, suppression of tears, rapid pulse) but the child is not shocked then 100 ml/kg WHO oral rehydration salts (ORS) solution is administered in frequent small aliquots over four hours.
4. If signs of dehydration are minimal or absent then 50 ml WHO ORS is administered over four hours.
5. If lower sodium concentration ORS (e.g. Dioralyte, Dextrolyte) are used, then correspondingly higher volumes of ORS solution will be required to correct electrolyte deficits.
6. Breast feeding may continue during this rehydration phase[2]. Non-breast-fed infants should have access to extra water.
7. Intravenous rehydration will be required for excessive vomiting or stool loss, ileus or when there is diagnostic doubt.
8. After successful rehydration, continue with breast feeding, or half strength formula after 24 hours. Continuing diarrhoeal losses may be replaced by offering 100 ml/kg/day ORS until the diarrhoea resolves or 10 ml/kg after each loose stool.

9. Antibiotics are only indicated for dysentery, systemic salmonellosis, cholera, giardiasis, amoebiasis, prolonged *Campylobacter* or *Yersinia* infections and where there is the possibility of septicaemia[3].

PROGNOSIS

- Among the 300 million children under the age of five years, 100 million attacks of diarrhoea occur every year, resulting in 5 million deaths from dehydration.
- If dehydration is accompanied by hypernatraemia (serum Na^+ > 150 mmol/l) brain damage may occur due to intracranial haemorrhage as a result of brain shrinkage or cerebral oedema due to rapid rehydration[4].

- In developing countries up to 15% attacks are prolonged resulting in malnutrition and growth failure[5].

FOLLOW-UP

The weight gain in one month should be checked. Secondary lactose intolerance may develop. Collaborate with public health authorities.

[1] WHO (1984) *A Manual for the Treatment of Acute Diarrhoea*. WHO/CDD/SER/80.2. Geneva: WHO.
[2] Kin-Maung-U et al. (1985) *Br. Med. J.*, **290**, 587.
[3] Levine M M (1986) *Rev. Inf. Dis.*, **8**, 5207.
[4] Pizarro D et al. (1983) *Am. J. Dis. Child.*, **137**, 730.
[5] Booth I W et al. (1987) *J. Trop. Pediatr.*, **33**, 69.

Toddler Diarrhoea

Toddler diarrhoea (chronic non-specific diarrhoea of infancy, irritable bowel syndrome of infancy) usually begins between the ages of six months and two years. The stool consistency is variable and diarrhoea may alternate with constipation. Stools contain undigested food, e.g. peas, carrots, and may contain mucus. Diagnosis is by exclusion (e.g. exclude giardiasis, carbohydrate intolerance)[1].

TREATMENT

1. No specific treatment is available or necessary.
2. Reassure parents that the underlying condition is probably based on disordered motility.

PROGNOSIS

- Affected children remain well and grow normally.
- Symptoms improve with age, they rarely persist beyond 6 years.
- There should be no delay in achieving continence.

FOLLOW-UP

Growth should be checked. Parents should be reassured that normal growth indicates normal gastrointestinal function. Acceptance of the child as healthy, albeit with loose stools should be emphasised. If growth velocity is suboptimal, investigate for malabsorption. If symptoms are causing distress try loperamide[2]. Frequent follow-up may emphasise the parents' suspicion of organic bowel disease.

[1] Walker-Smith J A (1984) In *Textbook of Gastroenterology*, p. 550. London: Ballière Tindall.
[2] Hamdi I et al. (1978) *Acta Paediatr. Belg.*, **31**, 106.

Protracted Diarrhoea

Protracted diarrhoea is defined as the passage of four or more loose stools a day, for more than two weeks associated with weight loss or failure of normal weight gain. In developed countries, dietary protein intolerance (coeliac disease, milk and soy intolerance) is likely to be the commonest cause, while in developing countries, bacterial and parasitic infections of the gastrointestinal tract predominate. In both environments the cause of many episodes of protracted diarrhoea remains unknown.

TREATMENT

1. Treatment should not be delayed while attempting to establish a diagnosis.
2. In the absence of a treatable cause, treatment is based on nutritional support while awaiting spontaneous recovery.
3. If the infant is grossly wasted, parenteral nutrition (PN) is introduced, after resuscitation, rehydration, correction of electrolyte disturbances and treatment of sepsis.
4. Once established on PN, a gluten free diet (e.g. Pregestimil, Pregomin, Pepdite) is introduced.
5. The milk substitute is commenced at 1 ml/hour by continuous rate enteral nutrition (CREN) via a nasogastric tube. As the infusion rate is increased, PN is withdrawn ml for ml.
6. In less malnourished infants, milk substitute may be introduced (40 ml/kg/24 hours as CREN) with the remainder of the fluid and electrolyte requirement being given i.v. The rate of CREN is then progressively increased (to 200 ml/kg/24 hours) and i.v. fluid decreased. If the infant fails to tolerate this regimen then PN is commenced.
7. If the semi-elemental diet is not tolerated then a modular diet based on comminuted chicken (Chix) is introduced[1].
8. When the infant is thriving, and is more than four months old, gluten free, milk free, soy free, disaccharide free solids are introduced (not more frequently than one new food per day) and the infant is discharged.
9. If the infant fails to respond, other empirical treatments may be tried: loperamide in high doses (may cause ileus), prednisolone 1–2 mg/kg/day for 10 days (withdraw if no response), sodium cromoglycate if the history suggests dietary protein intolerance, cholestyramine/trimethoprim/metronidazole.

PROGNOSIS

- The prognosis depends on the underlying cause.
- Mortality is 5% in developed countries[1]. It may be much higher in developing countries.
- The disorder may be familial if due to a recognised autosomal recessive gene (e.g. cystic fibrosis, congenital chloridorrhoea) or a familial disorder (coeliac disease). A small proportion of protracted diarrhoea of unknown origin may also be familial with an extremely poor prognosis[2].

FOLLOW-UP

Three months after discharge the infant is re-admitted for lactose and cow's milk challenge. If the infant is on a modular diet, lactose is progressively substituted for the carbohydrate module. If the infant is receiving a semi-elemental milk substitute, then a lactose challenge (0.5 g/kg) is administered. If lactose is tolerated, cow's milk is progressively introduced (commencing with an initial challenge of 1 ml or less) followed by sucrose containing solids and the child is discharged on a milk containing, gluten free diet. Three months after discharge, gluten is introduced. If there is a family history of coeliac disease, or symptoms followed the introduction of gluten then the challenge is controlled with pre and post-gluten challenge biopsies. Otherwise gluten is introduced in outpatients and the child's growth monitored.

[1] Larcher V F et al. (1977) Arch. Dis. Childh., 52, 597.
[2] Candy D C A et al. (1981) Arch. Dis. Childh., 56, 15.

Malrotation

Malrotation is due to disordered embryogenesis between the sixth and sixteenth weeks of gestation. There is failure of rotation of the caecum around the small intestine. The caecal mesentery fails to fuse with the parietal peritoneum, and Ladd's bands from the posterior abdominal wall and gallbladder cross the second part of the duodenum on their way to the caecum. The large intestine is on the left, and the small intestine on the right side of the abdomen[1].

TREATMENT

1. See Treatment of *Intestinal atresia* (p. 66).
2. Volvulus is a surgical emergency. Massive infarction may result if surgery is delayed. At laparotomy, Ladd's bands are divided, and the appendix is removed to attempt to fix the caecum to the posterior abdominal wall. Frankly infarcted gut is resected. Before massive intestinal resection, consider closure of abdomen with 'second look' laparotomy after 24 hours.
3. See also Treatment of *Protracted diarrhoea* (p. 73).

PROGNOSIS

- The abnormality may be an incidental finding at post-mortem[1].

- Duodenal obstruction due to Ladd's bands usually presents in the neonatal period.
- Partial, intermittent or complete duodenal or small intestinal obstruction may occur at any time, due to volvulus of the intestine which has a narrow pedicle.
- In up to 25% symptomatic cases severe associated congenital abnormalities, especially cardiac, are said to exist.

FOLLOW-UP

Follow-up is as for *Short bowel syndrome* (p. 76).

[1] Silverman A *et al.* (1983) In *Paediatric Clinical Gastroenterology*, p. 61. St Louis: Mosby.

Protein-losing Enteropathy

Excess protein loss into the gut may occur in any bowel condition associated with rapid intestinal mucosal cell turnover (e.g. Menétrièr's disease, coeliac disease), lymphatic stasis (e.g. intestinal lymphangiectasia, thoracic duct obstruction) or venous stasis (e.g. constrictive pericarditis, malrotation). Diagnosis is by exclusion of cirrhosis and nephrotic syndrome. If necessary, the condition can be confirmed by demonstrating excess faecal loss of ^{51}Cr-labelled albumin or α-1-antitrypsin[1].

TREATMENT

1. Correction of underlying disorder.
2. High protein diet.
3. In intestinal lymphangiectasia give a diet rich in medium chain triglycerides (MCT) which are absorbed via the portal venous system rather than intestinal lymphatics.
4. Dietary long chain triglycerides (LCT) are absorbed via the intestinal lymphatics. Hence decreasing LCT reduces lymphatic dilatation.
5. Only up to one-third of dietary fat should be replaced by MCT to avoid possible hepatotoxicity and essential fatty acid deficiency. Medium chain triglycerides are also unpalatable.
6. Portagen is a suitable MCT milk (not a highly modified formula); MCT oil (Mead Johnson, Cow & Gate, SHS) may be used in cooking.
7. A low fat diet is also effective, but less acceptable.

PROGNOSIS

- See *Prognosis* of underlying causes (e.g. coeliac disease, Crohn's disease, ulcerative colitis, malrotation).
- Intestinal lymphangiectasia may be localised. This is a rare finding but is amenable to correction by surgical resection.
- Generalised intestinal lymphangiectasia generally responds well to the dietary measures outlined below.

FOLLOW-UP

Check for fat soluble (A, D, E and K) vitamin deficiency if the child is on a low fat diet.

[1] Silverman A *et al.* (1983) In *Paediatric Clinical Gastroenterology*, p. 304. St Louis: Mosby.

Short Bowel Syndrome

Short bowel syndrome may follow massive intestinal resections, e.g. for volvulus or multiple atresias.

TREATMENT

Nutritional management of the short bowel syndrome, see *Protracted diarrhoea* (p. 73).

PROGNOSIS

- If the ileocaecal valve is preserved, then a total small bowel length of greater than 10 cm is compatible with survival.
- Ileum has a greater capacity to adapt than jejunum.

- If the ileocaecal valve has been resected then the prognosis is worse.

FOLLOW-UP

Height and weight centiles should be checked. Iron and vitamin absorption should be monitored, especially folic acid and vitamin B_{12} where the terminal ileum is involved. See follow-up for *Protracted diarrhoea*.

---

[1] Wilmore D W (1972) *J. Pediatr.*, **80,** 88.

Necrotising Enterocolitis

Since the introduction of intensive neonatal care, necrotising enterocolitis (NEC) has become the commonest indication for admission to neonatal surgical units. The incidence varies up to tenfold between units, and may occur in outbreaks. Segmental bowel necrosis occurs, with intramural gas formation which may be affected radiologically.

TREATMENT

1. Remove nasojejunal tube if present (leave nasogastric tube for aspiration of stomach).
2. Stop oral feeds or reduce to 0.5 ml/kg/hour fresh expressed breast milk if ileus not present.
3. Correct anaemia, hypovolaemia (using plasma 10–20 ml/kg), fluid and electrolyte imbalance.
4. Commence parenteral nutrition.
5. Start antibiotics (usually gentamicin and metronidazole).
6. Treat disordered coagulation (vitamin K, fresh frozen or fresh blood exchange transfusion as indicated).
7. Perform 12-hourly lateral decubitus x-rays to detect intestinal perforation.
8. Surgery is indicated if there is no improvement within 24 hours of medical treatment. Obviously non-viable gut is resected and the free ends brought out as temporary enterostomies rather than anastomosed.

PROGNOSIS

- Prognosis depends on the grade of disease[1], which is also a guide to treatment.
- Grading

		Score
a) Stools		
i) occult blood positive.		1
ii) bloody stools.		2
iii) shed mucosa and blood in stools.		3
b) Abdominal examination		
i) distension only.		1
ii) with tenderness.		2
iii) peritonism, oedema, erythema.		3

c) Abdominal x-ray (supine and lateral decubitus, left side uppermost)
   i) unilateral pneumatosis intestinalis.   1
   ii) bilateral pneumatosis intestinalis.   2
   iii) free intraperitoneal or intraportal venous gas.   3
d) Length of symptoms prior to presentation
   i) >24 hours.   1
   ii) 12–24 hours.   2
   iii) <12 hours.   3
e) Apnoea/bradycardia
   i) self-limiting.   1
   ii) prolonged.   2
   iii) requiring ventilation.   3

f) Score	Treatment	Mortality (%)
<10	Medical	5–10
11–12	Surgical	>40
>12	Immediate resuscitation/surgery	>90

FOLLOW-UP

Intestinal stricture is common after NEC, with or without surgery. This presents as subacute obstruction, or more often with symptoms of malabsorption.

---

[1] German J C et al. (1979) Pediatr. Surg., **14**, 364.

Intussusception

Intussusception is the slipping or invagination of one part of an intestine into another part just below it. It occurs usually in previously healthy infants in the first year of life, presenting with intermittent, severe pain and pallor, vomiting, lethargy and, usually as a late sign, blood in the stools (redcurrant jelly). Usually no underlying intestinal cause is found. It most commonly begins just proximal to the ileocaecal valve and progresses distally to the transverse colon or beyond.

TREATMENT[1,2]

1. Nasogastric suction and intravenous infusion is quickly established.
2. Hydrostatic barium reduction should be attempted initially. However, it is contraindicated if peritonitis is present. The presence of radiological intestinal obstruction, bleeding or clinical deterioration indicates that the attempted reduction should be brief. Success rate is 75% or more.
3. Surgery is indicated for failed hydrostatic reduction (25%), peritonitis, recurrence after barium enemas or when the patient's condition fails to improve following hydrostatic reduction.

PROGNOSIS

- The overall mortality is 1–2%.

- Unreduced, it has a mortality of 100%.
- Resection of more than 30 cm of terminal ileum leads to later vitamin B_{12} deficiency.
- The recurrence rate is 4–10%.

FOLLOW-UP

Long-term follow-up necessary only following loss of terminal ileum, when patients may need vitamin B_{12} replacement. A few patients may develop ulceration and bleeding at the site of an ileocolic anastomosis, but this is usually delayed by some years.

---

[1] Hutchison I F et al. (1980) Br. J. Surg., **67**, 209.
[2] Ein S H et al. (1971) J. Pediatr. Surg., **6**, 16.

Crohn's Disease

Crohn's disease is a transmural, focal subacute or chronic inflammatory disorder, affecting any part of the gastrointestinal tract from mouth to anus, but most commonly the distal ileum and proximal colon. It usually presents with colicky abdominal pain, diarrhoea, weight loss and fever. Growth failure occurs in 30% children.

TREATMENT

1. The aims of treatment are to induce and maintain remission, to correct malnutrition and restore growth. The choice lies between drugs and nutritional management.
2. Drugs do not alter the natural history of disease, but are useful in suppressing disease manifestations.

   a) Corticosteroids induce remission in 70% patients, but 70% relapse by 12 months, and there is no evidence that they fulfil a prophylactic role[1]. Prednisolone is begun in high dosage (2 mg/kg/day), reduced after 2–3 weeks. An alternate day regimen may subsequently control symptoms and avoid growth suppression.

   b) Immunosuppressives, azathioprine (1–2 mg/kg/day), or 6-mercaptopurine (starting dose 1.5 mg/kg/day, and adjusted to maintain white cell count over $4.5 \times 10^9/l$ and platelets above $100 \times 10^9/l$) may maintain remission, or reduce steroid requirements[2]. Monitor blood count closely.

   c) Sulphasalazine (30–50 mg/kg/day) is useful in the management of symptomatic Crohn's colitis but unlike in ulcerative colitis, has no prophylactic role[3]. Oligospermia is a recently recognised side-effect.

   d) Metronidazole (7.5 mg/kg t.d.s.) is useful in colonic and particularly perianal disease[4]. It is reserved for those failing to respond to sulphasalazine.

   e) Loperamide is useful in the control of diarrhoea following extensive ileocolic resection. The dose is titrated to provide freedom from diarrhoea at night and during school lessons (starting dose: 1–2 mg q.d.s.).

   f) Oral cholestyramine is indicated for bile acid induced diarrhoea following ileal resection.

3. Nutritional therapy

   a) Specific deficiencies are corrected (e.g. iron, folate, vitamin B_{12}, zinc).

   b) Remission can be induced by nutritional support, usually by enteral feeding with an elemental diet. Rarely, the parenteral route may be necessary if the enteral route is not tolerated. Elemental diet is at least as effective as steroids in inducing remission and is probably now the treatment of choice[5].

4. Correction of growth failure: a 40% increase in calorie and protein intake is recommended for the patient's height–age. This can be given as an elemental diet (initially) or solid food. Overnight tube feeds for many months may be necessary in some patients.

5. Surgery is indicated for the complications of Crohn's disease: obstruction, fistulae, toxic megacolon, haemorrhage, perforation, abscess, failed medical/nutritional management, growth failure (some prepubertal patients in whom nutritional support has been unsuccessful and complete resection is possible).

6. Psychosocial support.

PROGNOSIS

- Long-term prognosis when Crohn's disease begins in childhood is good. Morbidity during childhood may be high but most go on to experience good general health and to lead productive lives[6].
- Mortality is low in childhood (2.4% in a large series[7]). After 5 and 20 years of disease, the probability of survival was 98% and 89% of expected survival, respectively[7].
- Colonic disease is associated with more extraintestinal manifestations and a poorer prognosis[7,8].
- There is a slightly increased risk of colorectal carcinoma[9].

Lifelong follow-up is required, usually about three monthly. Important to monitor growth and nutritional status and full blood count if the patient is on sulphasalazine or immunosuppressive therapy.

[1] Jones J H et al. (1966) Gut, **7**, 488.
[2] Sleisenger M H (1980) New Eng. J. Med., **302**, 1024.
[3] Summers R W et al. (1979) Gastroenterology, **77**, 847.
[4] Gilat T (1982) Gastroenterology, **83**, 702.
[5] O'Morain C A et al. (1984) Br. Med. J., **288**, 1859.
[6] Puntis J et al. (1984) Gut, **25**, 329.
[7] Farmer R G et al. (1979) Dig. Dis. Sci., **24**, 752.
[8] Gryboski J D et al. (1978) Gastroenterology, **74**, 817.
[9] Weedon D D et al. (1973) New Eng. J. Med., **289**, 1099.

Ulcerative Colitis

Ulcerative colitis is a recurrent, inflammatory and ulcerative disease involving the mucous membrane of the colon. The rectum is involved almost invariably and disease may spread proximally to involve the entire colon. Characteristically, the disease presents with rectal bleeding, diarrhoea, colicky pain and weight loss.

TREATMENT

1. Prophylaxis

   a) Sulphasalazine (30–50 mg/kg/day) has a proven prophylactic role in ulcerative colitis but that of steroids seems limited.
   b) Melsalazine may be useful for those patients intolerant of sulphasalazine.
   c) Prednisolone 15 mg/day is a better choice than placebo in adults[1], but many develop symptoms when the dose is reduced.
   d) Azathioprine (1–2 mg/kg/day) may have a useful steroid-sparing role, but in childhood colectomy is usually the preferred choice in colitis requiring large, prolonged steroid dosage.

2. Mild attack

   a) Sulphasalazine (30–50 mg/kg/day) is usually successful.
   b) Proctosigmoiditis is best treated with topical steroids (e.g. Colifoam b.d.).
   c) Loperamide (starting dose: 1–2 mg q.d.s.) may be helpful in controlling frequency and urgency.

3. Moderate attack: bloody diarrhoea, more than six times per day, often nocturnal and with pain and tenesmus, plus low-grade fever, malaise, leucocytosis and mild anaemia.

   a) Admit the patient to hospital.
   b) Prednisolone (1–2 mg/kg/day orally) is commenced and progressively reduced after 1–2 weeks. ACTH (by i.v. infusion), may be more effective in the first attack or when the patient has been on steroids for some time[2].
   c) Avoid anticholinergic drugs, opioids and loperamide, as these may precipitate toxic megacolon.
   d) Correction of fluid, electrolyte, nutrient and blood deficits is essential. Maintain serum albumin above 25 g/l and haemoglobin above 9 g/dl (1.4 mmol/l). Magnesium deficiency is common.

4. Fulminating attack

   a) Consider urgent referral to a specialised centre.
   b) Hydrocortisone (10 mg/kg/day, to a maximum of 300 mg/day) or prednisolone (2 mg/kg/day) i.v.
   c) Administer parenteral, broad-spectrum

antibiotics (e.g. penicillin, gentamicin and metronidazole).

   d) Correct fluid, electrolyte, nutrient and blood losses.

   e) Close clinical, biochemical and radiological monitoring of patient is necessary, looking for the development of toxic megacolon in particular.

   f) Frequent changes of position in bed, and a long nasoenteric suction tube, may reduce risk of toxic megacolon[3].

5. Toxic megacolon is indicated by development of abdominal distention and tenderness, paucity of bowel sounds and persistence of colonic gas shadows on plain x-ray. Management is as for fulminating colitis, but in the absence of perforation, surgery should be considered after 48–72 hours' intensive medical treatment if there is no rapid improvement.

6. Surgery

   a) Emergency subtotal colectomy for fulminating colitis with no response to medical treatment within two weeks, toxic megacolon not improving after 48–72 hours intensive medical treatment, massive haemorrhage or colonic perforation.

   b) Elective proctocolectomy for failed medical treatment, 10 or more years of pancolitis where regular colonoscopy inappropriate, severe colonic dysplasia, severe intractable extracolonic manifestations.

7. Psychosocial support.

PROGNOSIS

- 10% children and adolescents with ulcerative colitis experience one episode only, 20% have intermittent symptoms and are well between flare ups, 50% have chronic but not incapacitating disease[4].
- One-third require a colectomy, with subsequent normal life expectancy[4].
- In ulcerative proctosigmoiditis extension to the transverse colon or beyond occurs in 38%, and colectomy is needed in 23%[5].
- The incidence of carcinoma of the colon complicating pancolitis is probably higher than previously suggested. It is 1 in 200 for each year of disease between the ages of 10 and 20 years, and 1 in 60 thereafter[6]. The risks for proctosigmoiditis are considerably less.

FOLLOW-UP

Three to six monthly. Full blood count necessary if on sulphasalazine. Patients seen more frequently when in relapse.

[1] Lennard-Jones J E et al. (1965) Lancet, i, 188.
[2] Meyers S et al. (1983) Gastroenterology, 85, 351.
[3] Kramer P et al. (1981) Gastroenterology, 80, 433.
[4] Michener W M et al. (1979) J. Clin. Gastroenterol., 1, 301.
[5] Mir-Madjlessi S H et al. (1986) J. Pediatr. Gastroenterol. Nutr., 5, 570.
[6] Lennard-Jones J E et al. (1977) Gastroenterology, 73, 1280.

Infantile Colic

Infantile colic is a common syndrome of recurrent non-pacifiable screaming and drawing up of the legs in babies otherwise well in the first few months of life. It is more common in the evening and appears to be helped by the passage of flatus.

TREATMENT

1. A full history and examination must precede any attempted reassurance. In particular, consider an incarcerated hernia, otitis media, urinary tract infection and anal fissures in the differential diagnosis.
2. Occasionally, 'colic' may be a symptom of cow's milk protein intolerance, particularly in the presence of a strong family history of atopy. A two-week trial of a cow's-milk free diet (in the mother if breast feeding) may be helpful[1].
3. Dicyclomine hydrochloride is sometimes useful[2] but very rare, unwanted effects have been described under the age of six months.
4. Parental behaviour modification[3].

PROGNOSIS

- The prognosis is excellent, with 100% resolution, although the condition may occasionally predispose to non-accidental injury.

FOLLOW-UP

Once the diagnosis has been made and explained to the parents, many parents need no further consultation although an occasional visit to the general practitioner may be helpful.

[1] Jakobsson I et al. (1978) Lancet, i, 437.
[2] Illingworth R S (1985) Arch. Dis. Childh., 60, 981.
[3] Taubman B (1984) Paediatrics, 74, 998.

Intestinal Polyposis[1]

Juvenile polyps'

Juvenile polyps are benign hamartomatous polyps, usually in the rectosigmoid, rare before one year of age and after 15. Inheritance is probably dominant. In 25%, more than one polyp is present, and very rarely, polyps present throughout the large and small bowel and stomach, causing anaemia, hypoproteinaemia and recurrent intussusception (familial multiple juvenile polyposis).

TREATMENT

Colonoscopic polypectomy if symptomatic.

PROGNOSIS

- The prognosis is usually excellent.
- There is no risk of malignancy, but a small risk of recurrence.
- The rare multiple juvenile polyposis has a high mortality and morbidity, but recently available fibreoptic endoscopy may improve upon this.

FOLLOW-UP

No regular follow-up needed although polyps may infrequently recur.

Adenomatous polyps

In familial adenomatous polyposis of the colon (dominantly inherited), the colon is carpeted by precancerous adenomatous polyps. When involving the colon and sometimes the small bowel and duodenum, the condition may be associated with soft tissue and bone tumours (Gardner's syndrome; dominant inheritance).

TREATMENT

1. Treatment is aimed at preventing colonic carcinoma by prophylactic colectomy as all affected individuals will eventually develop this complication.
2. Family members should be genetically counselled, and those at risk of developing polyposis colonoscoped every three years.

PROGNOSIS

- Cancer of the colon usually develops before 40 years of age with over 50% developing this complication after 15–20 years of polyposis.

FOLLOW-UP

No follow-up necessary after colectomy.

Peutz-Jeghers syndrome

The Peutz-Jeghers syndrome consists of dominantly inherited hamartomatous polyps, usually small and intestinal, in association with pigmentation of the lips and buccal mucosa.

TREATMENT

Those polyps causing symptoms (recurrent transient intussusception, vomiting, bleeding) are likely to be the larger ones, and should be removed, by endoscopy if possible or multiple enterotomies if necessary.

PROGNOSIS

- The lesions are probably not premalignant.
- Mortality is low, although morbidity, relating to the need for repeat laparotomy in some patients is appreciable.

FOLLOW-UP

Not believed to be a premalignant lesion and therefore patients seen only when symptomatic.

---

[1] Silverman A *et al.* (1983) *Pediatric Clinical Gastroenterology* 3rd edn. St Louis: Mosby.

Hirschsprung's Disease

Hirschsprung's disease is due to absence of ganglion cells in intramuscular and submucous plexuses of the intestine, extending proximally from the anus. Presentation usually occurs as neonatal large intestinal obstruction but diagnosis (by rectal biopsy) may be delayed, even into adult life.

TREATMENT

1. Acute enterocolitis requires relief of subacute obstruction and supportive care, as outlined for necrotising enterocolitis (see p. 76).
2. In those infants presenting with large intestinal obstruction, siting of enterostomy can be determined by frozen sections taken at surgery to determine the proximal extent of the aganglionosis.

PROGNOSIS

- Acute enterocolitis (severe diarrhoea and abdominal distension) complicating Hirschsprung's disease may be fatal[1].
- After surgery 70–90% achieve continence, but this may be delayed until adolescence.
- Permanent colostomy may be required in some patients.

- Very long segment Hirschsprung's disease involving the small intestine may be inherited as an autosomal recessive[2].

FOLLOW-UP

At one year, the aganglionic segment is bypassed by: (a) pull through anal anastomosis (Swenson procedure); (b) end-to-side anastomosis behind rectum (Duhamel); (c) resection, removal of anal mucosa and pull through operation (Soave). Older children may be treated by a single stage operation. Postoperatively, loperamide may assist the achievement of continence.

---

[1] Nixon H H (1964) *Arch. Dis. Childh.*, **39**, 109.
[2] McKinnon A E *et al.* (1977) *Arch. Dis. Childh.*, **52**, 898.

Constipation and Soiling

Constipation is the infrequent passage of abnormally large and/or hard stools, usually in the presence of a constantly full lower rectum. Soiling represents the involuntary passage of soft or liquid faeces as a result of overflow from the full rectum; it should be differentiated from encopresis, the voluntary passage of stool in socially unacceptable places in the absence of constipation.

TREATMENT[1,2]

1. Outpatient

   a) Explain the loss of normal rectal sensation, and the involuntary nature of soiling. Illustrate loss of sensation by showing the parents they cannot feel a ring on their finger.
   b) Increases in dietary fibre are traditionally recommended, but difficult to implement. That constipation in childhood is related to dietary fibre deficiency and is helped by supplementation is unproven.
   c) The combined use of a stool softener (e.g. lactulose 5–15 ml t.d.s.) and a stimulant (e.g. Senokot 2.5–20 ml nocte) is usually successful in mild to moderate constipation.
   d) Medication may be combined with an appropriate star chart, and advice to the parents to sit the child on the potty or lavatory in a relaxed environment for 5–10 minutes after each meal.

2. Inpatient

   a) Indicated usually for failed outpatient management, or poor home circumstances.
   b) Initially empty rectum with daily enemas until the rectum is empty, and follow-up with laxatives and other measures used in outpatients.

   c) In frequently relapsing or intractable cases, weekend leave initially may give family confidence to cope at home.

PROGNOSIS[3]

- The long-term prognosis is excellent in the absence of Hirschsprung's disease (suspected in the presence of severe, intractable constipation from infancy in the absence of soiling, a history of delayed passage of meconium, or abdominal distension, or recurrent severe unexplained diarrhoea).
- Relapses in childhood are not uncommon, and more likely to occur in children from socially disadvantaged groups[4].

FOLLOW-UP

Frequent follow-up (1–2 weekly) is important initially, until some success has been achieved. Thereafter see 4–6 weekly. Withdraw medications slowly over three months after normal bowel habit has been present for 8 weeks.

[1] Clayden G S et al. (1976) Arch. Dis. Childh., **51,** 918.
[2] Davidson M et al. (1963) J. Pediatr., **62,** 261.
[3] Bentley J F R (1971) Gut, **12,** 85.
[4] Taitz L S et al. (1986) Arch. Dis. Childh., **61,** 472.

6
Diseases of the Liver and Biliary System

M. S. Tanner

Neonatal Hepatitis

Defined as obstructive jaundice in the first four weeks, neonatal jaundice occurs in 1:6000 live births[1]; defined as jaundice for more than 2 weeks in the first four months of life, it occurs in 1:3000 live births[2]. 40% are due to an identifiable cause and 60% are idiopathic.

TREATMENT[3,4]

1. Differentiate from extrahepatic biliary atresia (EHBA), Alagille's syndrome.
2. Correct clotting disturbance (vitamin K 5 mg orally/day, i.v. if prothrombin time grossly prolonged; fresh frozen plasma if evidence of bleeding).
3. Exclude a treatable cause—galactosaemia, fructose intolerance, hypothyroidism, hypopituitarism, urinary tract infection, toxoplasmosis, syphilis.
4. Toxoplasmosis: sulphadiazine 25 mg/kg q.d.s. and pyrimethamine 1 mg/kg/day for 2–6 months[5].
5. Congenital syphilis: crystalline penicillin 50 000 U/kg/day in two doses for 10 days.
6. Exclude genetic causes: α-1-antitrypsin deficiency, chromosomal disorders, tyrosinaemia, Zellweger's syndrome.
7. Nutritional: continue breast feeding if possible, otherwise use a medium chain triglyceride (MCT) containing milk while jaundice persists. If rapidly resolving, use standard vitamin preparations; if persistent, management as for EHBA.

PROGNOSIS

- If secondary, prognosis depends on the cause[1,2].

- Idiopathic: if first and second week deaths are included and mild cases presenting after four weeks excluded, 18% die from liver damage, 6% from sepsis, and 14% from associated defects, with 25% mortality in the first year, and 9% later[1]. 12% survivors are severely retarded, 8% have liver disease. Including cases jaundiced for more than two weeks in the first four months, there is only a 7% mortality, only 7% survivors having liver disease, but 16% being educationally subnormal[2]. Familial cryptogenic neonatal hepatitis has a less favourable outcome than non-familial.

FOLLOW-UP

Measure clotting times daily while abnormal, then 2–4 weekly until jaundice resolved. After disappearance of jaundice, perform liver function tests (LFTs) 3 monthly during first year. If abnormal LFTs or splenomegaly at one year carry out a liver biopsy.

[1] Deutsch J et al. (1985) Arch. Dis. Childh., **60,** 447.
[2] Dick M C et al. (1985) Arch. Dis. Childh., **60,** 512.
[3] Alagille D (1985) Semin. Liver Dis., **5,** 254.
[4] Balistreri W F (1985) J. Pediatr., **106,** 171.
[5] Frenkel J K (1985) Pediatr. Clin. North Am., **32,** 917.

Alpha-1-antitrypsin Deficiency

Alpha-1-antitrypsin deficiency (AATD) is an autosomal recessive disorder, gene frequency for the PiZ allele being approximately 0.0125 in the UK (0.025 in Scandinavia)[1]. PiZZ,[1] Pi null, and rarely PiSZ individuals may develop liver disease in infancy, or occasionally in childhood, but have no respiratory complications in childhood[1]. Because AATD is difficult to distinguish from extrahepatic biliary atresia (EHBA) it is vital that AATD phenotype be obtained in cholestatic infants.

TREATMENT

1. No specific treatment is available.
2. Breast feeding may ameliorate the neonatal hepatitis[2].
3. Manage cholestasis as in EHBA (see p. 89).
4. Because AATD within a family tends to breed true, one severely affected infant may be an indication for fetal blood sampling with a view to termination in a subsequent pregnancy[3].

PROGNOSIS

- Of PiZZ neonates, 11% develop cholestasis, another 6% mild evidence of liver disease, and 50% the remainder have asymptomatic abnormalities of liver function tests[4].
- Of PiZZ cholestatic infants with cholestasis, about one-quarter die from cirrhosis by the second decade of life, one-quarter have cirrhosis in childhood, one-quarter have persistently abnormal liver function tests, and one-quarter are normal[5].
- Rarely liver disease due to AATD presents in older children, usually in association with other pathology.

FOLLOW-UP

AAT-deficient infants with neonatal hepatitis need monitoring in the first year as other neonatal hepatitides q.v. Thereafter, if there is apparent complete recovery, the child should be monitored 6 monthly till 5 years old then annually, checking for splenomegaly (developing portal hypertension) and measuring liver function tests. Ultrasound abdomen if abnormal (cirrhosis?). Continuing evidence of liver disease: monitor growth nutritional state, spleen size; consider for transplantation if deteriorating.

[1] Eriksson S G (1985) *Scand. J. Gastroenterol.*, **20,** 907.
[2] Udall J N *et al.* (1985) *J. Am. Med. Assoc.*, **253,** 2679.
[3] Psacharopoulos H T *et al.* (1983) *Arch. Dis. Childh.*, **58,** 882.
[4] Sveger T (1975) *New Eng. J. Med.*, **294,** 1361.
[5] Editorial (1981) *Br. Med. J.*, **ii,** 807.

Intrahepatic Biliary Hypoplasia

Two types exist: (a) *Syndromatic* (arteriohepatic dysplasia, Alagille's syndrome)[1,2]. The facial features (deep set eyes, mild hypertelorism, overhanging forehead, straight nose, small pointed chin) are less characteristic of Alagille's than was first thought[3]. Eye features include posterior embryotoxon, retinopathy. Other defects include pulmonary branch stenosis, butterfly vertebrae, mild retardation of growth, and of mental and sexual development. The condition presents with early cholestasis like extrahepatic biliary atresia (EHBA). The incidence is approximately 1:100 000 live births[4]. Inheritance is autosomal dominant, with variable penetrance. (b) *Non-syndromatic*. This presents with cholestasis in the first months without the above features. It may be seen with rubella, cytomegalovirus, α-1-antitrypsin deficiency, or trihydroxycoprostanic acid elevation. Diagnosis depends upon wedge biopsies in which the ratio of bile ducts to portal tracts is <0.45 (normal 0.9–1.8)[2].

TREATMENT[5]

1. Nutritional treatment is as for EHBA (see p. 89).
2. Fat soluble vitamins, A, D, and K, as for EHBA. Vitamin E supplementation is vital to prevent a neurological syndrome similar to abetalipoproteinaemia[6,7]. The first sign of neurological syndrome is areflexia appearing at 2–5 years, followed by:

   a) Peripheral neuropathy.
   b) Cerebellar dysfunction.
   c) Abnormalities of eye movements.
   d) Retinal degeneration.

   Treatment is by oral α-tocopheryl acetate 50–400 mg daily (monitor blood level) or, if absorption is poor, i.m. α-tocopheryl acetate 10 mg/kg up to 200 mg in total 2 weekly.
3. Phenobarbitone 5 mg/kg/day.
4. Cholestyramine 4–8 g/day.

PROGNOSIS[8]

- The syndromatic form has a good hepatic prognosis but in Alagille's series[5] 21 of 80 died, four from liver failure, the others from intercurrent infection or heart disease. Long-term survivors have minimal hepatic fibrosis and no cirrhosis.
- The non-syndromatic form has a worse prognosis, 50% developing cirrhosis and portal hypertension and dying from liver failure in the first few years[8].

FOLLOW-UP

During the first year, follow-up is as for neonatal hepatitis *q.v.* Thereafter frequency of follow-up depends on symptoms: (a) 6 monthly if well —check growth, nutrition, development, cardiac status, absence of splenomegaly or ascites, prothrombin time. (b) More frequently to optimise control of pruritus or if deteriorating and (if non-syndromatic) assessing for transplanation.

[1] Watson G H *et al.* (1973) *Arch. Dis. Childh.*, **48,** 459.
[2] Alagille D *et al.* (1975) *J. Pediatr.*, **86,** 63.
[3] Sokol R J *et al.* (1983) *J. Pediatr.*, **103,** 205.
[4] Danks D M *et al.* (1977) *Arch. Dis. Childh.*, **52,** 368.
[5] Alagille D (1985) *J. Hepatol.*, **1,** 561.
[6] Guggenheim M A *et al.* (1983) *J. Pediatr.*, **102,** 577.
[7] Rosenblum J L *et al.* (1981) *New Eng. J. Med.*, **304,** 503.
[8] Odievre M *et al.* (1987) *Hepatology*, in press.

Extrahepatic Biliary Atresia

Extrahepatic biliary atresia (EHBA) is a progressive fibrosing obliteration of extra- and intrahepatic bile ducts[1,2]. The incidence is approximately 1:12 000[3]. It is possibly related to reovirus type 3 infection[4], but associated in 10–15% with other abnormalities (approximately 6% have polysplenia syndrome)[5].

TREATMENT

1. Clinical and radiological criteria fail to discriminate intra- and extrahepatic cholestasis. Referral to a specialised unit is recommended. Early laparotomy is essential. A jaundiced infant with consistently acholic stools should have a laparotomy and operative cholangiogram unless:

   a) A cause of intrahepatic cholestasis (see p. 87) is present, in particular α-1-antitrypsin deficiency.

   b) A ^{99m}Tc-DISIDA scan shows the appearance of radioactivity in the gut[6]. Liver biopsy appearances contribute to the diagnosis but are less discriminatory at an early age.

2. Establishing bile drainage[1,7]: about 5% cases have a so-called 'correctable' lesion, i.e. a patent proximal common bile duct containing bile in continuity with intrahepatic ducts of diameter > 4 mm. Anastomosis to a Roux-en-Y jejunal loop achieves bile drainage. Surprisingly only half of such patients survive long term[1]. Hepatic porto-enterostomy is required in the remainder. Temporary exteriorisation of the bile conduit to reduce the risk of cholangitis is no longer deemed effective, and problems with exteriorisation include an unsightly stoma which increases parental distress and management difficulties, fluid loss, bleeding from stomal varices, and bile loss leading to fat malabsorption.

3. Postoperatively serum bilirubin falls over 6–12 weeks, occasionally considerably longer. Phenobarbitone increases bile salt independent bile flow, and hepatic bile acid synthesis. Give 5–10 mg/kg/day using crushed tablets in milk (not the elixir because of its unpleasant taste).

4. Re-operation should be considered in patients whose bile flow is initially good but falls after an episode of cholangitis. Less favourable results have been obtained for re-operation if the initial bile flow is poor.

5. Postoperative problems

   a) *Cholangitis*: there is a 40–60% risk of cholangitis during the first year. Presumptive diagnosis is based upon rising serum bilirubin, fever, leucocytosis, and decreasing bile flow from a conduit if present, and proved by positive blood culture or liver biopsy[8]. The incidence of cholangitis may be reduced by good surgical technique, by perioperative antibiotics (metronidazole and cephradine), but not by prophylactic antibiotics after surgery. It is important to have a high index of suspicion of cholangitis and to start intravenous antibiotics early, using an aminoglycoside, ampicillin or cephalosporin, and metronidazole. Steroids are not of proven efficacy and increase susceptibility to infection.

   b) Malnutrition[9]. Fat malabsorption causing steatorrhea and poor growth may be improved by continuing breast feeding if possible or using a low fat high carbohydrate diet with medium chain triglycerides (Pregestimil supplemented with glucose polymer). Vitamin supplements are also necessary — vitamin A: aqueous preparation (Aquasol A) 5000 IU daily; vitamin D: as vitamin D_2 (ergocalciferol) 5000–10 000 IU daily; vitamin K: as an oral preparation 5 mg daily; vitamin E: 50–400 mg/kg/day as oral α-tocopherol acetate while cholestasis continues.

   c) Portal hypertension: portal pressure is always raised at operation. Clinically apparent effects of portal hypertension may appear in the second year of life: increase in splenomegaly, hypersplenism, variceal haemorrhage from the oesophagus or from the stoma. Portal pressure subsequently falls and it is therefore usually possible to avoid shunt surgery while awaiting resolution. Aspirin in any form must be avoided. Variceal haemorrhage from the oesophagus should be treated with sclerotherapy. Rarely hypersplenism may be an indication for splenic embolisation. Splenectomy should not be performed.

PROGNOSIS

- Untreated, EHBA is invariably fatal. Mean age at death is 10 months[2].
- The success of hepatic porto-enterostomy (Kasai's operation) in the remainder depends upon surgical skill, histological findings at the hilum, but mainly upon age at surgery[7]:

Age (days)	Number achieving bile drainage (%)
<60	81
61–70	61
71–90	50
91–120	38
>120	15

- Five-year survival after porto-enterostomy is 60%[1,7]. Biopsies 5–8 years after successful surgery show that all are cirrhotic even though clinically well. Significant variceal bleeding occurs in about 20%.

- Later complications are more frequent in children who have troublesome cholangitis in the first year than in those who do not.

FOLLOW-UP

Frequent postoperative follow-up is necessary (a) to check that bilirubin is falling and (b) to maintain optimal nutrition, monitoring alkaline phosphatase (if rickets is suspected x-ray wrist 6 monthly or if clinically indicated). Tell parents/ GP that child is to be admitted immediately if febrile or if jaundice increases (which suggests cholangitis). In a child whose jaundice clears, see monthly for first year and 2 monthly in second year checking spleen size for portal hypertension. If spleen remaining or becoming large, ultrasound abdomen (portal vein diameter?). Warn parents of possibility of variceal bleed and admit immediately if haematemesis or melaena even if small. In a child whose jaundice does not clear, see at least monthly, maintaining optimal nutrition (coagulation, rickets) and assess for transplantation.

[1] Lilly J R et al. (1985) Pediatr. Clin. North Am., **32,** 1233.
[2] Mowat A (1982) Semin. Liver. Dis., **2,** 271.
[3] Dick M C et al. (1985) Arch. Dis. Childh., **60,** 512.
[4] Morecki R et al. (1982) New Eng. J. Med., **307,** 481.
[5] Paddock R J et al. (1982) J. Pediatr. Surg., **17,** 563.
[6] Gerhold J P et al. (1983) Radiology, **146,** 499.
[7] Ohi R et al. (1985) World J. Surg., **9,** 285.
[8] Kuhls T L et al. (1985) Pediatr. Infect. Dis., **4,** 487.
[9] Alagille D (1985) Semin. Liver Dis., **5,** 254.

Choledochal Cyst

A choledochal cyst is a cystic dilatation of part of the extrahepatic biliary system often associated with partial obstruction of the terminal common bile duct and intrahepatic cysts. It forms part of the spectrum of pancreaticobiliary malformations, the common feature of which is a long common bile duct/pancreatic duct junction[1-4]; this includes spontaneous perforation of the terminal bile duct. It presents at a variable age, with approximately 50% before the age of 10 years. Some cases present in infancy with cholestasis indistinguishable from biliary atresia, others at 1–3 years with intermittent jaundice and abdominal mass. Diagnosis is by ultrasound. The incidence is unknown. It comprises 1 in 13 000 hospital admissions in occidentals[5].

TREATMENT

1. Surgery

   a) Internal drainage by cholecyst jejunostomy gives temporary relief but has a high incidence of subsequent ascending cholangitis, stricture, hepatic fibrosis, and carcinoma.
   b) Radical excision of the cyst with hepaticojejunostomy is therefore indicated.

PROGNOSIS

- Operative mortality is <10%[2,4,5].
- Long-term prognosis depends upon intrahepatic pathology.

- The risk of malignancy in adult life is not totally abolished by cyst excision[6].

FOLLOW-UP

Following operation and resolution of jaundice, annual follow-up with LFTs to confirm that biliary obstruction is not recurring.

[1] Lilly J R (1985) *J. Pediatr. Surg.*, **20,** 299.
[2] Altman R P *et al.* (1985) *Surg. Clin. North Am.*, **65,** 1245.
[3] Lilly J R *et al.* (1985) *J. Pediatr. Surg.*, **20,** 449.
[4] Yamaguchi M (1980) *Am. J. Surg.*, **140,** 653.
[5] Saing H (1985) *J. Pediatr. Surg.*, **20,** 443.
[6] Nagorney D M *et al.* (1984) *Surgery*, **96,** 656.

Hepatitis A

Hepatitis A is spread by faecal/oral transmission. The incubation period is 15–40 days (mean 25 days). Nausea, vomiting, abdominal pain, malaise, fatigue, fever and chills are followed by jaundice with the onset of which the child begins to feel systemically better. Approximately one-third symptomatic children do not develop jaundice[1].

TREATMENT

1. There is no evidence that bed rest or diet alter the course of the disease.
2. Antiemetic drugs are best avoided since impaired hepatic metabolism will increase the risk of side-effects (extrapyramidal in the case of metoclopromide). If the severity of vomiting is sufficiently great to render antiemetics necessary, hospital admission and close surveillance to detect early liver failure is indicated.
3. Prevention of cross infection

   a) Maximum faecal infectivity is in the 2 weeks before jaundice appears. Gloved hands should be used for nappy changing and disposal of faeces.
   b) A single dose of gamma globulin 0.02 ml/kg i.m. should be given to household contacts unless more than 2 weeks has elapsed since exposure. In nurseries looking after infants in nappies, gamma globulin is recommended for all children and attendants if one or more cases occur among staff or children, or if cases are recognised in two or more households of attendees[1].
   c) Children travelling to endemic areas should receive gamma globulin 0.02 ml/kg if visiting for less than 2 months or 0.06 ml/kg every 5 months for prolonged visits.

PROGNOSIS

- Hepatitis A infection is asymptomatic in approximately 75% those infected under the age of two years, 60% those infected aged 4–6 years, compared with less than 30% infected adults. 70% cases show clinical and biochemical resolution within 30 days and 85% within 60 days. Three variants on this course exist[2]:

  a) Approximately 20% show a polyphasic course. Following symptomatic and biochemical recovery within 5–30 days, a second peak of elevated serum alanine aminotransferase (ALT) occurs 50–90 days after the onset and in a few children a third peak occurs 15–40 days later. This secondary rise in ALT is usually asymptomatic.
  b) Cholestatic hepatitis: a small number of cases show prolonged jaundice for more than 12 weeks with the bilirubin remaining high at a time when the serum aspartate aminotransferase (AST) has fallen to < 500 IU/l. Liver biopsy demonstrates marked centrilobular cholestasis with active portal inflammation. The prognosis is good.
  c) Fulminant hepatic failure (FHF): clinical signs which should alert attendants to this very rare complication are unremitting vomiting continuing after the onset of jaundice, disorientation, restlessness, irritability, hyperventilation and prolonged prothrombin time.

- Rare complications of hepatitis A are dermatological (Henoch–Schönlein purpura, papular acrodermatitis); neurological (Guillain–Barré syndrome, polyneuritis, mononeuritis, transverse myelitis); haematological (severe haemolysis in glucose-6-phosphate dehydrogenase deficiency, marrow aplasia); renal (acute renal failure, as part of FHF or in isolation).

FOLLOW-UP

No follow-up is required following clinical recovery if the acute hepatitis was proven to be virus A. If not serologically proven, follow until liver

Contd.

function tests normal because of risk of chronic hepatitis in non-A and non-B hepatitis.

[1] Lemon S M (1985) *New Eng. J. Med.*, **313**, 1059.
[2] Immunization Practices Advisory Committee (1985) *Morb. Mort. Week. Rep.*, **34**, 313.

Hepatitis B Infection

Hepatitis B virus (HBV) may be acquired perinatally, from a carrier or acutely affected mother; by child to child transmission within families or institutions; by blood products; by tattooing, drug abuse and venereal spread[1,2].

TREATMENT

1. For treatment of the acute hepatitis, see *Hepatitis A* (p. 92).
2. Treatment of babies born to mothers with acute perinatal hepatitis B, or who are HBeAg carriers comprises hepatitis B immune globulin 200 IU immediately after birth, followed by hepatitis B vaccine 10 µg at birth, 1 month, and 6 months. Treatment of babies born to antiHBe carrier mothers is controversial; hepatitis B vaccine is probably indicated.
3. Treatment for chronic HBV infection

   a) Steroids are usually ineffective, increase viral replication, may be associated with an increased frequency of complications and increased mortality, but may have a limited role in a sub-group with antiHBe. 'Rebound' activity after stopping steroids may cause an acute hepatitis with subsequent clearance of HBsAg.
   b) Antiviral agents are under study (adenine arabinoside monophosphate, interferon, acyclovir, and combinations of interferon and acyclovir[3]).

PROGNOSIS

- Transmission

   a) Perinatal transmission: the risk of transmission from a mother with acute hepatitis B in the third trimester or within 8 weeks of delivery, and the risk of transmission from an HBeAg carrier mother, is 80–90%.

   AntiHBe carrier mothers have a very low risk of transmission[2].
   b) Child to child: a mentally retarded HBV carrier child who may bite or drool over his siblings or peers constitutes a significant risk; those in close contact should have HB vaccine. A carrier child with normal behaviour constitutes a negligible risk in the home or school in the UK. Intrafamilial transmission is common in rural Africa[4-6].
   c) Haemophiliac boys treated with factor concentrates have a 40–60% incidence of past HBV infection[6].

- Acute hepatitis B: most HBV infections are asymptomatic. The risk of chronic HBV infection is less than 5% in adults and adolescents, is approximately 25% in pre-school children and is 90–95% in perinatally infected infants[8]. The risk of chronic infection is increased in immunosuppressed children or those with Down's syndrome.
- Chronic HBV infection: 25–30% children found to be HBV carriers have a past history of acute hepatitis[9]. Histologically, 3% carrier children had cirrhosis, 57% chronic active hepatitis (CAH), 35% chronic persistent hepatitis (CPH). None of those with CPH progressed to CAH, and those with CAH remained clinically well unless given steroids.
- Superinfection with delta virus may cause an acute hepatitis, or deterioration of chronic liver disease[10].
- Chronic carriers of HBV have an increased risk of hepatocellular carcinoma in adult life, and rarely in late childhood.

FOLLOW-UP

Of baby born to carrier mother and given vaccine: check antiHBs titre 1 year after last dose and give booster dose if < 100 IU/l. Of acute hepatitis B with clinical recovery and antiHBs in serum: no follow-up. Of asymptomatic carrier state with normal liver function tests: annual check of serology and LFTs. May enter antiviral treatment trial. Screening carriers for raised alphafetoprotein and liver ultrasound to detect early hepatoma is logical but not established. Of chronic hepatitis B: currently no treatment; monitor serology and LFTs 3–6 monthly.

[1] Brabin L et al. (1985) Am. J. Epidemiol., **122,** 725.
[2] Zuckermann A J (1984) Arch. Dis. Childh., **59,** 1007.
[3] Thomas H C et al. (1985) Br. Med. Bull., **41,** 374.
[4] Williams C et al. (1983) J. Pediatr., **103,** 192.
[5] McPhillips J C (1985) J. Pediatr. Gastroenterol. Nutr., **4,** 153.
[6] Whittle H C et al. (1983) Lancet, **i,** 1203.
[7] Nebbia G et al. (1986) Arch. Dis. Childh., **61,** 580.
[8] Beasley R P et al. (1982) J. Infect. Dis., **146,** 198.
[9] Bortolotti F (1981) Gut, **22,** 499.
[10] Farci P et al. (1985) Gut, **26,** 4.

Hepatosplenic Schistosomiasis

Schistosomal portal hypertension is the major complication of infection with *Schistosoma mansoni, S. japonicum* and *S. mekongi. S. mansoni* is widespread throughout Africa, South America, particularly Brazil, and in parts of the West Indies. *S. japonicum* is confined to the Far East, and *S. mekongi* occurs in the Mekong river basin in Kampuchea and produces a milder disease. *S. haematobium* and *S. intercalatum* usually do not produce liver disease[1,2]. Children who play in snail-infested water are at particular risk of heavy cercarial infection. The local reaction at the site of cutaneous penetration reaches a maximum in 24–36 hours and disappears within four days. During the subsequent three weeks, when migration of the worms is occurring, transient toxic and allergic symptoms such as malaise, fever, and giant urticaria may occur. Cough and haemoptysis result from migration through the lung, and acute hepatitis occurs when the schistosomes reach the liver. Egg laying within mesenteric venules commences 1–3 months after infection and may be associated with both gastrointestinal and systemic symptoms. *S. japonicum* infection is particularly associated with severe systemic reactions, with fever, rigours, malaise, and a significant mortality ('Katayama fever').

TREATMENT

1. Drugs

   a) Praziquantel is the treatment of choice for all schistosomal infections. It should be given in two oral doses of 25–30 mg/kg at an interval of 4 hours for *S. mansoni*, and 20 mg/kg three times in one day for *S. japonicum* and *S. mekongi*. Although side-effects are reported to be transient and mild (abdominal pain, fever, nausea, headache, dizziness), children in Zaire heavily infested with *S. mansoni* showed a high incidence of severe abdominal pain and bloody diarrhoea within hours of treatment.

   b) An alternative drug, oxamniquine, is effective only against *S. mansoni*. The dose is 20 mg/kg/day orally for 3 days. It causes drowsiness, dizziness, headache, and orange discoloration of the urine.

   c) Hycanthone should be avoided in the presence of liver disease because of reports of fulminant hepatic failure, and niridazole also produces unacceptable side-effects.

   d) Severe Katayama fever may respond to steroids.

2. Portal hypertension is managed with injection sclerotherapy or portal systemic shunting. The preservation of hepatocellular function would

be expected to allow portasystemic shunting without risk of hepatic encephalopathy, but in practice encephalopathy is common.

3. Control: attempts to eradicate the snail intermediate have been disappointing and have been superseded by the advent of new drugs. Following mass chemotherapy, or selective chemotherapy of those individuals with a high worm load, re-infection occurs at a low rate.

PROGNOSIS

- Symptoms of liver involvement may appear from 18 months to many years after infection. Most frequently, presentation is with abdominal discomfort associated with splenomegaly, or with variceal haemorrhage. Less than one-third give a previous history of dysentery. Children in whom hepatic schistosomiasis is detected because of asymptomatic hepatomegaly may have mild to moderate splenomegaly[3]. Liver enlargement affects the left lobe preferentially. As the disease progresses, the spleen may become massively enlarged. Enlargement results both from reticuloendothelial hyperplasia and from portal hypertension. Signs of hepatocellular failure are absent except in terminal disease or with coincident cirrhosis from another cause.

- The risk of progression of hepatomegaly and splenomegaly is greater if the faecal egg count exceeds 500 eggs/g, and is greater in children under 15 years. Faecal egg counts remain remarkably stable in untreated patients and, although the organisms' mean life span is approximately 5 years, egg excretion in individual patients may continue for more than 30 years.

- Complications include the nephrotic syndrome and chronic salmonella infection.

FOLLOW-UP

Following injection sclerotherapy of varices, 6 monthly repeat endoscopies seeking recurrence are required. After portasystemic shunting, 6 monthly review of spleen size (patency of shunt) and neurological examination (encephalopathy?) are indicated.

[1] Markell E K et al. (1986) In Medical Parasitology, 6th edn, p. 167. London: Saunders.
[2] Cock K M de (1986) Gut, 27, 734.
[3] Mackenjee M K R et al. (1984) Trans. R. Soc. Trop. Med. Hyg., 78, 13.

Hydatid Disease

Man is an accidental intermediate host of *Echinococcus granulosus* and most infections occur in children who may come into contact with dog faeces. Surveys in Wales before control schemes were started showed prevalences of *Echinococcus* in farm dogs of 25% and of cysts in adult sheep at abattoirs of 37%[1]. 20–25% patients in hospital cases of hydatid disease are aged less than 14 years[1,2].

TREATMENT

1. Surgical excision has, until recently, been the only available therapy. Following exposure of the cyst and careful packing of the surgical field, aspiration of cyst contents is followed by injection of a scolicidal agent. 10% formalin was frequently used but is toxic, has been associated with fatality, and has been replaced by 5% hypertonic saline or 0.5% silver nitrate. Following evacuation of the cyst and scooping out the germinal endothelium and daughter cysts, the cavity is obliterated or filled with an omentoplasty[2]. Large lesions may require lobectomy.

2. Three chemotherapeutic agents are available.

    a) Mebendazole has been associated with very variable results, relating to variable gastrointestinal absorption.
    b) Albendazole is well absorbed, and in doses of 10–14 mg/kg daily achieves good levels of the active metabolite (albendazole sulphoxide) in serum and hydatid cyst fluid[3].
    c) Praziquantel is active against *Echinococcus in vitro* and may prove to have a therapeutic role in amoebic liver abscess.

PROGNOSIS

- Hydatid disease has a long asymptomatic period of cyst growth.
- Presentations include asymptomatic hepatomegaly, or asymptomatic intrahepatic calcification noticed on x-ray; dragging right hypochondrial pain; rarely, obstructive jaundice due to biliary compression. Cyst rupture, either into the biliary system, causing features of cholangitis or obstructive jaundice, or into the peritoneum, causing catastrophic collapse with anaphylactic shock, is rare in childhood.
- Immune complex deposition may cause presentation with a membranous nephropathy.

FOLLOW-UP

Serial ultrasound confirms resolution, 1–2 monthly until resolved, then 6 months later seeking recurrence.

[1] Clarkson M J (1978) *Vet. Rec.*, **102,** 259.
[2] Elhamel A *et al.* (1986) *Br. J. Surg.*, **73,** 125.
[3] Saimot A G *et al.* (1983) *Lancet*, **ii,** 652.

Pyogenic Liver Abscess

Pyogenic liver abscess is rare in childhood, accounting for 3/100 000 paediatric hospital admissions in one series[1]. 20% are cryptogenic; 40% are associated with chronic granulomatous disease (CGD); others are associated with severe neutropenia, or other qualitative neutrophil defects such as 'Job's syndrome'. Neonatal cases are usually associated with generalised sepsis and multiple abscesses in other organs.

TREATMENT

1. Ultrasonically guided percutaneous drainage is the treatment of choice[2]. Under appropriate sedation a 20-gauge spinal needle is inserted. The mid-axillary approach should be avoided because this usually traverses the pleural space and may lead to development of an empyema. An anterior subcostal approach is preferable. Using angiographic guide wires and serial dilatation, a 7- or 8-Fr catheter is placed in the abscess cavity and allowed to drain. The catheter should be flushed 4–6 times per day but the abscess cavity should not be lavaged because this may increase the risk of septicaemia. The catheter is removed when drainage ceases and the abscess is seen to resolve on follow-up ultrasound and/or sinogram.

2. Broad spectrum antibiotics should be commenced before aspiration and continued during drainage and for several days following the removal of the catheter. Until cultures are available cover should include agents effective against anaerobes, gram-negative bacilli and *Staphylococcus aureus*.

3. Multiple abscesses in the newborn period require parenteral antibiotics. In CGD, multiple large abscess cavities have been effectively treated with catheter drainage of each cavity[3].

4. Open surgical drainage is indicated if percutaneous puncture is technically impossible or if there is failure to respond to the percutaneous drainage process.

PROGNOSIS

- The lack of specific features in the newborn and the associated generalised sepsis is responsible for the high mortality. A higher index of suspicion and more widespread use of abdominal ultrasound will probably increase both reported incidence and survival.

- In CGD, the majority of cases are boys aged between one and five years. Signs of liver abscess are non-specific, consisting of features of the predisposing pathology, fever, hepatomegaly, ileus with or without abdominal discomfort. The prognosis is that of the underlying condition.

FOLLOW-UP

Acutely, follow resolution with repeated ultrasound examination. Thereafter, follow-up determined by predisposing cause of liver abscess (see CGD p. 327): neonatal cases die or resolve.

[1] Chusid M J (1978) *Paediatrics*, **62**, 554.
[2] Vachon L *et al.* (1986) *J. Pediatr. Surg.*, **21**, 366.
[3] Skibber J M *et al.* (1986) *Surgery*, **99**, 626.

Hepatic Amoebiasis

The prevalence of infection with *Entamoeba histolytica* shows an early peak in childhood, infection often being 'handed on' from mother or siblings. Thereafter prevalence in childhood rises to a plateau at 15–20 years. In endemic areas, amoebic dysentery is approximately ten times as common as amoebic liver abscess. 70% paediatric cases are aged under three years, 30% below one year. While amoebic liver abscesses are usually single in adults, multiple lesions occur more commonly in children. Only 50% cases have a history of diarrhoea[1].

TREATMENT

1. Metronidazole is the drug of choice, effective both within tissues and, in adequate doses, in the gut lumen. Use 50 mg/kg/day in three doses for 8 days. Minor side-effects include a metallic taste in the mouth, nausea and dizziness. Prolonged courses are associated with leucopenia and peripheral neuropathy.

2. Tinidazole is equally effective in treating amoebic liver abscess and has fewer side-effects. It has a longer half-life and can, therefore, be given as a single daily dose of 60 mg/kg for 5 days. Its disadvantages are its cost and its failure to eradicate luminal amoebae.

3. Because treatment failures are reported with metronidazole it should be supplemented in severely ill cases with emetine or dihydroemetine. Emetine is highly effective but has cumulative cardiotoxicity. The dose should be limited to 1 mg/kg i.m. or deep subcutaneous injection daily for a maximum of 10 days. The course should not be repeated within 28 days. If dihydroemetine, which is less toxic, is available it should be used in a dose of 1.25 mg/kg/day.

4. Chloroquine, 10 mg/kg/day, has a limited role in the treatment of uncomplicated cases when other drugs are contraindicated, or in combination with emetine.

5. The luminal amoebicide diloxanide furoate should also be given to all patients with liver abscess, 20 mg/kg/day in three doses for 10 days.

6. Therapeutic needle aspiration of amoebic liver abscess is indicated only when the abscess is very large, is threatening rupture, or fails to improve after 5 days' chemotherapy.

PROGNOSIS

- Reported mortalities of 40–60% in young children in the mid-1970s have been markedly improved by earlier diagnosis using ultrasound[2] and by effective chemotherapy. The mortality in uncomplicated cases should be less than 3%, although rupture or extrahepatic spread is associated with mortalities of 10–15%.

- Various host factors may contribute to the occurrence of invasive amoebiasis. Reduced gastric acid secretion, mucosal integrity and cell-mediated immunity have been implicated in the increased incidence of hepatic amoebiasis in malnourished children. Steroid therapy, antimetabolites, radiotherapy, and concurrent infection with *Schistosoma mansoni*, *Trichuris*, *Shigella*, and *Strongyloides* are predisposing factors.

FOLLOW-UP

Follow resolution of abscess with ultrasound, repeated after 6 months if asymptomatic.

[1] Knight R (1984) *Semin. Liver Dis.*, **4**, 277.
[2] Merten D F *et al.* (1984) *Am. J. Radiol.*, **143**, 1325.

Autoimmune Chronic Active Hepatitis

Hepatitis should no longer be deemed 'chronic' on the basis of symptoms lasting for more than 6 months but on the histological appearance of the liver biopsy. Delay in diagnosis of chronic active hepatitis greatly increases the number who are cirrhotic at diagnosis[1]. Histologically, chronic hepatitis includes chronic active (CAH), chronic persistent (CPH), and chronic lobular (CLH) hepatitis, of which the latter two are benign and require no treatment. Chronic active hepatitis is defined as the presence of portal inflammation with piecemeal necrosis of adjacent hepatocytes and erosion of the limiting plate and may result from autoimmune disease, hepatitis B, non-A, non-B hepatitis, Wilson's disease, or drugs (nitrofurantoin, α-methyldopa, isoniazid). Autoimmune CAH is defined as the histological picture of CAH together with serological evidence of altered immunity, i.e. raised immunoglobulins, non-organ specific antibodies (antinuclear, smooth muscle, liver-kidney microsomal). It is associated with other autoimmune diseases, with coeliac disease and mesangiocapillary glomerulonephritis, and with the tissue type HLA-B8 drw 3.

TREATMENT

1. Exclude other forms of CAH, especially Wilson's disease and hepatitis B. Liver biopsy is essential, but may have to await improvement of blood clotting following steroid treatment.
2. Initial treatment with prednisolone 2 mg/kg/day, reducing over 12 weeks as the liver function tests improve. A maintenance dose is used to maintain serum transaminase levels at less than twice the upper normal value.
3. Alternate day steroids cannot be recommended because of proven inferiority in adult series. One paediatric study showing that alternate day steroids were effective and allowed catch-up and even supra-normal growth, may have studied a particularly favourable group of patients[2].
4. Azathioprine 1 mg/kg/day alone is ineffective but is steroid sparing. Restrict its use to those in whom biochemical normality cannot be achieved without unacceptably high steroid dosage.
5. In adults, penicillamine appears of comparable efficacy to steroids, but causes more side-effects[3]. In children, it is a therapeutic option if there are major steroid side-effects.

PROGNOSIS

- Untreated, 73% adults with CAH die within 10 years, with a median survival of 3.3 years[4]; no comparable figures are available for children.
- Features associated with poorer survival[1,2,5] are a longer history, and cirrhosis in the initial biopsy. Those with antinuclear factor only possibly have a better prognosis than those with liver–kidney microsomal antibody. Of 28 patients, 2 died, 13 went into remission, and 8 were able to stop therapy[1]. Cirrhosis was present in 8 of 10 of those with symptoms for more than 6 months before diagnosis, and in only 2 of 12 of those with symptoms for less than 6 months. Other series with a shorter mean duration of symptoms and mainly antinuclear antibody (ANA) positive children gave better results[5], while others with a longer duration of symptoms gave worse results[6].
- Following cessation of treatment, the relapse rate is lower than in adults[7]. It is higher if there is established cirrhosis, or if antibodies to liver-specific protein are present[8].

FOLLOW-UP

Steroid treatment should be continued for 12 months after the liver function tests return to normal. If a liver biopsy does not then show aggressive inflammation the steroids may be tailed off. Thereafter, check liver function tests, ESR, and globulin frequently in the first year and then six-monthly for five years.

[1] Vegnente A et al. (1984) Arch. Dis. Childh., **59,** 330.
[2] Fitzgerald J F et al. (1984) J. Pediatr., **104,** 893.
[3] Stern R B et al. (1977) Gut, **18,** 19.
[4] Kirk A P et al. (1980) Gut, **21,** 78.

[5] Arasu T S et al. (1979) *J. Pediatr.*, **95**, 514.
[6] Maggiore G et al. (1984) *J. Pediatr.*, **104**, 839.

[7] Silvermann A et al. (1983) *Pediatric Clinical Gastroenter ology* 3rd edn, p. 675. St Louis: C.V. Mosby.
[8] McFarlane I G et al. (1984) *Lancet*, **ii**, 954.

Wilson's Disease

Wilson's disease (WD) is an autosomal recessive disease, frequency approximately 5/million, gene frequency 1:200–1:400. Approximately 50% cases present by 15 years of age; 40% these with hepatic disease (fulminant hepatic failure with haemolysis, chronic active hepatitis, established cirrhosis and portal hypertension, or gallstones). Kayser–Fleischer (KF) rings, and neurological features, are absent in the first decade[1].

TREATMENT

1. Treatment of asymptomatic patients discovered while screening family members of index case:

   a) Establish the diagnosis unequivocally since life-long treatment will be required.
   b) Copper chelation
      i) *d*-Penicillamine is the drug of choice in a dose of 35 mg/kg/day initially with pyridoxine 50 mg/day. Monitor serum iron 6-monthly. Adverse effects include:
         1) Hypersensitivity reactions (rash, fever, lymphadenopathy). Temporarily withdraw penicillamine then reintroduce under the cover of a small dose of prednisolone.
         2) A lupus-like reaction may be controlled with prednisolone, but is often an indication to change to an alternative chelator.
         3) Proteinuria *per se*, is not an indication to discontinue but frank nephrosis is.
      ii) Second line chelating agents
         1) Triethylene tetramine dihydrochloride (trientine) has successfully been used in teenagers and young adults in a dose of 400–800 mg t.d.s. Most toxic effects of penicillamine do not recur on using trientine except for elastosis perforans and, in some patients, a drug-induced lupus reaction. Iron deficiency may occur.
         2) Zinc salts[2]: although remission may be maintained with oral zinc sulphate[3] liver copper concentration remains high, and results of long-term studies are awaited. Monitor serum zinc annually and if low supplement with oral zinc sulphate 150 mg t.d.s. after meals.
         3) Unithiol is a water-soluble analogue of dimercaprol with an unpleasant taste but promising results in limited use.
   c) Monitoring treatment
      i) Urinary copper excretion is expected to exceed 2 mg/24 hours in the first year, falling to 1 mg/24 hours thereafter.
      ii) Serum free copper should fall to $< 10\ \mu g/l$.
      iii) Doubt as to whether falling urinary copper values indicate a successful 'decoppering' or poor compliance with treatment, are an indication for repeat liver biopsy with copper estimation.
   d) A strict low copper diet is unnecessary, but high copper foods (shellfish, nuts, cocoa, liver, mushrooms, and broccoli) should be avoided.

2. Treatment of inactive cirrhosis consists of copper chelation as above together with management of complications of portal hypertension, hypersplenism, and ascites.

3. Treatment of patients with WD presenting with chronic active hepatitis (CAH).

    a) Distinguishing WD from other causes of chronic active hepatitis may be difficult:

        i) Urinary copper is elevated in approximately 50% non-Wilson's CAH and is in the range of WD in approximately 10%[4].

        ii) Serum caeruloplasmin levels are usually elevated in CAH.

        iii) Liver copper values may be elevated in CAH but rarely exceed 250 µg/g dry weight.

        iv) Radioactive copper studies clearly distinguish Wilson's from non-Wilson's CAH but are of limited availability because of the short half-life of the isotope (12.8 hours).

    b) Copper chelation therapy is given as in (1.) above.

4. Treatment of WD presenting as fulminant hepatic failure.

    a) The diagnosis of WD in liver failure is difficult. Features suggesting WD include haemolysis; elevation of bilirubin out of proportion to the level of the transaminases (because of haemolysis); raised serum copper (normal 60–110 µg/dl), the caeruloplasmin is low (but may be in other causes of liver failure because of reduced hepatic synthesis), calculated 'free' serum copper very high; screening siblings for reduced caeruloplasmin[3,5].

    b) Treatment for fulminant hepatic failure (FHF) (see p. 104) and commencement of d-penicillamine as in (1.) above.

    c) More active measures to remove copper are:

        i) Peritoneal dialysis, using enrichment of the dialysate alternately with albumin (10 g/l) and d-penicillamine (2 g/l)[6].

        ii) Emergency orthotopic liver transplantation.

PROGNOSIS

- Untreated, approximately one-third WD cases die from hepatic complications[7].
- Treated asymptomatic patients have remained well throughout childhood, even though most have abnormal liver biopsies at presentation (usually fatty change only). Treatment is required for life. Heterozygotes are asymptomatic and do not require treatment.
- Although it has been stated that most patients with a hepatic mode of presentation respond to penicillamine, those with CAH are an unfavourable group. In a study of 17 patients, 4 died within 3 weeks from FHF and 5 died within 2 years[7].
- Patients with fulminant hepatic failure and WD are unlikely to survive without emergency liver transplant.
- More than 50 pregnancies have been recorded in penicillamine treated women with WD with no problems, although there are reports of abnormal connective tissue changes in babies born to women treated with penicillamine for cystinuria and rheumatoid arthritis[7].
- Hepatocellular carcinoma is rare.

FOLLOW-UP

Measure the urine protein and FBC weekly during first 3 months of treatment, then 3 monthly. Monitor the 24 hour urine copper monthly during first year of treatment, 3 monthly thereafter. Measure the serum iron and zinc 6 monthly.

[1] Sternlieb I et al. (1985) In Liver and Biliary Disease (Wright R, Millward-Sadler E H, Alberti K G M M, Karran S eds), p. 949. London: Baillière Tindall.
[2] van Caillie-Bertrand M et al. (1985) Arch. Dis. Childh., 60, 656.
[3] Kraut J R et al. (1984) Clin. Pediatr., 23, 637.
[4] LaRusso N F et al. (1976) Gastroenterology, 70, 653.
[5] McCullough A J et al. (1983) Gastroenterology, 84, 161.
[6] De Bont B et al. (1985) J. Pediatr., 107, 545.
[7] Arima M et al. (1977) Eur. J. Pediatr., 126, 147.

Portal Hypertension

Extrahepatic portal hypertension (EPH) may be a result of congenital or thrombotic portal vein occlusion. It usually presents with variceal haemorrhage (often precipitated by salicylates) before the age of five years; 20% present with asymptomatic splenomegaly. Intrahepatic portal hypertension (IPH) is a result of hepatic cirrhosis or fibrosis (especially in extrahepatic biliary atresia (EHBA), cystic fibrosis (CF), hepatic fibrosis with polycystic kidneys)[1].

TREATMENT[1,2]

1. Acute variceal haemorrhage: if acute bleeding has stopped, endoscopy may be delayed until clotting derangements and blood loss have been corrected. At endoscopy the source of bleeding will usually be apparent, and injection of varices be commenced. Much more difficult is the child who is actively bleeding on arrival. Immediate measures are:

   a) Transfusion: whole blood or its equivalent as red cells and colloid (saline, plasma equivalent, or if clotting times are prolonged, fresh frozen plasma).
   b) Monitoring: it is vital that the child be observed in an intensive care environment with facilities for monitoring heart rate, respiration, blood pressure through an arterial line, blood gases, and central venous pressure.
   c) A nasogastric wide bore tube should be passed to aspirate blood and clot from the stomach.
   d) Arrange emergency endoscopy for variceal injection. Since this requires an experienced endoscopist it may be necessary to resuscitate a child and transfer him to a unit with this facility. During this delay vasopressin and if necessary balloon tamponade should be used.
   e) Vasopressin in effective dose (0.4 units/minute in 5% dextrose, i.e. 200 units of vasopressin in 500 ml of 5% dextrose running at 1 ml/minute), will produce abdominal cramps, defaecation, and pallor. Beware of infiltration of vasopressin at the infusion site since it will cause local necrosis and gangrene. Infusion should be continued for 24 hours, or until endoscopy. If, at the end of 24 hours, bleeding has stopped, as judged by the nasogastric aspirate, the dose should be halved for 6 hours, quartered for 6 hours, and then stopped. The long-acting analogue glypressin (triglycyl lysine vasopressin) 2 mg i.v. 6-hourly is an alternative but there is little experience of its use in childhood. Somatostatin remains unproven in variceal haemorrhage. Propranolol is of no benefit in acute variceal haemorrhage. Cimetidine is often given since there may be initial confusion as to whether the bleeding is coming from gastric erosions; it does not reduce variceal bleeding.
   f) Balloon tamponade is an effective but potentially hazardous manoeuvre. Hazards include inflation of the gastric balloon in the oesophagus, causing rupture; failure to keep the oesophagus empty, leading to aspiration; the gastric balloon being allowed to ride up into the oesophagus or pharynx; the child may bite through the tube, causing deflation or difficulty in deflating; rebleeding on removal of the tube (approximately 60%).
   g) If at endoscopy it is impossible to visualise the source of bleeding, or to arrest haemorrhage, a Sengstaken tube is inserted in theatre and endoscopy repeated 12–24 hours later. In the rare event that acute haemorrhage is not controlled at a second endoscopy, the Sengstaken tube is again replaced; the safest therapeutic option at that point is oesophageal transection using the staple gun, rather than emergency portacaval shunt or percutaneous transhepatic variceal obliteration.

2. Management after a bleed controlled by acute sclerotherapy: varices may be obliterated by repeated injection, three to five sessions being required, and follow-up endoscopies being required at approximately 6-monthly intervals[3,4]. An alternative policy, that of waiting for repeat haemorrhage and then responding acutely to it by further injection, is unacceptably hazardous. Sclerotherapy has reduced the requirement for portasystemic shunting. In EPH, successful shunting is usually curative and encephalopathy is rare, but shunt thrombosis is common. Vessels for anastomosis should be > 1 cm diameter. In IPH, the prognosis for hepatic encephalopathy depends upon parenchymal function—poor in cirrhosis, good in cystic fibrosis or congenital hepatic fibrosis. Propranolol does not significantly reduce rebleeding rates.

3. Although it has been generally felt that varices which have not bled should be left alone that view has been questioned[2,5].

4. Massive splenic enlargement: hypersplenism is unlikely to cause clinical problems and does not require splenectomy[6]. Massive splenic enlargement may cause respiratory embarrassment or episodic abdominal pain (splenic infarction) and be an indication for splenectomy combined with a splenorenal shunt. Partial splenic embolisation is an alternative[7].

PROGNOSIS

- Conservative management of EPH has a high (about 19%) mortality if patients live remote from medical care centres[8].
- The best results for shunt surgery achieve a > 90% patency rate; average figures are much lower than this. Rebleeding rates even with successful surgery may be about 20%.
- Injection sclerotherapy achieves about 65% freedom from rebleeding in the first year, although the risk of rebleeding is increased during treatment[1], and repeat annual check endoscopies are necessary seeking recurrence.
- The prognosis of IPH depends upon the parenchymal disease.

FOLLOW-UP

Of EPH treated with sclerotherapy: repeat endoscopies 6 monthly seeking recurrent varices. Of EPH treated surgically: if well check spleen size, and neurological examination 6 monthly. Ultrasound abdomen checking shunt patency. Of portal hypertension with cirrhosis: as above and as necessary, for intrahepatic disease (e.g. see EHBA, Wilson's, CAH).

[1] Howard E R (1985) In *Liver and Biliary Disease* (Wright R, Millward-Sadler G H, Alberti K G M M, Karran S, eds.), p. 1355. London: Baillière Tindall.
[2] Tanner M S (1986) *J. Roy. Soc. Med.*, **79**, 38.
[3] MacDougall B R D et al. (1982) *Lancet*, **i**, 124.
[4] Stamatakis J D et al. (1982) *Br. J. Surg.*, **69**, 74.
[5] Paquet K J (1982) *Endoscopy*, **14**, 4.
[6] El Kishen M A et al. (1985) *Surg. Gynecol. Obstet.*, **160**, 233.
[7] Moses M F et al. (1984) *Surgery*, **96**, 694.
[8] Mitra S K et al. (1978) *J. Pediatr. Surg.*, **13**, 51.

Fulminant Hepatic Failure

Fulminant hepatic failure (FHF) is defined as the onset of hepatic encephalopathy within eight weeks of the first evidence of hepatocellular disease[1-4]. It is to be distinguished from a) hepatic encephalopathy in chronic liver disease, in which complete recovery cannot be expected, and b) Reye's syndrome and the other microvesicular fat disorders.

TREATMENT

1. The aim is to support the patient until liver function recovers or transplantation is performed, to anticipate and prevent features associated with deterioration, and to prevent further iatrogenic damage.
2. Assess the coma grade:

Grade	Mental state
I = prodrome	Behavioural changes, agitation, restlessness, mild confusion, slowness of mentation, slurred speech, disordered sleep.
II = impending coma	Accentuation of I; drowsiness, inappropriate behaviour, loss of sphincter control.
III = stupor	Sleeps most of the time but rousable; incoherent speech, marked confusion.
IV = coma	May (IVA) or may not (IVB) respond to painful stimuli.

Patients in grades III and IV, and those in grade II who are rapidly deteriorating, should be transferred to an intensive care unit and preparations made for ventilation and insertion of central venous pressure line, arterial line, urinary catheter, and intracranial line.

3. Reduce enteric production of nitrogenous toxins.

   a) Stop protein feeds.
   b) Give neomycin 25 mg/kg 8-hourly orally, unless parenteral broad spectrum antibiotics are being given.
   c) Give lactulose as an enema, 300 ml lactulose syrup made up to 1000 ml with water, given in appropriate volume for age, 4 times over first 24 hours and 1 ml/kg orally 4 times in first 24 hours, thereafter titrated to give 2–3 stools/day.

4. Give carbohydrate to limit catabolism, as glucose polymer orally if tolerated (Hycal, Maxijul), otherwise intravenous glucose. Monitor BMstix regularly; give 10% dextrose, increasing to 15% if serum glucose is low, with boluses of 50% dextrose as necessary.
5. Prevent iatrogenic insults known to increase mortality. Avoid barbiturates (increased encephalopathy), paraldehyde (lactic acidosis), and diazepam (respiratory depression). Small doses of promethazine hydrochloride, lorazepam or oxazepam may be used. Trials of steroids have shown a marginally worse survival in treated patients[5].
6. Monitor electrolytes twice daily, more frequently if abnormal. Hypokalaemia is to be anticipated and very large amounts of potassium may be required; monitor ECG. Be prepared to stop if renal failure develops. Hyponatraemia is usually a result of water overload, not sodium deficiency; restrict water if serum sodium < 125 mmol/l but monitor central venous pressure to prevent hypovolaemia. Anticipate hypocalcaemia, hypomagnesaemia.
7. Monitor the neurological status using a coma scale. Take daily EEG.
8. Acid–base status: respiratory alkalosis is common in stage I and requires no action. Respiratory acidosis, either cerebral or due to respiratory infection requires early intervention with nasotracheal intubation, paralysis, and mechanical ventilation. Metabolic acidosis requires correction with sodium bicarbonate.
9. Raised intracranial pressure (ICP): ICP monitoring is desirable but often precluded by coagulation disorder. Dexamethasone does

not reduce raised ICP. Mannitol 0.25–1.0 g/kg as 20% solution should be given i.v. if ICP rises above 20 mmHg. Avoid fluid overload and hypercapnia. Mechanical ventilation should be commenced early, and PCO_2 maintained at 25–30 mmHg.

10. Bleeding: give vitamin K 5 mg daily i.v. Measure prothrombin time daily; give fresh frozen plasma if prolonged more than 5 seconds. Give cimetidine 20 mg/kg daily i.v.

11. Sepsis: nurse the patient in protective isolation. Take blood cultures (aerobic, anaerobic, and fungal), blood for WBC, and chest x-ray if pyrexial or unexplained deterioration develops and commence parenteral antibiotics. If ascites is present, fever or clinical deterioration may represent spontaneous bacterial peritonitis; take 5 ml ascitic fluid from right iliac fossa (using fine needle) for microscopy and culture. Attendants should assume that stool and blood samples are contaminated with hepatitis viruses.

12. Uraemia may be prerenal, due to dehydration or nitrogen absorption following gastrointestinal haemorrhage; renal, due to acute tubular necrosis (urine contains granular and cellular casts, urine sodium >20 mmol/l, urine/plasma urea ratio <10); or 'functional renal failure' (urine sodium <20 mmol/l, no urinary sediment), often proceeding to acute tubular necrosis. Renal failure should be treated promptly with peritoneal or haemodialysis, both of which have a high complication rate in FHF. It is therefore extremely important to anticipate and prevent renal shutdown by monitoring urine output and central venous pressure and rapidly correcting hypovolaemia with salt-poor albumin or fresh frozen plasma[2,3].

13. Pancreatitis may be clinically inapparent or cause vomiting and ileus. Stop oral intake, avoid laparotomy, feed parenterally.

14. Hepatic support: exchange transfusion has given variable results in different series; at best it produces a temporary neurological improvement. Peritoneal dialysis is of no value, except possibly in Wilson's disease to remove copper by including d-penicillamine in dialysate[6]. Plasmapheresis has recently been reported to maintain a patient in FHF await-ing transplant[7]. Haemoperfusion using the 'Haemacol' coated charcoal column with prostacyclin infusion has produced an improved survival in adult series, particularly if commenced in stage III[8], and is currently the best alternative: transfer to a specialised unit is therefore required early. Cross circulation using a volunteer or baboon has been successful in very small numbers of patients.

15. Liver transplantation has been successfully performed in FHF; donor availability usually precludes. A theoretical alternative is splenic injection of viable hepatocytes whose survival may be adequate to maintain function during liver recovery.

PROGNOSIS

- Although children were previously reported to have better survival figures than adults[1], recent studies show a mortality of 65–72% in grade III, and 85–94% in grade IV[4].
- Survival is unlikely if the prothrombin time is prolonged by >90 seconds, if grade IV coma lasts for >24 hours, if convulsions, myoclonic jerks, or apnoea occur, or if major complications (renal failure, gastrointestinal haemorrhage, pancreatitis, sepsis) arise.
- A rising serum α-fetoprotein is favourable, suggesting regeneration.

FOLLOW-UP

Recovery from FHF is associated with complete restoration of normal liver histology, and thus where the cause of FHF is clear (e.g. paracetamol, halothane, *Amanita phalloides*), long-term follow-up is not required. If LFTs do not return to normal, liver biopsy is indicated seeking features of chronic active hepatitis *q.v.*

[1] Trey C et al. (1970) In *Progress in Liver Disease III* (Popper H, Schaffner S eds.), p. 282. New York: Grune and Stratton.
[2] Riely C A (1984) *Yale J. Biol. Med.*, **57**, 161.
[3] Kirsch R E et al. (1985) In *Liver and Biliary Disease* (Wright R, Millward-Sadler G H, Alberti K G M M, Karran S eds.), p. 659. London: Baillière Tindall.
[4] Psacharopoulos H T et al. (1980) *Arch. Dis. Childh.*, **55**, 252.
[5] EASL (1979) *Gut*, **20**, 620.

[6] De Bont B et al. (1985) J. Pediatr., **107**, 545.
[7] Winikoff S et al. (1985) J. Pediatr., **107**, 547.
[8] Gimson A E S et al. (1982) Lancet, **ii**, 681.

Benign Liver Tumours

One-third of liver tumours are benign and principally comprise vascular tumours (60%), mesenchymal hamartoma (30%), focal nodular hyperplasia and adenomas associated with glycogen storage disease[1,2].

Vascular tumours

Infantile haemangioendotheliomas and cavernous haemangiomas consist of anastomosing vascular channels lined by endothelial cells. Cavernous haemangiomas are often incidental autopsy findings. Vascular tumours presenting symptomatically do so in the first six months of life. They may be associated with cutaneous haemangiomas, with or without multiple other visceral haemangiomas (diffuse neonatal haemangiomatosis). Arteriovenous shunting through the haemangioma may produce high output cardiac failure. Thrombocytopenia or disseminated intravascular coagulation may cause bleeding or anaemia. Obstructive jaundice and portal hypertension rarely occur. Plain x-rays may show calcification, and ultrasound and CT define the tumour. Selective hepatic arteriography is indicated if resection, embolisation or hepatic artery ligation are being considered.

TREATMENT

1. If a vascular tumour is discovered asymptomatically or if cardiac failure can be managed medically then spontaneous resolution should be awaited.
2. Radiotherapy should not be used.
3. Prednisolone 2–4 mg/kg/day is associated with a more rapid involution by sensitising blood vessels to endogenous circulating vasoconstrictors and should be given in infants aged more than six weeks in congestive heart failure.
4. If steroids do not control heart failure or if the infant is under six weeks of age a direct attack on the tumour is necessary. Hepatic artery

ligation or embolisation have now superseded lobar resection[3].

PROGNOSIS

- The natural history of vascular liver tumours is of enlargement during infancy with later spontaneous regression after the first year.
- Neonates with large or multiple haemangiomas have a high mortality while those in whom cardiac failure can be controlled have an excellent prognosis.
- Rarely, resolution of infantile haemangioendothelioma is followed by angiosarcoma development.

Mesenchymal hamartoma

These tumours consist of multiple cysts with a greyish smooth lining filled with clear fluid or mucoid material separated by myxoid fibrous tissue containing proliferating bile ducts, blood vessels and lymphatic channels.

TREATMENT

1. Definitive diagnosis requires surgical biopsy. Total resection of the tumour is usually possible. The tumour is usually confined to one lobe and may be pedunculated facilitating excision.
2. Very large lesions may however require a difficult right lobectomy for total excision and some have been successfully treated by simply unroofing cysts allowing contents to drain to the peritoneum, although this has been

reported as causing intractable ascites. Others have suggested anastomosis of the opened cyst to a Roux-en-Y loop of bowel.

PROGNOSIS

- 77% occur under the age of two years[2,4]. They usually present with abdominal distension, and rapid enlargement of the liver, as fluid accumulation within cysts is a characteristic feature.
- In neonates they may present with congestive heart failure or disseminated intravascular coagulation.
- Malignant change of hepatic mesenchymal hamartoma has not been reported.

Focal nodular hyperplasia

Focal nodular hyperplasia (FNH) is a discrete usually subcapsular nodule in an otherwise normal liver, multiple in 15% cases, occurring throughout the paediatric age range, girls outnumbering boys by three to one. It usually presents as an asymptomatic non-tender mass noted on routine examination.

TREATMENT

While resection is not necessary for this benign lesion any diagnostic uncertainty after biopsy should lead to resection[5].

PROGNOSIS

- The prognosis is good; malignant transformation is not reported.

Hepatic adenomas

Spontaneous liver cell adenomas are rare in children but develop in up to 50% patients with type I glycogen storage disease. Distinction from well differentiated hepatocellular carcinoma and from regenerating cirrhotic nodules may be difficult. They are usually asymptomatic.

TREATMENT

In glycogen storage disease excellent dietary control may achieve resolution.

PROGNOSIS

- Malignant transformation is recorded in multiple adenomas[6].

[1] Ehren H (1983) *Am. J. Surg.*, **145,** 235.
[2] Weinberg A G et al. (1983) *Hum. Pathol.*, **14,** 512.
[3] Vomberg P P et al. (1986) *Eur. J. Pediatr.*, **144,** 472.
[4] Alkalay A L et al. (1985) *J. Pediatr. Surg.*, **20,** 125.
[5] Stocker J T et al. (1981) *Cancer*, **48,** 336.
[6] Wheeler D A et al. (1986) *Am. J. Clin. Pathol.*, **85,** 6.

Malignant Tumours

Among children presenting with hepatomegaly and found to have a hepatic malignancy, primary liver tumours are outnumbered by secondary involvement from neuroblastoma, Wilm's tumour, lymphoma or leukaemia. Primary liver tumours constitute 0.5–2% paediatric malignancies. Primary hepatic malignancies include hepatoblastoma (64%), hepatocellular carcinoma (27%), and mesenchymal tumours[1–4].

Hepatoblastoma

Males predominate by two to one. 63% hepatoblastoma (HB) occur before the age of two years. The epithelial cells of HB may be 'fetal' or 'embryonal'. Approximately 20% HB are 'mixed', i.e. contain mesenchymal elements, in particular osteoid, cartilage or muscle. Anaplastic and indeterminate varieties are less common. Hepatoblastoma usually presents with systemic symptoms (anorexia, weight loss, nausea, vomiting) in a male infant with abdominal distension and a palpable abdominal mass. Rare clinical associations include precocious puberty in males, hypercholesterolaemia, and hemihypertrophy. Serum α-fetoprotein (AFP) is elevated 1000 to 10 000-fold above normal in 80–90% HB. Abdominal x-ray, intravenous pyelogram (IVP), ultrasound and CT scan enable a pre-laparotomy diagnosis and determination of resectability in most cases. Percutaneous liver biopsy is hazardous in this vascular tumour and arteriography has been superseded by CT scanning.

TREATMENT

1. Total primary resection offers the best chance of survival.
2. Radiotherapy is ineffective.
3. Chemotherapy is indicated for: unresectable tumours which may be rendered resectable; metastatic disease or residual hepatic disease after primary resection; adjuvant treatment after apparently successful resection. It is now clear that those regimens including doxorubicin (adriamycin) and cisplatin are the most effective[5].

PROGNOSIS

- Total primary resection offers the best chance of survival, is possible in 50–70% cases and in the absence of metastatic disease has achieved 'cure' in 30–50%.
- Adjuvant chemotherapy may improve prognosis.
- Pure fetal type HB has a relatively favourable outcome, but any embryonal or undifferentiated tissue implies a less favourable prognosis, emphasising the need for extensive histological sectioning of excised tissue[1].

Hepatocellular carcinoma

Hepatocellular carcinoma (HCC) is usually extensively invasive or multicentric or both at presentation. Males outnumber females by two to one. Most HCC occur in children over the age of five years but infantile and even congenital cases occur. Most present with abdominal swelling, pain and constitutional symptoms and 25% have lung metastases at presentation. Conditions associated with an increased risk of HCC include hepatitis B virus infection, pre-existing hepatic adenoma (including glycogen storage disease), tyrosinaemia, Fanconi's anaemia treated with androgenic steroids. In known HBV carriers, serial α-fetoprotein measurement and high resolution ultrasonography may enable detection of early and resectable HCC.

TREATMENT

1. As with hepatoblastoma primary surgical resection offers the best hope of survival and radiation is ineffective. An unresectable tumour may be rendered resectable by prior chemotherapy.
2. The excellent results reported for hepatic artery embolisation in adults[6] have yet to be matched in paediatric series.

3. Encouraging results from chemotherapy using adriamycin and cisplatin dictate that adjuvant chemotherapy should now be given even if the tumour is deemed resectable.
4. Liver transplantation has been associated with a high incidence of subsequent metastatic recurrence with the exception of tumours arising in tyrosinaemia[7].

PROGNOSIS

● The median survival from diagnosis to death (4.2 months)[3] is only slightly better than in adult series (1.6 months) despite the lower incidence of pre-existing cirrhosis. Approximately 30% are resectable and these patients have a five-year survival of approximately 30%[8].
● Prognosis in the fibrolamellar variant is better—48% resectable, average survival 32 months, two- and five-year survivals 82% and 62% respectively[1,9,10].
● In tumours related to prior androgen therapy, cessation of androgens has been associated with tumour regression.

FOLLOW-UP

The child should be followed-up by the specialist centre.

[1] Weinberg A G et al. (1983) Hum. Pathol., **14,** 512.
[2] Lack E E et al. (1983) Cancer, **52,** 1510.
[3] Giacomantonio M et al. (1984) J. Pediatr. Surg., **19,** 523.
[4] Mahour G H et al. (1983) Am. J. Surg., **146,** 236.
[5] Quinn J J et al. (1985) Cancer, **56,** 1926.
[6] Allison D J et al. (1985) Lancet, **i,** 595.
[7] Starzl T E et al. (1985) J. Pediatr., **106,** 604.
[8] Exelby P R et al. (1974) J. Pediatr. Surg., **10,** 329.
[9] Craig J R et al. (1980) Cancer, **46,** 372.
[10] Alkalay A L et al. (1985) J. Pediatr. Surg., **20,** 125.

7
Diseases of the Genitourinary Tract

S. P. A. Rigden

Congenital Abnormalities of the Genitourinary Tract

Congenital abnormalities of the genitourinary tract are relatively common, occurring in 1 in 1–2000 live births. They may be detected by antenatal ultrasound examination[1], routine examination in the neonatal period or later in childhood, or by investigation following presentation with urinary tract infection or renal impairment.

Bilateral renal agenesis

This rare condition is three times more common in boys than girls. The associated oligohydramnios results in the typical Potter facies (flattened nose, receding jaw, prominent epicanthic folds, hypertelorism with eyes with an 'anti-mongolian' slant and folded low set ears with little cartilage).

TREATMENT

Active treatment is inappropriate in view of the associated pulmonary complications and abnormalities of the lower urinary tract.

PROGNOSIS

- Bilateral renal agenesis is invariably fatal, with affected infants usually dying of the associated pulmonary insufficiency.
- If respiratory function is sufficient to maintain life, then death from renal failure ensues in approximately 7–10 days.

Unilateral renal agenesis

Unilateral renal agenesis is relatively common and is associated with hypertrophy of the contralateral kidney. The single kidney may be subject to other congenital abnormalities, e.g. ectopia, vesicoureteric reflux, pelviureteric junction obstruction.

TREATMENT

No treatment is required for an otherwise normal, solitary kidney.

PROGNOSIS

- A single normal kidney is compatible with a normal life span; if associated with another congenital abnormality, the prognosis is dependent on the severity of that abnormality.

Renal hypoplasia, dysplasia and multicystic kidney

True renal hypoplasia implies a kidney which is normal in all respects apart from its diminutive size. Dysplasia is strictly a histological term used when non-renal elements (e.g. cartilage, smooth muscle) are present in a disorganised kidney. Variable sized cysts are common. Dysplasia may occur with urethral obstruction, vesicoureteric reflux or ureteric atresia. Multicystic kidney is pathologically an extreme form of dysplasia, associated with an atretic ureter. The cysts are large and there is no functional renal tissue.

TREATMENT

1. Renal hypoplasia: unilateral hypoplasia requires no treatment; bilateral requires chronic renal failure management.
2. Dysplasia: there is no specific treatment, but associated abnormalities must be sought and treated. Chronic renal failure management may be necessary (see p. 129).
3. Multicystic kidney: unilateral multicystic kidneys should be removed surgically, particularly if the contralateral kidney is normal, as the child can then be discharged from further follow-up.

PROGNOSIS

- If the hypoplasia is unilateral it is of no consequence except that blood pressure should be monitored for life, as renal hypoplasia may be the result of renal arterial or renal venous thrombosis which may also cause hypertension. If the hypoplasia is bilateral and the total number of nephrons is therefore reduced, there is hypertrophy of the nephrons and the condition of oligomeganephronia results. There is renal impairment which is usually progressive.
- The prognosis for a child with dysplastic kidneys depends on the amount of functional renal tissue present and on the presence of associated abnormalities, e.g. vesicoureteric reflux, obstruction. If the glomerular filtration rate (GFR) is < 40 ml/minute/1.73 m^2 surface area, progressive renal failure is likely.
- Multicystic kidney: this condition is rarely bilateral, when it is fatal: usually it is unilateral, although the other kidney may be dysplastic or hydronephrotic. Multicystic kidneys may cause hypertension.

Posterior urethral valves

Posterior urethral valves are the commonest obstructive lesion in male children. Severe cases usually present in infancy with urinary tract infection (UTI) and renal failure or may be detected antenatally by ultrasound scanning[2]. Less severe cases present with UTI, and a history of a poor urinary stream.

TREATMENT

1. The definitive treatment is surgical ablation of the valve, but in very young children this may have to be deferred until some growth has occurred in which case temporary bladder drainage via a vesicostomy is recommended.
2. If there is vesicoureteric obstruction, upper tract drainage via percutaneous nephrostomy tubes or loop ureterostomies is indicated until ureteric reimplantation is feasible. Catheter drainage using a small feeding tube, provides temporary emergency relief to allow treatment of infection and correction of metabolic abnormalities before surgery. Postoperatively continuous low dose prophylactic antibiotics should be given to prevent further infection.
3. If the child has renal impairment this should be managed as for chronic renal failure.

PROGNOSIS

- Prognosis depends on the degree of any associated renal dysplasia, vesicoureteric reflux or vesicoureteric obstruction and on successful surgery to relieve the original obstruction.
- 50% boys with obstructive uropathy secondary to posterior urethral valve have an elevated plasma creatinine[3] and the majority of these show progressive decline in renal function and ultimately require renal replacement therapy.

Pelviureteric junction obstruction

Pelviureteric junction (PUJ) obstruction causing hydronephrosis occurs more commonly in boys than girls and, in unilateral cases, more commonly affects the left kidney. Hydronephrosis due to PUJ obstruction is now quite frequently detected by antenatal ultrasound examination[2]. If this is not the case it may present in infancy with a loin mass or later in childhood with abdominal or loin pain, or may remain asymptomatic. Haematuria, hypertension and urinary tract infection may complicate PUJ obstruction.

TREATMENT

1. Treatment of unequivocal PUJ obstruction is surgical. If renal function is good or moderately impaired (> 20% of total GFR) pyeloplasty is performed. If renal function is severely reduced nephrostomy drainage may allow surprising improvement such that pyeloplasty is indicated. If no improvement occurs nephrectomy is performed.
2. If obstruction is equivocal or intermittent it should be further investigated by a ^{99m}Tc diethylene triamine pentacetate (DTPA) renal scan under diuretic conditions or with frusemide to produce a diuresis, or intravenous urography (IVU) under diuretic conditions or at the time of pain, if confusion remains an antegrade pressure-flow study is indicated.

PROGNOSIS

- Prognosis is dependent on the amount of pressure-induced parenchymal damage. Even if renal function is reduced to <20% total GFR as demonstrated by radioisotope imaging, improvement sufficient to avoid nephrectomy may occur with percutaneous nephrostomy drainage.

Vesicoureteric junction obstruction (obstructed megaureter)

Vesicoureteric junction (VUJ) obstruction is also more common in boys and more commonly affects the left ureter. The pathogenesis is unclear but there is a functional obstruction of the intravesical and intramural parts of the ureter. Presentation is often in early childhood with urinary tract infection (UTI) or haematuria.

TREATMENT

Treatment is surgical to excise the segment of ureter causing the obstruction followed by ureteric reimplantation.

PROGNOSIS

- Prognosis depends on whether the VUJ obstruction is unilateral or bilateral or affects a solitary kidney and on the extent of renal damage due to infection and back pressure.
- Renal function may be normal or impaired.

---

[1] Innes Williams D, Johnston J H (1982) *Paediatric Urology* 2nd edn. London: Butterworths.
[2] Thomas D (1984) *Arch. Dis. Childh.*, **59,** 913.
[3] Barratt T M *et al.* (1979) Obstructive uropathy in children. In *Renal Disease* (Black D, Jones N F eds.), pp. 804–24. Oxford: Blackwell Scientific.

Polycystic Disease

The polycystic diseases of the kidney include two principal forms: infantile polycystic disease and adult polycystic disease. However renal cysts occur in many other conditions, the most important of which are cystic dysplasia, multicystic kidney, medullary cystic disease (familial juvenile nephronophthisis), simple cysts and those associated with hereditary syndromes, e.g. tuberous sclerosis.

Infantile polycystic disease

Infantile polycystic disease is inherited as an autosomal recessive condition and usually presents in infancy with large kidneys and renal impairment. Occasionally the condition may not present until later in childhood. There is an almost invariable association with hepatic fibrosis.

TREATMENT

The treatment is that of progressive renal insufficiency (see *Chronic renal failure*, p. 129) proceeding to renal replacement therapy when indicated in suitable children. There are four points of special note:

a) Salt replacement – a minority of infants pass through a salt-losing phase and require sodium chloride supplements to prevent chronic dehydration, to optimise renal perfusion (and therefore function) and to promote growth. This phase is of variable duration but is almost always superseded by hypertension.
b) Hypertension may be severe and require treatment with a combination of hypotensive agents.
c) Portal hypertension may require surgery.
d) Antenatal diagnosis using ultrasound is possible from approximately 16 weeks' gestation and should be offered to parents who already have an affected child, together with appropriate genetic advice.

PROGNOSIS

- Delivery of affected infants may be obstructed by the enormous renal enlargement.
- The most severely affected infants have oliguria *in utero* and therefore oligohydramnios and at birth have a Potter's facies and compression deformities. These infants usually die in the neonatal period due to respiratory insufficiency, secondary to pulmonary hypoplasia consequent on oligohydramnios.
- Most affected infants survive the neonatal period with a variable degree of renal impairment, which gradually deteriorates through childhood. The rate of progression is extremely variable but end stage renal failure commonly occurs towards the end of the first decade.
- Hepatic fibrosis may be progressive causing hepatomegaly, splenomegaly, and portal hypertension in some children. Often severe renal disease is associated with mild liver disease and vice versa, although this is not invariably so.

Adult polycystic disease

Adult polycystic disease is inherited as an autosomal dominant condition and despite its name may present in childhood, either with symptoms (haematuria, hypertension, renal masses) or as a result of family screening. Renal functional impairment is rare in childhood.

TREATMENT

1. In childhood the most important aspect is the control of hypertension.
2. Progressive renal impairment in later life should be managed in the standard way with renal replacement therapy when necessary.

PROGNOSIS

- Renal failure usually becomes symptomatic in the fifth decade of life and is progressive.
- Approximately 10% adults with adult polycystic disease have berry aneurysms of the cerebral arteries, but these are rare in children.

Medullary cystic disease (familial juvenile nephronophthisis)

Familial juvenile nephronophthisis is an autosomal recessive disorder, which is sometimes associated with non-renal abnormalities, e.g. retinitis pigmentosa[1]. It typically presents in childhood with growth failure, polyuria, anaemia and progressive renal failure. There are cysts in the renal medulla morphologically indistinguishable from those found in medullary cystic disease, which occurs in older patients.

TREATMENT

Treatment is that of progressive renal impairment with renal replacement therapy when indicated.

PROGNOSIS

- Children with juvenile nephronophthisis usually reach end stage renal failure towards the end of their first decade.

---

[1] Donaldson M D C (1985) *Arch. Dis. Childh.*, **60**, 426.

Undescended Testis

An empty scrotum may be due to the testis being undescended, ectopic, retractile or absent. The incidence of undescended testes varies from 17.2% in preterm to 1.2% in full term babies. It falls further to 0.8% by one year of age but then remains constant, i.e. if spontaneous descent of a testis is going to occur it will do so before one year of age.

TREATMENT

Treatment is by orchidopexy, ideally performed between 4 and 24 months of age[1] and certainly before 5 years of age. If the testis is palpable it is usually possible for surgery to be undertaken as a day case. Patients with a high undescended testis may require a two-stage operation.

PROGNOSIS

● The undescended testis is at risk of:

a) Degenerative change leading to defective spermatogenesis. These changes are present from as early as 2 years of age and are progressive.

b) Malignancy. Tumours of the testis are extremely rare in childhood, whatever the position of the testis. In the adult with an undescended testis the risk of testicular cancer is increased 50-fold. Orchidopexy probably does not reduce this risk significantly, as the predisposition to neoplasia seems to be inherent in the testis itself. Orchidopexy does however expedite diagnosis of the tumour, thereby increasing the likelihood of successful treatment.

c) Torsion and trauma.

[1] Atwell J D (1985) *Hosp. Update*, **11**, 761.

Urinary Tract Infection

Urinary tract infection (UTI) is common in infants and children with a strong female preponderance except during early infancy. It has been estimated that 3–5% girls and 0.5–2.0% boys will have UTI during childhood. Without adequate investigation and treatment 75% children will have recurrent UTI. All infants and children with a proven UTI should be investigated in order to discover the underlying cause of infection, to assess the extent of renal damage, to plan appropriate management and to predict the prognosis[1].

TREATMENT

1. First acute episode

   a) Following the collection of a satisfactory urine sample (or preferably two samples from a child who is not acutely ill) antibiotic therapy should be started without delay.

   b) In the acutely ill child who may have an accompanying septicaemia, gentamicin 2 mg/kg per dose is the drug of choice despite its potential nephrotoxicity, which should be avoided by relating the interdose interval to the level of renal function and by measuring serum gentamicin levels.

   c) In the less ill child, co-trimoxazole (20 mg sulphamethoxazole:4 mg trimethoprim/kg/day) divided into two doses is the drug of choice.

   d) Antibiotic therapy should be reviewed when the results of the urine specimen and sensitivities of the organism become available. Full therapeutic dosage should be continued for 5–7 days, after which the dose should be reduced to a prophylactic level or an alternative prophylactic antibiotic substituted until investigations are complete. If infection persists despite appropriate antibiotic therapy or is replaced by a resistant organism, urgent investigation is required.

   e) Useful antibiotics in the management of urinary tract infection in children include:

	Therapy		Prophylaxis
	Dose (mg/kg/day)	Dose interval (hours)	(mg/kg/day)
Co-trimoxazole	20	12	5–10
(sulphamethoxazole and trimethoprim)	4		1–2
Trimethoprim	4	12	1–2
Nitrofurantoin	3–5	6	1–2
Nalidixic acid	50	6	20
Amoxycillin	20	8	——
Cefadroxil	25	12	——
Gentamicin	2 mg/kg/dose	*	——

*varies with level of renal function —imperative to measure blood levels

118

2. Vesicoureteric reflux (VUR)

   a) The options are either conservative management until the VUR disappears spontaneously with age, or surgical correction of the VUR.
   b) Conservative management requires careful attention to the general measures set out below and continuous low dose antibiotic prophylaxis to prevent further UTI. Meticulous follow-up is required with regular urine cultures and biennial investigations to monitor renal growth, detect fresh scarring and whether the VUR has ceased.
   c) Surgical correction of VUR is indicated if break-through infections occur. These usually occur because of poor compliance with medical management due to social reasons, in the presence of large paraureteric diverticula or when there is gross VUR with intrarenal reflux in a young child.
   d) Neither conservative nor surgical management has yet been shown to be superior in terms of recurrence of infection, renal growth or new scar development. Controlled trials are currently in progress to answer these questions.

3. Obstructive lesions

   a) Anatomical lesions require surgical correction (see *Congenital anomalies*, p. 112).
   b) Functional lesions: the most satisfactory treatment for the child with a neuropathic bladder is intermittent catheterisation.
   c) Stones:
      i) Mixed infective stones must be removed surgically with appropriate antibiotic therapy to sterilise the urinary tract.
      ii) Metabolic stones should only be operated on if causing obstruction; otherwise treatment is that of the underlying metabolic disorder.

4. There are certain general supportive measures applicable to all children with UTI:

   a) Ensure a high urine flow rate by encouraging a high fluid intake.
   b) Ensure regular, complete bladder emptying at intervals of two to three hours.
   c) Prevent the child becoming constipated.
   d) Encourage double micturition. This can be helpful even in children who do not have VUR to correct careless bladder emptying habits.

5. In addition to the general measures outlined above, continuous nightly low dose antibiotic prophylaxis given over 6–12 months may be helpful for recurrent UTI in the child with an anatomically normal urinary tract.

PROGNOSIS

- The prognosis of UTI in childhood depends on whether there is an associated urinary tract abnormality (present in 25–55% infants and children with UTI) and on the extent of renal parenchymal damage.
- Vesicoureteric reflux (VUR:reflux nephropathy):

   a) Approximately 30% children investigated for UTI are found to have VUR on micturating cystourethrography and approximately one-third of these will have already sustained parenchymal scarring, as demonstrated by intravenous urography (IVU) or dimercaptosuccinic acid (DMSA) renal scan. If the damage is sufficient to reduce the glomerular filtration rate (GFR) to < 30–40 ml/minute/1.73 m^2 surface area, progression to end stage renal disease (ESRD) is likely, even in the absence of further infection, vesicoureteric reflux or hypertension.
   b) VUR is the commonest cause of ESRD in children aged < 15 years in the UK and accounts for 20% patients aged under 40 years developing ESRD in Europe[2]. Lesser degrees of scarring will cause milder degrees of renal impairment.
   c) 10% children with renal scarring due to VUR will develop hypertension.
   d) VUR, but not its consequences, disappears spontaneously with time in up to 80% children.

- Obstructive lesions are found in approximately 7% children with UTI:

a) Anatomical obstructive lesions, e.g. posterior urethral valve, vesicoureteric junction obstruction, ureterocoele, pelviureteric junction obstruction, require surgical correction (see *Congenital anomalies of the genitourinary tract*, p. 112).

b) Functional lesions, e.g. neuropathic bladder: the prognosis for children with neuropathic bladders depends on the degree of renal parenchymal damage caused by VUR under high pressure or obstruction.

c) Stones[3]

  i) Mixed infective stones occur as a result of infection (usually due to *Proteus*) and are often associated with structural anomalies of the urinary tract. Prognosis varies with the extent of the renal parenchymal damage.

  ii) Metabolic stones resulting from hypercalciuria, acidification defects, primary hyperoxaluria, cystinuria and disorders of purine metabolism are not commonly associated with urinary tract infection unless causing obstruction. The prognosis is that of the underlying disease.

- Some children have either no structural abnormality of the urinary tract or minor abnormalities such as duplex kidney or horse-shoe kidney with no reflux or obstruction: such children with UTI (about 50% those presenting with UTI) have a good prognosis.

---

[1] Smellie J et al. (1986) *Med. Int.*, **2,** 1344.
[2] Broyer M et al. (1984) *Proc. EDTA*, **5,** 55.
[3] Ghazali S et al. (1973) *Arch. Dis. Childh.*, **48,** 291.

Glomerular Disorders

Disorders of the glomeruli may manifest either as leakage of blood constituents normally retained by the glomerular basement membrane (e.g. proteins, red blood cells), by impaired filtration causing retention of metabolites which are normally excreted, or by a combination of both features. Proteinuria (normal < 200 mg/24 hours) may be asymptomatic but if persistent and in excess of 1 g/24 hours should be investigated by renal biopsy. Heavy proteinuria (> 3 g/24 hours) usually results in hypoalbuminaemia and oedema, i.e. the nephrotic syndrome.

Minimal change nephropathy

Minimal change nephropathy (MCN) i.e. normal histology on light microscopy but fusion of podocyte foot processes on electron microscopy, is the commonest cause of the nephrotic syndrome in childhood, accounting for about 90% cases. It is rare in the first year of life and reaches a peak incidence at 2–3 years when it is twice as common in boys as girls. By puberty the sex incidence is equal. It is associated with normal renal function, normal blood pressure, microscopic or no haematuria, highly selective proteinuria and normal C3 levels.

TREATMENT

1. Prednisolone 60 mg/m²/day will induce remission in 95% children with MCN within 4 weeks. After three days of protein free urine (Albustix negative or trace only on first morning urine specimen) the dose is tapered and discontinued. If a further relapse occurs the same treatment schedule is followed. If two relapses occur within six months alternate day prednisolone is given in the smallest dose necessary to maintain remission. If this proves impossible or signs of steroid toxicity develop the child should receive a course of cyclophosphamide. If at any stage, remission is not achieved with prednisolone 60 mg/m²/day for four weeks, the nephrotic syndrome is deemed steroid resistant and a renal biopsy should be performed.
2. Cyclophosphamide given in a dose of 3 mg/kg/day for eight weeks will induce remission for at least a year in 75% children with steroid dependent MCN and for 5 years in 50% patients. The risks of bone marrow depression

(weekly full blood count required during treatment course), alopecia (usually mild and always reversible) and infertility (very unlikely in this dose given before puberty) have to be balanced against those of steroid toxicity.
3. Other therapies include:

   a) Chlorambucil is as effective as cyclophosphamide, but probably more toxic.
   b) Azathioprine is not effective in preventing relapse.
   c) Cyclosporin A and levamisole are currently under evaluation.

PROGNOSIS

- Prognosis is good. About one-third of children will only have a single attack and a further third suffer only infrequent relapses during childhood. The remaining third have frequent relapses, but even so almost all remit before adulthood. Renal function and life expectancy are then normal.
- Two serious complications may occur:

   a) Hypovolaemia due to heavy proteinuria and rapid accumulation of oedema fluid may lead to life-threatening venous and arterial thromboses.
   b) Infection, particularly pneumococcal, may present as primary peritonitis and also be life threatening.

FOLLOW-UP

Children with frequently relapsing MCN or on continuous therapy should have their first morning urine sample tested with albustix and the parents instructed to report for advice if there is

+ + or + + + proteinuria for three consecutive days, or if the child is unwell, becomes oedematous, develops diarrhoea or vomiting, or complains of abdominal pain (a hallmark of hypovolaemia).

Focal segmental glomerulosclerosis

Focal segmental glomerulosclerosis (FSGS) is the most common histological pattern found in steroid-resistant nephrotic syndrome in childhood. It is frequently associated with haematuria, renal impairment, hypertension and poorly selective proteinuria.

TREATMENT

1. Treatment is generally unrewarding.
2. Prednisolone (60 mg/m²/day until remission + 3 days). A minority of patients with FSGS will respond to prednisolone at least initially.
3. Cyclophosphamide (3 mg/kg/day for 8 weeks) will induce remission in a small proportion of children with FSGS.
4. Other therapies include:

   a) Cyclosporin A is presently being evaluated.
   b) Combination chemotherapy with vincristine, cyclophosphamide and prednisolone is currently under trial.

5. Symptomatic treatment for hypertension, oedema and progressive renal failure is indicated.

PROGNOSIS

- About one-third of children with FSGS will remit spontaneously, although the time course may be prolonged.
- A further one-third continue with proteinuria and haematuria but normal renal function.
- One-third will have a persistent severe nephrotic syndrome and progress to end stage renal failure.

FOLLOW-UP

Children with frequently relapsing FSGS or on continuous therapy should have their first morning urine sample tested with albustix and the parents instructed to report for advice if there is + + or + + + proteinuria for three consecutive days, or if the child is unwell, becomes oedematous, develops diarrhoea or vomiting, or complains of abdominal pain (a hallmark of hypovolaemia).

Acute nephritic syndrome

Acute nephritic syndrome is characterised by a sudden onset of a variable combination of haematuria (usually macroscopic), proteinuria (usually mild), oedema as a consequence of sodium and water retention, hypertension and impaired GFR. There are many causes of acute nephritic syndrome, which in childhood include postinfectious glomerulonephritis (commonly group A streptococcal infection), shunt nephritis and the nephritis associated with subacute bacterial endocarditis, Henoch-Schönlein purpura, mesangiocapillary glomerulonephritis, systemic lupus erythematosus (SLE), antiglomerular basement membrane antibody nephritis (Goodpasture's syndrome) and Wegener's granulomatosis.

TREATMENT

1. General measures

   a) To combat salt and water overload, due to low GFR and increased proportional reabsorption of glomerular filtrate in the proximal tubule, sodium should be restricted to 1 mmol/kg body weight/day and if oliguria is present the fluid intake restricted to the insensible loss (300 ml/m² body surface area/day) plus the urinary output. If the child is hypertensive, frusemide should be given to increase urinary sodium loss as first treatment (1–5 mg/kg i.v. depending on renal function). If there is severe renal impairment and no response to frusemide, dialysis will be necessary.

b) Hypertension: if restriction of sodium and water and i.v. frusemide do not control hypertension, hydralazine 0.2–0.5 mg/kg i.m. or i.v. should be given. If this is insufficient an intravenous infusion of labetalol (1–3 mg/kg/hour) is indicated. Dialysis may be required.

c) Renal failure: see *Acute renal failure* (p. 127).

2. Specific measures

a) It is usual to give a course of penicillin to eradicate streptococcal infection.

b) Crescentic nephritis in association with post-streptococcal glomerulonephritis, Henoch–Schönlein nephritis, SLE, mesangiocapillary glomerulonephritis, anti-GBM nephritis, Wegener's granulomatosis may respond to intensive treatment with immunosuppression with or without plasma exchange.

PROGNOSIS

- Prognosis depends on aetiology and histological changes.
- Post-streptococcal glomerulonephritis: the overall prognosis is good with complete recovery being the rule if the biopsy shows only endothelial proliferative glomerulonephritis. By 10 years after the acute episode > 90% children have normal renal function and normal urine, while about 5% have persistent proteinuria and haematuria. The prognosis is poor if the biopsy shows epithelial proliferation with crescents.
- Henoch–Schönlein purpura nephritis: generally the prognosis is good. Children with asymptomatic haematuria and proteinuria on the whole do well, although 20% may develop permanent renal damage. Up to 50% those who present with acute nephritic syndrome or nephrotic syndrome are well with reasonable renal function 10 years later[1]. Crescentic nephritis carries a bad prognosis but may be amenable to treatment (see above).

FOLLOW-UP

All patients with acute nephritic syndrome should have their blood pressure and renal function checked regularly, until the urine is free from blood and protein.

---

[1] Counahan R *et al.* (1977) *Br. Med. J.*, **2**, 11.

Alport's syndrome

Alport's syndrome (familial nephritis plus nerve deafness) typically presents with microscopic haematuria with macroscopic exacerbations.

TREATMENT

Unfortunately no specific treatment is available. Hypertension should be treated rigorously and the usual measures to manage chronic renal failure applied.

PROGNOSIS

- Affected males usually develop end stage renal failure during the second or third decade of life.
- Affected females are carriers and usually only have mild renal disease, although this may be exacerbated by pregnancy.

IgA nephropathy (Berger's disease)

Berger's disease is one of the principal causes of the syndrome of benign recurrent haematuria. It presents with recurrent bouts of haematuria, often precipitated by intercurrent viral infections, with completely normal urine between attacks. Renal biopsy shows focal proliferative glomerulonephritis or only very trivial changes but immunofluorescence reveals mesangial IgA.

TREATMENT

No specific treatment is available.

PROGNOSIS

- The prognosis of childhood IgA nephropathy is usually good. Onset in later life may be associated with progressive renal impairment in a minority of cases.

Tubular Disorders

Disorders of tubular function result in abnormal or inappropriate composition or volume of the final urine. In the normal kidney approximately 98% the glomerular filtrate is reabsorbed.

Cystinosis

Cystinosis is the commonest cause of the Fanconi syndrome in children. It occurs in about 1 in 40 000 live births and is inherited as an autosomal recessive disorder. The primary defect is a failure in the transport system to remove cystine from lysosomes, resulting in accumulation of cystine and crystal formation in all cells[1].

TREATMENT

1. Antenatal diagnosis is possible using cultured amniotic fibroblasts.
2. Early treatment is directed towards compensating for the abnormal tubular losses:

   a) Sodium bicarbonate up to 10 mmol/kg/day.
   b) Potassium and phosphate supplements are usually necessary.
   c) Vitamin D supplements to prevent or treat rickets.
   d) High calorie/high fluid intake.

3. Prostaglandin synthetase inhibitors, e.g. indomethacin reduce renal blood flow and GFR, resulting in less sodium and water loss[2].
4. Cysteamine[3] or phosphocysteamine reduce the intracellular cystine concentration by binding with it to form a mixed disulphide which leaves the lysosome through a cationic amino acid transport system. Therapy is monitored by measuring white blood cell cystine levels.
5. As renal failure progresses, chronic renal failure management should be applied (see p. 129).
6. Renal replacement therapy is suitable in some children.

PROGNOSIS

- End stage renal failure usually develops before 10 years of age.

- The disease does not recur in transplanted kidneys.
- Hypothyroidism develops as a consequence of cystine deposition in the thyroid gland.
- Corneal cystine deposition causes photophobia.
- An associated retinopathy may lead to gradual visual failure.

[1] Schneider J A (1985) *New Eng. J. Med.*, **313**, 1473.
[2] Haycock G B et al. (1982) *Arch. Dis. Childh.*, **57**, 934.
[3] da Silva V A et al. (1985) *New Eng. J. Med.*, **313**, 1460.

Distal renal tubular acidosis

Hydrogen ion homeostasis requires bicarbonate reabsorption in the proximal tubule and the excretion of net hydrogen ion in the distal renal tubule. Failure of either or both these mechanisms results in acidosis. The most common form is distal renal tubular acidosis (type 1, classical). Most cases are sporadic, although dominant and recessive forms have been described. Children present between two and four years of age with failure to thrive, rickets and nephrocalcinosis. Hypokalaemia and hyperchloraemic metabolic acidosis are found with urine pH always greater than 6.

TREATMENT

Treatment consists of alkali 1–3 mmol/kg/day in divided doses.

PROGNOSIS

- Prognosis is dependent on the extent of the nephrocalcinosis at diagnosis. If this is not severe the long-term prognosis can be favourable.

Proximal renal tubular acidosis (type 2)

Pure primary proximal renal tubular acidosis is very rare and may be permanent or transient. It presents in infancy with failure to thrive, vomiting and a hyperchloraemic acidosis. Urine acidification is normal when the plasma bicarbonate is below threshold.

TREATMENT

Sodium bicarbonate (>10 mmol/kg/day) is required to restore the plasma bicarbonate to normal.

PROGNOSIS

- Prognosis is good.

Nephrogenic diabetes insipidus

Nephrogenic diabetes insipidus (NDI) is inherited as a sex-linked recessive defect. Affected male infants present with marked polyuria and polydipsia frequently leading to episodes of hypernatraemic dehydration. Constipation and intermittent fevers also occur. Female heterozygotes are less severely affected but can be detected as they have reduced concentrating ability.

TREATMENT

1. Adequate water intake is important particularly when the child does not have free access to fluids, e.g. during infancy or the unconscious patient.
2. Thiazide diuretics, e.g. hydrochlorothiazide 1–2 mg/kg/day improve polyuria by reduction of extracellular volume and increased proximal tubular reabsorption.
3. Reduction of the solute load the kidney has to excrete.

PROGNOSIS

- Prognosis is good so long as a high fluid intake is maintained. Some patients are developmen-

tally delayed, which may be secondary to repeated episodes of hypernatraemic dehydration.

Bartter's syndrome

Bartter's syndrome, which may be inherited as a recessive disorder, usually presents in childhood with failure to thrive, polyuria and polydipsia. There is also hypokalaemic metabolic alkalosis, high plasma renin and a normal plasma aldosterone, which usually rises when the plasma potassium is normalised. Blood pressure is normal.

TREATMENT

Treatment with indomethacin[1] with or without potassium supplements has been successful in normalising plasma chemistry and improving growth.

PROGNOSIS

- Few data are available on the long-term prognosis of Bartter's syndrome. It is a chronic disease and its course may be complicated by episodes of dehydration and vascular collapse, acute electrolyte imbalance, intercurrent infection or side-effects of treatment.

---

[1] Dillon M J et al. (1979) Q. J. Med., **48**, 429.

Cystinuria

Cystinuria is inherited as an autosomal recessive disorder and is characterised by excessive urinary excretion of cystine, lysine, ornithine and arginine. Cystine stones may form causing obstruction.

TREATMENT

1. A high fluid intake (3–5 litres/day) will help prevent cystine stone formation and aids dissolution of stones already present.
2. Alkalinisation of the urine to pH >8 with

sodium bicarbonate also improves cystine solubility.

3. Penicillamine 0.25–1.5 g/day contributes to stone dissolution and prevents recurrence.

4. Surgery may be required to remove or dislodge stones causing acute obstruction.

PROGNOSIS

• Prognosis is good if stone formation is prevented. However multiple episodes of obstruction may finally progress to end stage renal failure.

Acute Renal Failure

Acute renal failure (ARF), defined as the sudden inability of the kidneys to maintain body homeostasis, may result from impaired renal perfusion, disease or damage of the renal parenchyma or obstruction to urine flow. The causes of ARF are diverse and vary with age and geographical area; e.g. in Third World countries dehydration secondary to diarrhoeal illnesses is the commonest cause of ARF, whereas in Western countries cardiopulmonary bypass surgery is now one of the commonest causes[1].

TREATMENT

1. The diagnosis and management of ARF should proceed simultaneously and the most important clinical problems sought and treated in the following order.
2. Ventilation

   a) Salt and water overload may result in life-threatening pulmonary oedema, recognised by:
      i) Cyanosis, restlessness, tachypnoea, orthopnoea, crepitations, gallop rhythm usually associated with other signs of saline overload – arterial hypertension, raised jugular venous pressure, hepatomegaly, peripheral oedema.
      ii) Arterial hypoxaemia.
      iii) Chest x-ray – cardiomegaly with 'bat's wing' appearance of pulmonary oedema.
   b) Inadequate ventilation may result from:
      i) Severe illness, e.g. meningitis, septicaemia.
      ii) Convulsions due to the primary disease, biochemical abnormalities, hypertension or their treatment.
   c) If the child is cyanosed and restless and/or has arterial hypoxaemia, give oxygen and proceed immediately to elective ventilation with positive end expiratory pressure (PEEP) followed by arrangements for dialysis.

3. Circulatory state

   a) Assess by pulse rate, blood pressure, central venous pressure measurement (CVP) or clinical assessment of jugular venous pressure, peripheral circulation using central-peripheral temperature gap[2], urine output measured hourly with indwelling catheter.
   b) Hypovolaemia, recognised by raised pulse rate, low blood pressure, low CVP, wide central–peripheral temperature gap and oliguria (the production of < 0.5 ml/kg/hour of urine) with sodium concentration of < 10 mmol/l, urine to plasma urea ratio of > 4:1 and urine to plasma osmolality ratio of > 1.3:1, requires urgent correction with appropriate i.v. fluid, 20 ml/kg of plasma, whole blood or saline. The adequacy and effect of this replacement must be monitored carefully using the above signs.
   c) Impaired cardiac output causing raised pulse rate, low blood pressure, high CVP, wide central–peripheral temperature gap and oliguria with concentrated urine should be treated with inotrope infusion, e.g. dopamine, dobutamine.
   d) Poor peripheral circulation with a normal or raised blood pressure and CVP and oliguria may be improved by giving hydralazine 0.1–0.2 mg/kg i.v. or i.m. or chlorpromazine 0.25 mg/kg i.v. Note i.v. fluids may also be required.
   e) Circulatory overload with raised blood pressure, raised CVP, signs of cardiac failure, pulmonary oedema (see above), may respond to i.v. frusemide 5 mg/kg. If a satisfactory response is obtained repeat frusemide 2 mg/kg i.v. 4–6 hourly. If there is not a satisfactory response urgent arrangements for dialysis must be made and fluid intake restricted to absolute minimum. Mannitol is contraindicated because it will exacerbate volume overload if it is not excreted. Hypertension unresponsive to frusemide, should be treated with hydralazine 0.2–1.0 mg/kg i.v.

4. Biochemistry

   a) Hyperkalaemia ($K^+ > 6.0$ mmol/l) requires urgent treatment and ECG monitoring.
      i) 10% calcium gluconate 0.5 ml/kg i.v. slowly.
      ii) Calcium/potassium cation exchange resin 1 g/kg orally or rectally.
      iii) Correction of acidosis (see below).
      iv) Intravenous 50% glucose (0.5 g/kg). If blood glucose > 10 mmol/l, soluble insulin 1 unit:4 g glucose will be required. Check blood glucose frequently.
   b) Dialysis is needed in addition to the above measures if $K^+ > 7.0$ mmol/l.
   c) Metabolic acidosis should be half corrected with i.v. 8.4% sodium bicarbonate (1 mmol/ml) using the formula $\frac{1}{2} \times 0.3 \times$ body weight (kg) $\times$ base deficit. It should be noted that this dose may need to be reduced in severe circulatory overload because of the sodium load and correction of acidosis may precipitate tetany.

5. Sepsis: if suspected of causing or complicating ARF, sepsis should be treated aggressively with a loading dose of gentamicin 2 mg/kg i.v. Further doses will depend on level of renal function and trough blood levels.

6. Dialysis: apart from exceptional circumstances, a child requiring dialysis should, after necessary emergency measures have been carried out, be transferred to a unit with experience of dialysing children.

   a) Indications:
      i) Hyperkalaemia, $K^+ > 7.0$ mmol/l recorded before emergency treatment.
      ii) Circulatory overload unresponsive to frusemide causing pulmonary oedema or systemic hypertension.
      iii) Severe acidosis.
      iv) Severe biochemical disturbance causing neurological symptoms.
   b) Peritoneal dialysis is suitable for most children with ARF, exceptions being burns involving the anterior abdominal wall or recent abdominal surgery, when haemodialysis is indicated via a temporary central venous catheter or an arteriovenous shunt.

7. Specific investigation may be necessary to establish the underlying cause of ARF leading to definitive treatment, e.g. septicaemia or pyelonephritis, needing appropriate antibiotic therapy or posterior urethral valve requiring surgical relief of obstruction.

8. Conservative management: if dialysis is not indicated and the circulatory status is satisfactory, fluid balance is most easily maintained by giving the child hourly fluid, calculated by adding 1/24 the daily insensible losses to the previous hour's urine output. Calculate insensible losses as 300 ml/m² surface area. As recovery proceeds this can be calculated from a 12- or 24-hour period.

9. Nutrition is vital for recovery and may necessitate dialysis or haemofiltration to make the required 'space'. The aim should be to provide 100–150 kcal/kg body weight and 1 g/kg body weight of first class protein per day orally if tolerated or intravenously if necessary.

PROGNOSIS

- The prognosis of ARF is largely dependent on its cause, e.g. in a prospective study of ARF in the newborn infant, the mortality was 45%, but all of the babies had more than one life-threatening problem[3]. Acute renal failure complicating trauma or cardiac surgery has in most series a mortality of at least 50%[1].

FOLLOW-UP

In patients who survive, recovery of renal function is usually good, but should be checked by determination of glomerular filtration rate (GFR) and dimercaptosuccinic acid (DMSA) renal scan some months after the acute episode.

[1] Rigden S P A et al. (1982) Arch. Dis. Childh., **57,** 425.
[2] Aynsley–Green A (1974) Arch. Dis. Childh., **49,** 477.
[3] Norman M E et al. (1979) Pediatrics, **63,** 475.

Chronic Renal Failure

Chronic renal failure (CRF), defined as the clinical state resulting from a reduced number of functioning nephrons, may result from a variety of primary renal diseases. In children the most common causes of CRF are reflux nephropathy, chronic glomerulonephritis, congenital and inherited forms of renal disease.

TREATMENT

1. Conservative management

   a) The objectives of conservative therapy are to prevent uraemic symptoms, to promote normal growth, and to preserve renal function.

   b) Provision of adequate energy: children with CRF spontaneously have low energy intakes. Energy intakes of 150–180 kcal/kg actual body weight/day in infants and 100–120 kcal/kg/day in older children are necessary to prevent catabolism and to maximise growth. Most children require calorie supplements to meet these aims and infants and young children may require nasogastric tube feeding, which can be performed at home.

   c) Protein restriction: there is evidence in adults that protein restriction retards the progression of CRF[1]. Children have an increased protein requirement because of the demands of growth and protein restriction should only be employed if the blood urea remains above 20 mmol/l after ensuring an adequate energy intake as above. Total protein intake should not be restricted to less than 6% of total calories. Essential amino acid and keto acid supplements have been used in conjunction with very low protein diets, but are unpalatable, expensive and rarely indicated.

   d) Phosphate control: reduction in GFR causes phosphate retention, which directly and indirectly leads to secondary hyperparathyroidism. Excessive parathyroid hormone (PTH) causes renal osteodystrophy (osteitis fibrosa cystica) and may also play a role in growth failure, glucose intolerance in CRF, the anaemia of CRF and progression to end stage renal failure. Plasma phosphate concentration should be kept at the lower end of the normal range for age[2] by:

      i) Reduction of dietary phosphate to about 600 mg/day. This can usually be achieved by restriction of dairy products especially milk, cheese and yoghurt.

      ii) The use of calcium carbonate with meals as a phosphate binder[3]. Aluminium hydroxide should not be used as a long-term phosphate binder because of its toxic effects on bone, brain and bone marrow.

   e) Prevention and treatment of renal osteodystrophy:

      i) Phosphate control (see above).

      ii) Hydroxylated vitamin D supplements. In CRF, endogenous levels of 1,25-dihydroxycholecalciferol are low because of reduced activity of the renal enzyme 1α-hydroxylase. This can be overcome by lowering the plasma phosphate and the administration of 1α-hydroxycholecalciferol or 1,25-dihydroxycholecalciferol (starting dose 20 ng/kg/day).

      iii) Plasma calcium and phosphate must be closely monitored to avoid hypercalcaemia and metastatic calcification. If available, serum PTH levels are invaluable in assessing progress[3] and an x-ray of left hand and wrist should be checked 3–4 monthly for evidence of renal osteodystrophy.

   f) Hypertension:

      i) Hypertension may be the consequence of underlying renal pathology, e.g. reflux nephropathy, chronic glomerulonephritis, in which case hypotensive agents should be prescribed to maintain the blood pressure within the normal range for age.

ii) Alternatively it may be the result of sodium and water retention in advanced CRF and may respond to sodium restriction or diuretic therapy, but may require dialysis.

iii) In general, children with CRF and hypertension should not receive more than 1–2 mmol/kg/day of sodium.

g) Sodium and water balance: in contradistinction to those underlying conditions causing hypertension, many causes of CRF in childhood are associated with excessive sodium loss, resulting in contraction of the extracellular fluid (ECF) volume and further impairment in renal function, e.g. renal dysplasia, obstructive uropathy, nephronophthisis. If there are signs of ECF depletion, particularly postural hypotension, sodium supplements should be given to the limit of tolerance, i.e. the appearance of hypertension or peripheral oedema.

h) Control of acidosis requires monitoring with venous blood gas determinations and treatment with sodium bicarbonate supplements as required.

i) Hyperkalaemia is usually responsive to dietary manipulation and correction of acidosis. If these measures are insufficient, Calcium Resonium (1 g/kg/dose) may be given as an emergency measure but arrangements for dialysis must be made.

j) Infection: children with an underlying urological abnormality predisposing to recurrent urinary tract infection must have a urine sample checked regularly for infection and may require low dose prophylactic antibiotic therapy.

k) It is vitally important that sufficient time and opportunity are given to the family to discuss the child's likely future treatment and outlook. The management of a child with CRF progressing to end stage renal failure can be extremely stressful even to the best adjusted families. They require, and should be offered the help of a medical social worker, psychologist and/or psychiatrist as part of an integrated team.

l) If possible immunisations should be completed before end stage renal failure is reached.

m) Vascular access for haemodialysis should be established in most older children once the plasma creatinine has risen above 500 µmol/l.

2. Transplantation: a detailed account is beyond the scope of this chapter; the general principles will be briefly described.

a) Transplantation is the preferred treatment for children with end stage renal disease (ESRD), because this offers the best prospect of rehabilitation to a near normal life style. However, it is likely that most children with ESRD will require treatment by dialysis before or between transplants.

b) Transplantation is performed using a cadaveric kidney or a kidney from a living relative over the age of consent: for children this usually means a parent. With recent improvements in immunosuppression and cadaveric graft survival, the indications for live donor transplantation are diminishing. Compatible blood group and negative cross-match are essential prerequisites for transplantation but HLA matching is less important.

c) Following transplantation immunosuppressive therapy must be given meticulously and indefinitely. Immunosuppressive agents in use include:

i) Cyclosporin A is the most effective immunosuppressive agent presently available but is difficult to use because of its nephrotoxic side-effects. The dose for each patient has to be determined by blood levels. In some units it is used as the sole immunosuppressive drug but more often in combination with one or more others.

ii) Prednisolone regimens vary between different transplant units; in the Guy's Hospital paediatric unit the prednisolone dosage has been reduced to 10 mg/m² body surface area on alternate days by six months after transplantation.

iii) Azathioprine is used either in combination with prednisolone or with low dose prednisolone and low dose cyclosporin A.

iv) Antithymocyte globulin or antilymphocyte globulin may be given i.v. either to treat acute rejection episodes or in an attempt to prevent rejection in highly sensitised patients.

d) In addition to immunosuppression transplant patients may require:
  i) Hypotensive therapy especially within the first six months or if it has been required before transplantation.
  ii) Prophylactic antibiotic therapy to prevent urinary tract infection.

3. Haemodialysis has to be performed three times a week for 3–5 hours per session depending on the patient's size. Vascular access for long-term haemodialysis is best achieved by an arteriovenous fistula preferably in the forearm. Surgically placed, double lumen central venous catheters have now been used successfully in small children for short to moderate term haemodialysis. For short-term dialysis percutaneously positioned temporary venous catheters or arteriovenous shunts are used.

4. Peritoneal dialysis may be performed either intermittently (IPD) or continuously (continuous ambulatory peritoneal dialysis, CAPD) or by a combination of these techniques (continuous cycling peritoneal dialysis, CCPD). Access to the peritoneum is by a soft, surgically placed peritoneal catheter. If a child with ESRD requires a period of dialysis therapy, CAPD is the treatment of choice as this can be performed entirely at home or school without the need for complex machinery and allows the child and family the most normal life style. Four exchanges a day usually provide better biochemical control with a less severe degree of anaemia than thrice weekly haemodialysis. The major potential problem is peritonitis and the technique may prove impossible in patients who have had previous intra-abdominal surgery resulting in adhesions.

PROGNOSIS

● Progression to end stage renal failure is inevitable in some diseases, e.g. malignant focal segmental glomerulosclerosis, Alport's syndrome in boys, infantile polycystic disease.

● The prognosis of chronic pyelonephritis due to reflux nephropathy, congenital abnormalities and of finite episodes of acute glomerulonephritis causing parenchymal damage, e.g. Henoch–Schönlein purpura nephritis, depends on the residual number of normal nephrons.

● About 75% children treated for end stage renal disease by transplantation and, if necessary, dialysis will be alive 4 years after commencing treatment[4].

● Patient survival from the registry of the European Dialysis and Transplant Association (EDTA) was 67.9% in the 5–10 year age group, and in the 10–15 year age group 77.7% 5 years following first cadaveric transplantation. It was 82.2% at 4 years and 83.6% at 5 years respectively following transplantation from a living related donor[4].

● In the Guy's Hospital series 88% of the first 144 children treated by transplantation were alive at 5 years and 78% of the 28 children aged less than 5 years at the time of transplantation, were alive 5 years later.

● The survival of first live related grafts from the EDTA registry was 64.4% at 3 years in children aged 5–10 years and 50.8% at 5 years in children aged 10–15 years[4]. For first cadaveric grafts the 5-year survival was 47% in children aged 5–10 years and 50.8% in the 10–15 year group[4].

● In the Guy's Hospital series 72% 58 live related grafts and 46% 86 cadaveric grafts were functioning at 5 years, 64% the 28 grafts (3 live related, 25 cadaveric) given to recipients aged less than 5 years were functioning 5 years later.

● Patient survival on hospital haemodialysis is 66.3% at 5 years and on home haemodialysis is 84.6%[5].

● Patient survival on continuous ambulatory peritoneal dialysis (CAPD) is 85% and 80% at 1 and 2 years respectively[4].

FOLLOW-UP

Patients are usually followed closely by the transplant unit (in the Guy's Hospital unit daily for the first six weeks, tapering to weekly by 3–4 months and monthly by one year), but may present elsewhere with a rejection episode, which may be recognised by one or more of the following: tender graft, hypertension, pyrexia, vague 'flu-like' symptoms. If the patient has any of the above, even if there appears to be an adequate alternative explanation, the plasma creatinine must be checked and the transplant unit contacted. All children with ESRD treated by dialysis require regular review of all of the points listed under conservative management (see above) and in addition will require an individually adjusted fluid restriction depending on their residual urine output, if any, and their mode of dialysis. Insensible fluid losses should be calculated as 300 ml/m^2 body surface area per day.

[1] Rosman J B et al. (1984) Lancet, **ii**, 1291.
[2] Clayton B E et al. (1980) Paediatric Chemical Pathology, p. 125. Oxford: Blackwell Scientific.
[3] Tamanaha K et al. (1987) Paediatr. Nephrol., **1**, 45.
[4] Donckerwolcke R A et al. (1982) Proc. Eur. Dialysis Transplant Assoc., **19,** 60.
[5] Donckerwolcke R A et al. (1980) Proc. Eur. Dialysis Transplant Assoc., **17,** 87.

8
Diseases of the Endocrine System

J. A. Hulse

Short Stature

Non-endocrine causes of short stature include chronic renal failure, congenital heart disease, chromosomal abnormalities (e.g. Turner's or Down's syndromes), coeliac disease, Crohn's disease, poor nutrition and psychosocial deprivation. Endocrine causes include hypothyroidism, Cushing's syndrome and growth hormone (GH) deficiency. A child with a height velocity (HV) below 25 percentile or a declining HV (growth failure) is more likely to have an identifiable cause for the short stature.

TREATMENT

1. Growth hormone deficient children can be treated with biosynthetic GH 0.5 U/kg/week s.c. or i.m. divided into three doses. Height velocity should have been measured over at least a 6-month period before treatment is started. Treatment should continue until fusion of the epiphyses has occurred.
2. It is essential that any thyroid or adrenal insufficiency should also be identified and treated.
3. It is likely that many short children with other abnormalities of GH control or metabolism will be treated with GH in the future.

PROGNOSIS

- Early diagnosis is critical for treatment to be effective. This is particularly true for GH deficiency[1].
- While a significantly delayed 'bone age'[2] is more likely to be associated with an identifiable cause, it also occurs in idiopathic delay of growth and development.
- Charts are available for children aged between two and nine years which allow for mid-parent height and help in the diagnosis of genetic short stature[3].
- Tables are available for prediction of adult height[2].
- Delayed puberty is an important cause of short stature.

FOLLOW-UP

Measurement of HV before and after treatment with GH is a vital part of the diagnostic process. Thyroid function tests should be repeated after starting treatment in idiopathic GH deficiency. The possibility of gonadotrophin deficiency should be considered in a GH deficient child who fails to enter puberty.

[1] Burns E C et al. (1981) Eur. J. Pediatr., 137, 155.
[2] Tanner J M et al. (1984) Assessment of Skeletal Maturity and Prediction of Adult Height. London: Academic Press.
[3] Tanner J M et al. (1970) Arch. Dis. Childh., 45, 755.

Tall Stature

Excessive growth is a less common childhood problem than short stature. It may be part of a syndrome such as Klinefelter's, Marfan's or Soto's syndromes, each having its own distinguishing features. Endocrine causes include thyrotoxicosis, congenital adrenal hyperplasia (CAH), precocious puberty and rarely a growth hormone (GH)-producing adenoma. Other causes include obesity and genetic tall stature.

TREATMENT

1. Precocious puberty can be arrested by medroxyprogesterone acetate (Provera) 5–20 mg/day orally, cyproterone acetate 75–100 mg/m^2/day or by luteinising hormone releasing factor (LRF) analogues[1]. These analogues are now the treatment of choice. Not all patients need treatment but an underlying CNS lesion or an adrenal or ovarian tumour must be excluded.
2. Girls with an excessive height prediction may be treated with cyclical oestrogen therapy to induce premature fusion of the epiphyses.

PROGNOSIS

- Final height is influenced considerably by the 'bone age' and tables are available for prediction of adult height[2].

- Bone age is considerably advanced in CAH and precocious puberty so that adult height may be considerably compromised.

FOLLOW-UP

Six monthly follow-up of height velocity and yearly bone ages is necessary. An accelerating bone age suggests pathology or poor endocrine control, e.g. non-compliance in a thyrotoxic child.

[1] Styne D M et al. (1985) J. Clin. Endocrinol. Metab., **61**, 142.
[2] Tanner J M et al. (1984) Assessment of Skeletal Maturity and Prediction of Adult Height. London: Academic Press.

Diabetes Mellitus

Diabetes mellitus (DM) has a prevalence of 1:500 in children under 16 years of age and the great majority are insulin dependent (IDDM). Evidence suggests that both genetic and environmental factors are involved in the aetiology; there is an association with the D locus of the HLA system and serological evidence of recent coxsackie virus infections in many children[1]. Presentation is usually with polyuria, polydipsia, enuresis or weight loss. In the precoma stage there may be acute abdominal pain, vomiting and hyperventilation from the metabolic acidosis. Diagnosis is confirmed by blood glucoses over 10 mmol/l, glycosuria and ketonuria. A formal glucose tolerance test is only needed when the diabetes is detected at a presymptomatic stage or in the maturity onset diabetes of the young (MODY) form.

TREATMENT

1. Acute ketoacidosis

a) Rehydration
   i) Give 0.9% saline at 20 ml/kg over 1–2 hours to correct hypovolaemia.
   ii) Give maintenance fluid and deficit replacement (usually about 10% body weight divided over 48 hours)
   iii) Change from 0.9% saline to 0.45% saline and 4% dextrose when blood glucose is below 12 mmol/l.
   iv) KCl is added after 1 hour (20 mmol/ 500 ml fluid).
b) Insulin
   i) Give 0.1 U/kg/hour soluble human insulin in 0.9% saline at 1 U/ml by a syringe pump or in the burette for at least 24 hours.
   ii) Monitor blood glucose by chemical strips every 1–2 hours.
   iii) Hypoglycaemia can be prevented by slowing the rate of the insulin infusion and/or giving 10% dextrose.

2. Maintenance therapy

a) Insulin
   i) Human insulin U–100 (100 units/ml) as a mixture of soluble and medium acting (e.g. isophane) is given twice daily in divided doses, two-thirds in the morning and one-third in the evening. The total daily dose is 0.5–1.0 unit/kg.
   ii) The insulin regimen may be simplified by giving a premixed soluble/isophane preparation reducing the chance of errors. An alternative is to give ultra lente once daily and soluble insulin before each meal.
b) Diet
   i) Traditional diets allow carbohydrate as 100 g + (age in years × 10) spread through the day. Highly refined carbohydrates should be discouraged. The diet should be based on the existing family life style.
   ii) The concept of carbohydrate 'exchange' lists is probably still of value. However, an increase in fibre content and the use of unrefined carbohydrate (wholemeal flour, soya beans, lentils, etc.) give better control with higher carbohydrate content[2] and reduced fat intake.

PROGNOSIS

- Childhood DM is a serious condition which reduces life expectancy and has considerable morbidity. Both early death and the complication rate can be reduced by good diabetic control which begins in childhood[3].
- Diabetic ketoacidosis may recur usually because of infection in a poorly controlled diabetic. Death from ketoacidosis should be very rare.
- Hypoglycaemia is a common problem of childhood DM: nocturnal hypoglycaemia may present as enuresis. Severe recurrent hypoglycaemia may result in epilepsy or learning difficulties.

- Infection is more common in poorly controlled diabetics, for example at injection sites, in the ear or urine.
- There is a higher than normal incidence of emotional problems, especially in adolescence.
- Some young diabetics develop cataracts very early in their disease.
- Long-term complications such as retinopathy, neuropathy and nephropathy are related to the length of time from diagnosis and degree of control.
- After 5–9 years 10% diabetics have retinopathy, rising to 70% after 15 years[4].
- After 4–17 years 50% diabetics have evidence of a sensory neuropathy (delayed nerve conduction velocity or high threshold to vibration[5].
- It is less common in childhood than adult diabetics to find albuminuria suggestive of early severe diabetic nephropathy.
- 6% siblings of diabetic children will themselves be diabetic by 16 years – a 30-fold increase in risk.

FOLLOW-UP

Diabetic children are best seen in a special clinic where they can meet and learn from each other. Education is an important part of management. Diabetic holiday camps are also useful for helping young diabetics learn about their disease. Monitoring diabetic control is essential. Home blood-glucose monitoring with test strips, an automatic 'finger-pricker' and a reflectance meter is the best method. Tests are performed at different times on different days to build up a profile. Some children may still use urine glucose methods. In the clinic haemoglobin A1$_c$ provides an integrated measure of glycaemic control over the preceding weeks. Optic fundi should be re-examined every 6 months.

[1] Banatvala J E et al. (1985) Lancet, **i,** 1409.
[2] Kinmonth A-L et al. (1982) Arch. Dis. Childh., **57,** 187.
[3] Dornan T L et al. (1982) Br. Med. J., **285,** 1073.
[4] Hamilton W et al. (1984) Disorders of the endocrine glands. In Textbook of Paediatrics (Forfar J O, Arneil G C eds.). Edinburgh: Churchill Livingstone.
[5] Ludvigsson J et al. (1979) Acta Paediatr. Scand., **68,** 739.

Diabetes Insipidus

Diabetes insipidus (DI) may result from antidiuretic hormone (ADH, vasopressin) deficiency (central DI) or from renal unresponsiveness to ADH (nephrogenic DI). Central DI may be due to head injury, neurosurgery, tumours (e.g. craniopharyngiomas) or infiltrative lesions such as histiocytosis. In children, many cases are idiopathic. Presentation may be with polyuria, polydipsia, failure to thrive, enuresis or dehydration. Severe hypernatraemia may lead to neurological damage in the young child. Nephrogenic diabetes insipidus must be distinguished from the urine concentrating defect of chronic renal failure and from compulsive water drinking.

TREATMENT

1. Drinking should not be restricted in DI and extra fluid should be given as water, not milk.
2. The long-term treatment of choice for central DI is a synthetic ADH analogue, DDAVP. It is usually administered nasally in a dose of 5–20 µg b.d. Oral treatment in a dose of 100–400 µg may soon be available[1].
3. Chlorpropamide 100–300 mg once daily increases the sensitivity of the renal tubules to ADH and may be useful in partial DI. Hypoglycaemia may be a serious side-effect.
4. Nephrogenic DI does not respond to pitressin or DDAVP. Thiazide diuretics or a low-salt diet may increase proximal tubular reabsorption of salt and water. Indomethacin may also be effective.

PROGNOSIS

- The prognosis depends on the underlying cause. After head injury or surgery four different patterns are seen:

a) Transient polyuria starting after 1–3 days and lasting up to one week.
b) Permanent polyuria starting after 1–3 days.
c) Permanent polyuria with a partial decrease in urine output after a few days.
d) A triphasic pattern with an intermediate period of normal urine output.

- Central DI resulting from tumours or histiocytosis is usually permanent.
- Nephrogenic DI, although permanent, may become less severe with age.

FOLLOW-UP

Idiopathic cases need careful prolonged follow-up as DI may precede the appearance of a cranial tumour by several years. The dosage of DDAVP is variable and is controlled by the clinical state and urine output aiming for a urine volume of 500–1000 ml.

---

[1] Westgren U et al. (1986) Arch. Dis. Childh., **61,** 247.

Congenital Hypothyroidism

In developed countries, congenital hypothyroidism (CH) occurs sporadically (incidence 1:4000). The commonest aetiology is thyroid ectopia and dysplasia resulting from maldescent in early gestation[1]. In other cases there is thyroid aplasia or a recessively inherited dyshormonogenesis. In underdeveloped countries, iodine deficiency is an important cause of CH. Neonatal screening for CH is now widely practised throughout the world.

TREATMENT

1. Treatment should be with L-thyroxine, given once daily. Treatment should continue for life.
2. Thyroxine dosage

Age	Dose/kg/day (μg/kg)	Dose/day (μg)
0–6 months	8–10	25–50
6–12 months	6–8	50–75
1–5 years	5–6	75–100
6–12 years	4–5	100–150
> 12 years	2–3	150–200

PROGNOSIS

- Thyroid hormones are vital for normal brain development. Since almost no thyroxine (T4) crosses the placental barrier the fetus is dependent on its own pituitary–thyroid axis[2].
- If treatment is delayed beyond 6 weeks of age, permanent intellectual impairment may occur[3].
- In a study of English hypothyroid children diagnosed on clinical grounds, 33% were detected by three months and 66% by one year; 25% were mentally retarded and 29% attended special schools[3].
- Neonatal screening for CH using filter paper blood-spot specimens analysed for T4 or thyroid stimulating hormone (TSH) almost entirely prevents the above complications[4].

FOLLOW-UP

Follow-up should be 6-weekly to 3-monthly during the first year; 6-monthly until 5 years and yearly thereafter. Accurate growth and growth velocity charts should be kept. Thyroid function tests (TFTs) (total serum T4 or free T4, triiodothyronine (T3) resin uptake and TSH) are useful to detect non-compliance. Even with adequate treatment, serum TSH may take 3–6 months to return to normal values[4]. In screening cases, the diagnosis should be reviewed after 1–2 years to exclude transient neonatal hypothyroidism. A 'T3 withdrawal test' should be carried out; TFTs are measured before and after 3 weeks of T3 substitution (20 μg/day) followed by one week without any treatment[4].

[1] Hulse J A et al. (1980) Br. Med. J., **280,** 675.
[2] Fisher D A et al. (1964) J. Clin. Endocrinol. Metab., **24,** 393.
[3] Hulse J A (1984) Arch. Dis. Childh., **59,** 23.
[4] Hulse J A (1983) Br. Med. J., **284,** 1435.

Acquired Hypothyroidism

Acquired hypothyroidism (AH) is usually the end result of chronic lymphocytic thyroiditis (CLT or Hashimoto's disease), an autoimmune process. As in congenital hypothyroidism (CH), twice as many girls are affected as boys. Presentation is often with growth failure and most patients will have a palpable goitre and positive microsomal thyroid antibodies. Other causes of AH include late-presenting CH and secondary or tertiary hypothyroidism resulting from TSH or TRH deficiency.

TREATMENT

1. Use L-thyroxine once daily (see *Congenital hypothyroidism* (p. 139) for dosage).
2. Secondary or tertiary hypothyroidism is also treated with L-thyroxine but with smaller doses (50–100 µg/day)[1]. Many children are also growth hormone deficient and need treatment with both thyroxine and growth hormone to achieve full growth potential.

PROGNOSIS

- Acquired hypothyroidism does not have the serious neurological consequences of CH.
- Complete catch-up growth is usually achieved after two years of treatment.
- Cases of secondary or tertiary hypothyroidism should have a full evaluation of anterior pituitary function since isolated TSH deficiency is uncommon.

- Autoimmune thyroiditis may be associated with other autoimmune diseases, especially diabetes mellitus, and is more common in Down's, Turner's and Noonan's syndromes.

FOLLOW-UP

Follow-up should be 6-monthly until catch-up growth is completed; then yearly. Accurate growth charts should be kept and TFTs measured regularly. A rise in TSH indicates under-treatment. Some children may exhibit behaviour changes after starting treatment[2]. Parents should be warned about this problem, but it usually resolves within a few months.

---

[1] Preece M A (1982) *Clin. Endocrinol. Metab.*, **11**, 1.
[2] Barnes N D (1983) *Paediatric Endocrinology in Clinical Practice*. Lancaster: MTP Press.

Non-Toxic Goitre and Thyroid Cancer

A goitre is found in 3.9–6.0% teenage children and is two to three times more common in girls[1]. The commonest causes are chronic lymphocytic thyroiditis (CLT or Hashimoto's disease) and colloid goitre. Auto-antibodies are usually present in CLT. The rare possibility of malignancy must always be considered, especially in nodular goitre. Medullary thyroid carcinoma (MTC) may be associated with phaeochromocytomas or parathyroid tumours.

TREATMENT

1. If treatment is necessary, a goitre may be shrunk by TSH suppression using L-thyroxine 100–150 µg daily.
2. 'Cold' nodules found on thyroid scanning should be removed surgically.
3. Thyroid cancer: treatment is by total thyroidectomy with block dissection of the cervical lymph glands if they are involved. In differentiated tumours, surgery is followed by therapeutic doses of ^{131}I.
4. Doxorubicin (adriamycin) may be used in metastatic disease.
5. Treatment for MTC is by total thyroidectomy but the tumour is resistant to radio- or chemotherapy.

PROGNOSIS

- Simple goitre may lead to multinodular goitre in adulthood.
- In CLT there is often gradual onset of hypothyroidism. Other autoimmune diseases such as Addison's disease, pernicious anaemia, hypoparathyroidism or ovarian failure may also develop.

- Thyroid carcinoma is usually papillary or follicular; survival is good even when metastases are present and the 20-year survival is 83%[2].

FOLLOW-UP

For goitre, follow-up is 6-monthly with annual TFTs. Auto-antibody tests should also be repeated as they may later become positive. For thyroid cancer follow-up should be for life as metastases may develop late. Differentiated tumours may be followed-up by radio-iodine scanning for metastases, chest x-ray and measurement of serum thyroglobulin (Tg) – a useful marker for the presence of thyroid tissue[3]. For MTC calcitonin is a useful tumour marker. In familial cases, all family members should be followed-up and total thyroidectomy performed at the first signs of disease.

---

[1] Peden V H et al. (1975) J. Pediatr., **86,** 816.
[2] Winship T et al. (1970) Clin. Proc. Child. Hosp. DC., **26,** 327.
[3] Black E G et al. (1981) Br. Med. J., **3,** 443.

Hyperthyroidism

Transient neonatal thyrotoxicosis results from transplacental transfer of thyroid-stimulating immunoglobulins (TSIs) from a mother who has or has had Graves' disease. Acquired hyperthyroidism is common in young teenage girls and is usually also a manifestation of Graves' disease. Presenting features include exophthalmos, excessive growth and deteriorating school performance. Findings include a diffuse goitre, advanced bone-age and raised serum T4 and/or T3.

TREATMENT

1. Neonatal thyrotoxicosis: if symptoms demand treatment give carbimazole 1.25–2.5 mg b.d. or t.d.s. (0.75–1.0 mg/kg/day). Propranolol 2.5–5.0 mg t.d.s. (0.75–2.0 mg/kg/day) may be added for rapid control of symptoms. Treatment is for 2–3 months.
2. Acquired hyperthyroidism: usually also treated with carbimazole in the UK. In the USA propylthiouracil (PTU) 100–150 mg t.d.s. is more commonly used. The starting dose for carbimazole is 30–40 mg t.d.s. or q.d.s. After control is achieved (usually about 3 weeks) the dose may be reduced by 50%.
3. If control proves difficult a higher dose may be considered and L-thyroxine 50–100 µg/day added. When there is marked T3 toxicosis, propranolol 30–40 mg t.d.s. will block peripheral conversion of T4 to T3 but it should never be used on its own. Consider non-compliance when there are problems with control.
4. Surgical treatment is by subtotal thyroidectomy. Vascularity of the gland is reduced preoperatively with Lugol's iodine solution 3–5 drops in water b.d. for 2 weeks. Indications for surgical treatment include antithyroid drug toxicity, failure of medical treatment with poor prognostic indicators, non-compliance, or a large goitre resistant to medical treatment.

PROGNOSIS

- Neonatal thyrotoxicosis is usually self-limiting; treatment is only required for tachycardia or diarrhoea. Rare long-term effects include craniosynostosis and neurological problems.
- Acquired hyperthyroidism: medical treatment gives long-term remission in 25–61% cases after 2–3 years[1]. Persistently elevated serum thyroid stimulating immunoglobin titres, HLA type DRw3[2] and persistent goitre are poor prognostic indicators.
- Surgical treatment is effective in controlling hyperthyroidism permanently but an experienced surgeon is required. Complications include recurrent laryngeal nerve palsy, haemorrhage, transient or permanent hypoparathyroidism and keloid formation.

FOLLOW-UP

Follow-up should be every 1–2 months. Check signs, symptoms, growth, bone-age and TFTs. Measure the antinuclear factor (ANF) titre before and after treatment. Remember that carbimazole and other antithyroid agents have significant toxicity, the most important being neutropenia. Patients must be warned to seek medical advice should they develop sore throats or rashes when the FBC can be performed. Other complications include hepatitis and a lupus-like syndrome. The use of radioactive iodine ^{131}I in children is controversial and the only major studies on this are from the USA[3]. Treatment is simple and effective but the prevalence of subsequent hypothyroidism is 92%. Doubts also remain about the long-term neoplastic and genetic effects. In all cases long-term follow-up is essential as hypothyroidism may occur in up to 50% cases of acquired hyperthyroidism.

[1] Barnes H V et al. (1977) J. Pediatr., **91,** 313.
[2] McGregor A et al. (1980) Lancet, **i,** 1101.
[3] Safe A M et al. (1975) New Eng. J. Med., **292,** 167.

Abnormal Sexual Differentiation

Disorders of sexual differentiation are usually classified as female pseudohermaphroditism, male pseudohermaphroditism and mixed or dysgenetic gonadal development. Female pseudohermaphrodites have a 46XX karyotype with normal internal genitalia and the commonest cause is congenital adrenal hyperplasia (CAH). Male pseudohermaphrodites (karyotype 46XY) may have an inborn error of testosterone biosynthesis or impaired metabolism or response of the peripheral tissues to testosterone (androgen insensitivity). An important cause of micropenis is hypopituitarism which may be associated with other abnormalities such as septo-optic dysplasia[1].

TREATMENT

1. Female pseudohermaphrodites usually undergo clitoroplasty in the first year with further surgery at puberty. They may also require steroid treatment (see *Congenital adrenal hyperplasia* (p. 145) for details).
2. Males with defects of testosterone biosynthesis will respond to androgens at puberty, but in androgen insensitivity the response is poor.
3. In mixed gonadal dysgenesis and complete androgen insensitivity, intra-abdominal gonads should be removed because of the risk of malignancy[2].

PROGNOSIS

- Diagnosis may not be possible on the basis of phenotype alone. When there is doubt, gender choice should be delayed until investigations are completed and should not be made solely on the basis of karyotype.
- Parental opinions and cultural values need to be considered in gender assignment.
- Female pseudohermaphrodites are usually raised as females.
- Male pseudohermaphrodites may be raised as males or females. A trial of testosterone treatment (testosterone enanthate 25–50 mg monthly for three months) may indicate the potential for penile growth at puberty.

FOLLOW-UP

Close follow-up is required throughout childhood and until completion of puberty. Long-term emotional and psychiatric support may be needed for the child and family.

[1] Hoyt W F *et al.* (1970) *Lancet*, **i,** 893.
[2] Aarskog D (1971) *Birth Defects*, **7,** 122.

Adrenal Insufficiency

Adrenal insufficiency is uncommon in childhood. Congenital adrenal hypoplasia occurs in X-linked and autosomal recessive forms[1] and may present with a salt-losing crisis or hypoglycaemia. Acquired adrenal insufficiency (Addison's disease) usually results from autoimmunity and is often associated with other autoimmune diseases such as diabetes mellitus or thyroiditis. The usual presentation is with lethargy, pigmentation and salt-losing crises. Tuberculosis is now a rare cause of Addison's disease.

TREATMENT

1. Chronic glucocorticoid replacement therapy is given in childhood as hydrocortisone 10–20 mg/m²/day in three divided doses.
2. Once growth is completed, a long-acting steroid such as dexamethasone or prednisolone may be used.
3. During times of illness, infection or surgery the dose of steroid should be tripled. In the acute crisis a saline infusion may be needed.

PROGNOSIS

- Acute adrenal insufficiency in infancy is easily missed since both hypoglycaemia and hypo-natraemia are common. The outcome may be fatal.
- Addison's disease may also be missed for years but should be considered when there is hypo-natraemia in an acute illness. With steroid replacement, the prognosis is excellent.
- Treatment should continue for life.

FOLLOW-UP

Symptoms, pigmentation, growth velocity and bone-age should be monitored. Growth failure usually indicates over-treatment.

---

[1] Brook C G D (1978) *Practical Paediatric Endocrinology.* London: Academic Press.

Congenital Adrenal Hyperplasia

Congenital adrenal hyperplasia (CAH) is an autosomal recessive disorder of adrenal corticosteroid metabolism. In over 90% cases, there is a defect of the 21-hydroxylase enzyme giving rise to intrauterine stimulation of ACTH production and hence over-production of the adrenal androgen, androstenedione. This is converted to testosterone which virilises the female fetus. Two-thirds of cases also have a defect of mineralocorticoid production and so are salt-losers. In the rarer forms of CAH with defects early in the pathways of steroid metabolism, males may be inadequately virilised and females have normal genitalia.

TREATMENT

1. Initial resuscitation in a salt-losing crisis is with normal saline. Dextrose is also needed to prevent hypoglycaemia.
2. Mineralocorticoid can be given initially as deoxycorticosterone pivalate (DOCP) (Percorten M Cystules) 12.5–25 mg every 2–4 weeks[2]. Subsequently 9α-fludrocortisone (Florinef) 0.05–0.2 mg daily orally can be given. Salt supplementation (2–3 g/day) may also be needed at first.
3. Only replacement doses of glucocorticoids, given as hydrocortisone 20–25 mg/m²/day, are needed to suppress ACTH.
4. Clitoroidectomy is performed at 6–12 months, but further vaginoplasty may be needed later.
5. Once growth is completed, adrenal suppression may be achieved with dexamethasone 0.25–0.75 mg/day.

PROGNOSIS

- Unrecognised CAH in the neonatal period may be fatal. Females usually present with variable degrees of virilisation but in males virilisation is difficult to detect, so they present with a salt-losing crisis – hyponatraemia, hyperkalaemia, acidosis and often hypoglycaemia. A raised plasma 17-OH-progesterone (17-OH P) is diagnostic.
- Late complications include persistent virilisation, advanced bone-age, precocious puberty and short adult stature. Prevention of these complications depends on meticulous control throughout childhood.
- Females with CAH have normal internal genitalia and are fertile.
- The clinical spectrum of CAH is more variable than was previously thought and may not present until adult life with hirsutism[1].

FOLLOW-UP

Growth velocity, bone-age and blood pressure must be checked regularly. Plasma 17-OH P (pre-dose), testosterone and plasma renin activity (PRA) are useful biochemical parameters. Salt-losers should continue on mineralocorticoid replacement. Menstrual irregularities in girls may be managed by changing to once daily dexamethasone. Both at diagnosis and subsequently, detailed counselling on gender identity and sexual orientation is needed.

[1] Levine L S et al. (1980) *J. Clin. Endocrinol. Metab.*, **51**, 1316.
[2] Hughes I A (1983) *Paediatric Endocrinology in Clinical Practice*. Lancaster: MTP Press.

Cushing's Syndrome

Glucocorticoid excess is uncommon in childhood and most cases are iatrogenic. Growth is profoundly affected by excess cortisol so Cushing's syndrome should be considered when obesity is accompanied by short stature since most obese children are tall. Children may also present with psychological symptoms or school problems. There may be truncal and facial obesity, a 'buffalo hump', bruising, striae, hypertension and glycosuria. Cushing's syndrome may arise from adrenal hyperplasia due to hypothalamic pituitary dysfunction, adrenal adenoma or carcinoma, or an ectopic ACTH secreting tumour. A primary adrenal tumour may also present with signs of virilisation resulting from excessive adrenal androgens.

TREATMENT

1. The treatment of choice for Cushing's disease is trans-sphenoidal pituitary microsurgery leaving the rest of the pituitary intact. However this does require a skilled, experienced surgeon.
2. External beam irradiation with 3500–5000 cGy gives good results with preservation of pituitary function[1]. It takes up to 9 months before this becomes effective and initial treatment with metyrapone, an inhibitor of steroid biosynthesis, may also be needed.
3. Adrenal tumours are treated by adrenalectomy. Preoperative preparation with steroids is needed as the contralateral adrenal may be suppressed.
4. Metastasising adrenal carcinoma has been treated with *op'*-DDD, an adrenolytic agent.
5. Iatrogenic Cushing's syndrome is managed by a gradual transfer to alternate-day steroid therapy, but pituitary–adrenal function may remain abnormal for up to a year[2].

PROGNOSIS

- Prognosis depends on the aetiology, treatment method and the length and severity of the glucocorticoid excess. Severe complications may occur such as vertebral collapse or necrosis of the head of the femur. Posterior subcapsular cataracts are also common.

- In Cushing's disease (ACTH dependent Cushing's syndrome), bilateral adrenalectomy often leads to Nelson's syndrome[3].
- Excision of an adrenal adenoma results in complete cure and restoration of catch-up growth. Adrenal carcinoma, on the other hand, has a poor prognosis and metastasises to the liver and lungs. Histological differentiation between the two may be difficult.

FOLLOW-UP

Bilateral adrenalectomy requires life-long steroid replacement therapy with hydrocortisone 10–20 mg/m^2/day in three divided doses. Mineralocorticoid replacement may be given as 9α-fludrocortisone (Florinef) 0.05–0.2 mg/day. With pituitary microsurgery there is a risk of recurrence so that periodic postoperative reassessment of adrenal function is needed. Recovery of adrenal function in iatrogenic Cushing's syndrome may be assessed by measuring early morning cortisol. Values below 200 nmol/l suggest adrenal suppression[2]. This can be followed by a Synacthen test.

[1] Jennings A S et al. (1977) New Eng. J. Med., **247**, 957.
[2] Hughes I A (1982) Clin. Endocrinol. Metab., **11**, 116.
[3] McArthur R G et al. (1979) J. Pediatr., **95**, 214.

Phaeochromocytoma

Tumours of chromaffin tissues are rare in childhood and although most arise in the adrenal glands, they can arise wherever there is sympathetic tissue. They may be associated with neurofibromatosis or with the inherited multiple endocrine neoplasia (MEN) syndromes. Paroxysmal attacks of hypertension may present with pallor, sweating, headache and chest pain. Hypertension may also be sustained between attacks.

TREATMENT

1. Once identified, the tumour should be removed surgically. Multiple tumours may be present.
2. Depending on the type of catecholamines produced by the tumour, α-blockade with phenoxybenzamine 20–50 mg b.d. or β-blockade with propranolol 10–30 mg q.d.s. for 2 weeks before surgery may be needed.
3. Postoperatively, pressor agents such as noradrenaline or metaraminol tartrate may be needed.

PROGNOSIS

- 2.4% phaeochromocytomas are malignant[1].

- Severe complications may occur such as retinal or subarachnoid haemorrhages and left ventricular hypertrophy.

FOLLOW-UP

In the week after surgery, hypotension and hypoglycaemia may occur. Urinary catecholamines should be followed 6-monthly to detect recurrence. Children with phaeochromocytomas should be followed throughout childhood; those with the MEN syndrome should be followed for life as new tumours may arise.

---

[1] Stackpole R H et al. (1963) J. Pediatr., 63, 315.

Neuroblastoma and Ganglioneuroma

Neuroblastoma is a neural crest tumour which usually arises in the adrenal medulla but may also be found in other sites such as the thorax or pelvis. It usually presents in children under the age of 2 years and may be highly malignant. The tumour usually excretes catecholamines as excess vanillylmandelic acid (VMA) (or in 15% as homovanillic acid (HVA). Histologically more mature forms of the tumour are known as ganglioneuroblastoma, and benign ganglioneuromas of sympathetic tissue are also found which do not excrete catecholamines. Presentation may be with an abdominal mass, painful metastases or with the 'dancing eyes' syndrome (a syndrome of rapid irregular movements of the eyes and limbs).

TREATMENT

1. Stages I and II: surgical resection and local radiotherapy.
2. Stages III and IV have been treated with high-dose melphalan followed by autologous bone-marrow replacement with some success[1].
3. Neuroblastoma cells will react with specific monoclonal antibodies which can be used to detect and possibly treat diseased tissues such as bone-marrow.

PROGNOSIS

● Staging[2]

I   Confined to organ of origin.
II Extension beyond organ but not over the midline.
III Extending over midline and/or nodal involvement.
IV Metastatic to liver, bone (especially skull), marrow, nodes.
IVS Stage I or II plus involvement of liver/ marrow, skin (infant under one year).

● Stages I and II have a good prognosis with local therapy.
● Stages III and IV have a poor prognosis except following treatment with intensive chemotherapy regimens.
● Stage IVS has a good prognosis because of spontaneous regression.
● Survival decreases with increasing age.
● Over 60% patients have metastatic disease at presentation.

FOLLOW-UP

Follow-up should be at least 6-weekly to 3-monthly in the first year and 6-monthly to annually thereafter. A 24-hour urine collection for VMA estimation should be collected at each visit; a rise in VMA may be the earliest sign of a recurrence.

[1] Pritchard J et al. (1982) Br. J. Cancer, **45,** 86.
[2] Evans A E (ed.) (1979) Advances in Neuroblastoma Research. New York: Raven Press.

9

Metabolic Diseases

J. A. Hulse

Hyperphenylalaninaemia

Since the introduction of neonatal screening, it has been recognised that many conditions may result in hyperphenylalaninaemia (HP) but classical phenylketonuria (PKU) remains the most important condition as it can be treated so successfully. In classical PKU there is almost complete absence of the enzyme phenylalanine hydroxylase which converts phenylalanine to tyrosine; the defect is inherited as an autosomal recessive and the incidence ranges from 1:4000 (Eire) to 1:100 000 (Japan)[1]. Less severe forms with some enzyme activity ('atypical' or 'mild' HP) are also recognised. Much less common are disorders of the various cofactors involved in phenylalanine metabolism which lead to tetrahydrobiopterin (BH_4) deficiency. Acquired HP may present transiently in infancy or arise as a result of liver disease or drugs.

TREATMENT

1. *Classical PKU*

a) Most centres would treat infants whose phenylalanine levels were above 900 µmol/l (15 mg/dl) while on a normal protein intake.

b) The treatment consists of dietary restriction of phenylalanine intake with milk substitutes such as Minafen or Lofenalac which are low in phenylalanine and high in tyrosine. Ordinary formula is added to give adequate phenylalanine levels.

c) Weaning with low protein foods is encouraged but the special formula needs to be continued.

d) The aim of treatment is to keep blood phenylalanine between 150–500 µmol/l (2.5–8 mg/dl).

e) Dietary phenylalanine requirements are around 50–80 mg/kg/day falling to 15–25 mg/kg/day by 6 years. Infants with less severe enzyme defects need more phenylalanine as some is converted to tyrosine.

2. *BH_4 deficiency*

a) Giving amine precursors such as L-dopa, carbidopa and 5-hydroxytryptophan helps control clinical symptoms in many forms of BH_4 deficiency.

b) A low phenylalanine diet will help control the HP which may be supplemented with oral BH_4 (1–2 mg/kg/day).

PROGNOSIS

● *Classical PKU*

a) Untreated classical PKU results in severe mental retardation, microcephaly and convulsions. Infants may vomit, the hair is fair and skin pale and eczematous.

b) The high plasma phenylalanine levels are directly toxic to the brain and affect production of proteins, amine neurotransmitter substances and myelin[2].

c) The signs and symptoms of HP only develop once a baby starts on milk feeds.

d) Successful treatment depends on early diagnosis; this can only be achieved by neonatal metabolic screening of a filter-paper blood-spot specimen taken at about 7–10 days of age. Despite screening, the possibility of 'missed cases' (where screening was omitted) or false negative screening results must always be remembered.

e) Any infant found to have HP must be rapidly traced and fully investigated.

f) Since the onset of screening in the UK in the mid-1960s there has been a steady rise in the mean IQ of annual cohorts from 85.1 (1964) to 104.4 (1979) (Stanford–Binet at 4 years)[1]. Final IQs tend to be just a few points lower than sibling or parent controls[3].

g) Behavioural disorders are also more common in treated PKU children.

h) If the special diet is completely stopped at 6–8 years, there is evidence of behavioural changes, neurological signs and in some studies a fall in IQ of 6–8 points[5].

- BH₄ deficiency

a) Only 1–3% children with HP have defects of biopterin metabolism (1:500 000 births)[1].
b) The neurological disease of BH₄ deficiency is more severe than untreated classical PKU and there may be marked hypotonia leading to choreiform movements and infantile spasms[6]. However, the clinical presentation may be quite variable.
c) Control of the HP with a low phenylalanine diet alone does not prevent progression of the disease.

FOLLOW-UP

The correct diagnosis and treatment for patients with HP should be undertaken in centres with experience in treating metabolic disorders. In particular an expert dietician is very important. After three months of dietary treatment the diet should be stopped for 2–4 days to determine the severity of the HP. Blood phenylalanine levels should be monitored frequently; initially twice weekly reducing to monthly by one year. Filter-paper specimens may be used. After the age of eight years the diet may be relaxed aiming to keep phenylalanine levels at 900–1200 µmol/l (15–20 mg/dl). Maternal HP may lead to severe fetal damage (microcephaly, mental retardation and congenital heart disease). Dietary treatment should start before conception and a level of 250 µmol/l (4 mg/dl) is needed. Prenatal diagnosis is now becoming possible for families who already have one child with PKU.

[1] Smith I (1985) *Genetic and Metabolic Disease in Pediatrics* (Lloyd J K, Scriver C R eds.). London: Butterworths.
[2] Patel M S et al. (1975) *Am. J. Clin. Nutr.*, **28**, 183.
[3] Williamson M L et al. (1981) *Paediatrics*, **68**, 161.
[4] Stevenson J E et al. (1979) *Arch. Dis. Childh.* **54**, 14.
[5] Smith I et al. (1978) *Br. Med. J.*, **2**, 723.
[6] Smith I et al. (1975) *Lancet*, **i**, 1108.

Tyrosinaemia

Transient hypertyrosinaemia is quite common in many newborn infants especially when preterm[1]. This may result from immaturity of liver enzymes or a high protein intake and needs to be distinguished from true hereditary tyrosinaemia which is a serious neonatal disease leading to liver failure and renal tubular damage. These complications result in failure to thrive, hepatosplenomegaly and ascites, thrombocytopenia, rickets and the Fanconi syndrome. The differentiation from neonatal hepatitis may be difficult.

TREATMENT

1. Treatment consists of a special low tyrosine formula.
2. The Fanconi syndrome (renal tubular leak) may be treated with sodium and potassium citrate (5–10 mmol/kg/day), 1,25-dihydroxy vitamin D 0.05 µg/kg/day.
3. The hepatocellular damage may be treated with vitamin K 1 mg/day and a controlled protein diet.

PROGNOSIS

- Untreated tyrosinaemia will lead to death in a few weeks.
- The coagulation disorder may be particularly severe[2].
- Less severe forms of the disease exist which are compatible with survival into adult life.

FOLLOW-UP

Infants with tyrosinaemia are best managed in a unit with experience of metabolic diseases. The advice of an experienced dietician is vital. Growth, renal and liver function need close and frequent monitoring.

[1] Avery M E et al. (1967) *Paediatrics*, **39**, 378.
[2] Evans D I K et al. (1984) *Arch. Dis. Childh.*, **59**, 1088.

Homocystinuria

Homocystinuria results from a defect on the pathway of the conversion of homocysteine to cystathionine, usually as a result of cystathionine synthetase deficiency. A defect in the metabolism of the cofactors of vitamin B_{12} may also lead to homocystinuria but is also associated with methylmalonic aciduria and megaloblastic anaemia. The clinical appearance is similar to Marfan's syndrome with arachnodactyly, kyphoscoliosis, pes cavus and eye complications including lens dislocation and retinal detachment. There may be osteoporosis, vertebral collapse and intravascular thrombosis. Cardiac problems include aortic incompetence and dissecting aortic aneurysms. Homocysteine appears to disrupt collagen cross-links. Plasma methionine may be raised but neonatal screening does not appear to be effective[1].

TREATMENT

1. All patients should be treated with pyridoxine 100–500 mg/day. Response may be monitored by plasma methionine or urinary homocystine.
2. Folic acid is also a cofactor and should be given in both pyridoxine responders (10–20 mg/day) and non–responders (50–100 mg/day).
3. Patients who do not respond to vitamins can be treated with a low methionine diet. Infants may be given special formulae (Methionaid).
4. Patients with vitamin B_{12} cofactor deficiency can be treated with hydroxo-B_{12} 1–2 mg/day i.m.

PROGNOSIS

- About 50% patients are mentally retarded and many of those with normal intelligence have psychiatric problems including schizophrenic-like states[2].
- There is considerable morbidity especially from thrombosis. Homocystinuria should always be considered in 'idiopathic' hemiplegia in childhood.
- There is a very high spontaneous abortion rate in homocystinuric women, but in the pyridoxine responsive group normal pregnancy is possible with treatment[3].
- Treatment will prevent further complications from developing.

FOLLOW-UP

All homocystinuric subjects need regular ophthalmic and cardiac examinations. Homocystinuric women should be advised of the importance of taking treatment during pregnancy. Siblings should be carefully examined and screened for homocystinuria.

[1] Whiteman P D et al. (1979) Arch. Dis. Childh., 54, 593.
[2] Buist N R M et al. (1984) Metabolic disorders. In Textbook of Paediatrics (Forfar J O, Arneil G C eds.). Edinburgh: Churchill Livingstone.
[3] Mudd S H et al. (1985) Am. J. Hum. Genet., 37, 1.

Cystinosis

Cystinosis is an autosomal recessive inherited disorder in which cystine is deposited throughout the tissues. For diagnosis cystine crystals may be seen in the cornea on slit-lamp examination and in the bone marrow. The main presentation is with the Fanconi syndrome (renal tubular leak) of which it is the commonest cause. Affected individuals present in the first year with failure to thrive, vomiting, lethargy, rickets, polyuria and polydipsia. The hair is blond and there is photophobia.

TREATMENT

1. The Fanconi syndrome: sodium and potassium citrate solution is given (5–10 mmol/day), oral phosphate (1–2 g/day) and 1,25-dihydroxy vitamin D (0.05 µg/kg/day).
2. Reducing agents such as ascorbic acid and cysteamine have been shown to work *in vitro* and have been tried.
3. Indomethacin 3 mg/kg improves the polyuria and polydipsia[1].

PROGNOSIS

- Even with treatment there is progressive deterioration and death usually occurs in early childhood.
- Renal failure may be treated by transplantation since the transplanted kidney does not accumulate cystine crystals.
- Other tissues continue to deteriorate; the thyroid for example often fails and patients become hypothyroid[2].
- Less severe forms of cystinosis are known with better prognoses.

FOLLOW-UP

Cystinotic patients need close supervision and frequent biochemical monitoring. Thyroid function, creatinine clearance and wrist x-rays (to assess the degree of rickets) should be repeated every 6 months. Preparations need to be made for renal transplantation.

[1] Haycock G B et al. (1982) *Arch. Dis. Childh.*, **57**, 934.
[2] Buist N M R et al. (1984) Metabolic disorders. In *Textbook of Paediatrics* (Forfar J O, Arneil G C eds.). Edinburgh: Churchill Livingstone.

Amino Acid Transport Defects

Both the kidney and gut may be affected by inherited defects of amino acid transport across cell membranes. In cystinuria there is a transport defect of the basic amino acids, cystine, lysine, ornithine and arginine. Since cystine is insoluble in urine, renal stones develop. Hartnup disease is caused by a defect of neutral amino acids and leads to massive urine and gut losses. The symptoms are those of tryptophane deficiency (pellagra) and include photosensitivity, ataxia, and mental symptoms. Generalised amino aciduria may also occur in renal tubular defects together with bicarbonaturia, glycosuria and phosphaturia (Fanconi's syndrome; see *Cystinosis*, p. 153).

TREATMENT

1. *Cystinuria*

   a) A high urine flow is important and if possible some fluid should be drunk at night.
   b) Alkalinisation of the urine (to pH 8) with sodium or potassium citrate solution (5–10 mmol/day) reduces cystine solubility.
   c) Penicillamine (25 mg/kg/day) combines with cystine and makes it more soluble.
   d) Established renal stones may be dissolved by perfusion through a nephrostomy with tromethamine (THAM), an alkaline buffer[1] or by lithotripsy.

2. *Hartnup disease*: tryptophane deficiency may be treated with nicotinic acid (100–250 mg/day)[2].

PROGNOSIS

- The prognosis for amino and transport defects is very variable depending on the underlying type of defect.
- Cystinuria accounts for 1% renal stones.

FOLLOW-UP

The development of renal stones may be assessed by 6-monthly ultrasound examinations.

---

[1] Buist N M R *et al.* (1984) Metabolic disorders. In *Textbook of Paediatrics* (Forfar J O, Arneil G C eds.). Edinburgh: Churchill Livingstone.
[2] Smith I *et al.* (1982) Disorders of amino acid metabolism. In *Textbook of Paediatric Nutrition* (McLaren D S, Burman D eds.). Edinburgh: Churchill Livingstone.

Hyperammonaemia and Urea Cycle Defects

Hyperammonaemia is a feature of urea cycle defects (UCD) but may also occur as a secondary phenomenon in liver failure, Reye's syndrome and the organic acidaemias. Unlike UCD or transient hyperammonaemia, organic acidaemias are associated with a metabolic acidosis. Clinical features of patients with hyperammonaemia include failure to thrive, mental retardation, ataxia and convulsions. Hyperammonaemia may present acutely with neurological signs and coma in the neonatal period. Less severely affected subjects may have attacks of cyclical vomiting associated with intermittent hyperammonaemia and a dislike for protein.

TREATMENT

1. Neonatal hyperammonaemic coma

   a) Attempts should be made to reduce the ammonia levels to normal by haemodialysis or peritoneal dialysis[1].
   b) When there is no metabolic acidosis 10% arginine hydrochloride (4 mmol/kg over 1 hour) may be given.
   c) Correction of the arginine deficiency in UCD helps to prevent proteolysis.

2. Treatment of UCD

   a) Protein is limited to 1–2 g/kg/day.
   b) Arginine may be given at 2–4 mmol/kg/day.
   c) Sodium benzoate 250 mg/kg/day helps excretion of nitrogen by transacylation of glycine to hippuric acid which is excreted by the kidney.
   d) Sodium phenylacetate 250 mg/kg/day has a similar effect through glutamine.

PROGNOSIS

- Neonatal hyperammonaemic crises are rapidly fatal unless quickly recognised and treated. Provided the infants survive, the prognosis is good in those infants without inherited enzyme defects (transient hyperammonaemia of the newborn).
- Before the use of benzoate and phenylacetate the one year mortality for patients with neonatal onset of UCD was 90%[2]. 80% survivors of neonatal hyperammonaemia have developmental disabilities with a mean IQ of 46. However infants treated prospectively have done well[3].
- Ornithine transcarbamylase deficiency (OTCD) is an X-linked UCD. Males are severely affected in the neonatal period[4]. Females are either asymptomatic or have periodic hyperammonaemic crises[5].
- Citrullinaemia (argininosuccinate synthetase deficiency) may vary from severe neonatal coma to being virtually asymptomatic. Many patients are mentally retarded.
- Ornithinaemia (ornithine mitochondrial transport defect) may occur with or without hyperammonaemia. The latter presents with gyrate atrophy of the choroid and retina and progressive blindness in adult life.

FOLLOW-UP

Treatment and follow-up of UCD is extremely demanding of families, doctors, nurses and the laboratory, and should only be undertaken by those with experience of the problems.

---

[1] Donn S M et al. (1979) J. Pediatr., **95,** 67.
[2] Shih V E (1976) Hereditary urea cycle defects. In The Urea Cycle (Grisolia S et al. eds.). New York: John Wiley.
[3] Brusilow S W (1985) Inborn errors of urea synthesis. In Genetic and Metabolic Disorders in Pediatrics (Lloyd J K, Scriver C R eds.). London: Butterworths.
[4] Kendall B E et al. (1983) Neurol. Neurosurg. Psychiatr., **46,** 28.
[5] Glasgow A M et al. (1978) Paediatrics, **62,** 30.

Maple Syrup Urine Disease

Maple syrup urine disease (MSUD) results from a deficiency of branched-chain ketoacid decarboxylase resulting in high levels of the amino acids leucine, isoleucine and valine and their respective ketoacids in blood, urine and CSF. The disease varies in its severity from a severe neonatal form to an intermittent form with symptoms precipitated by illness or a high-protein diet. A common but not invariable feature is a severe metabolic acidosis. In the neonatal form there is progressive vomiting, convulsions and coma often with associated ketotic hypoglycaemia. The urine has a sweet malt-like smell. The condition can be detected by neonatal screening.

TREATMENT

1. The main treatment is dietary using a mixture of synthetic amino acids without the branched chain amino acids (MSUD-aid). Small amounts of natural protein provide 25–60 mg/kg/day of branched chain amino acids. Levels of the amino acids are altered individually as an excess or deficiency of any one may be damaging[1].
2. Catabolism of endogenous protein during illness may lead to high amino acid levels. Dehydration must be avoided.
3. The aim is to keep plasma leucine at 100–700 μmol/l (1.3–9.1 mg/dl) and isoleucine and valine at 50–400 μmol/l (0.65–5.2 mg/dl)[2].
4. Most patients with MSUD are also treated with thiamine 10–20 mg/day.

PROGNOSIS

- Untreated, severe neonatal MSUD may lead to early death or survival with severe mental retardation.
- In a study of 12 patients with the severe neonatal form, 25% had spastic quadriplegia, 50% had abnormal neurological signs while 25% had normal intelligence[2]. Only one child was unequivocally normal.
- Outcome is best when MSUD is diagnosed within 24 hours of symptoms. A delay of 2 weeks is always associated with cerebral palsy and retardation[2].
- The possibility of MSUD should be considered in any neonate with an unexplained neurological illness and poor feeding, even if they are not initially acidotic.

FOLLOW-UP

Management of MSUD should only be undertaken in an experienced metabolic unit with good laboratory facilities capable of giving rapid results. Close liaison is needed between the parents, doctor and dietician. Most children with MSUD need frequent admission to hospital during intercurrent illnesses. Treatment is needed for life.

---

[1] Francis D E M (1987) *Diets for Sick Children*, 4th edn. Oxford: Blackwell.
[2] Naughten E R *et al.* (1982) *Arch. Dis. Childh.*, **57,** 918.

Organic Acidaemias

The organic acidaemias are a group of inherited disorders similar to MSUD resulting from inherited defects on the pathways of leucine, isoleucine, methylmalonate or propionate metabolism. They may present in the neonatal period with acidosis and hyperventilation, hypoglycaemia, hyperuricaemia, ketotic hyperglycinaemia, convulsions and coma. They may also present less acutely with intermittent acidosis, failure to thrive and vomiting. Many produce a characteristic odour.

TREATMENT

1. A high calorie, low protein diet should be used[1]. Specific amino acid supplementation may be needed. Dehydration must be avoided.
2. Some forms of methylmalonic acidaemia respond to vitamin B_{12} 1–2 mg/day. Carnitine supplementation has also been used[2].
3. Some forms of propionic acidaemia respond to biotin 10 mg/day.
4. Added alkali may be needed if there is persistent acidosis.

PROGNOSIS

- Untreated cases of methylmalonic and propionic acidaemia may be lethal, or have severe failure to thrive with motor and mental handicap.
- Less severe variants and transient cases have also been recognised.

FOLLOW-UP

Close, detailed follow-up by an experienced team is vital for successful treatment of the organic acidaemias.

[1] Francis D E M (1987) *Diets for Sick Children*, 4th edn. Oxford: Blackwell.
[2] Roe C R *et al.* (1983) *Arch. Dis. Childh.*, **58**, 916.

Hyperuricaemia

Primary hyperuricaemia leading to gout is extremely rare in childhood. There is a sex-linked form (Lesch-Nyhan syndrome)[1] in which there is absence of the enzyme hypoxanthine-guanine phosphoribosyl transferase. Secondary hyperuricaemia may occur during treatment of leukaemia (tumour lysis syndrome) and result in acute renal failure.

TREATMENT

1. The hyperuricaemia in Lesch-Nyhan's syndrome can be controlled with allopurinol 10–20 mg/kg/day.
2. Restraint and dental extraction may be needed to control the self-mutilation.
3. Secondary hyperuricaemia can be prevented by use of allopurinol, a high fluid intake and alkalinisation of the urine.

PROGNOSIS

- The Lesch-Nyhan syndrome results in mental retardation, self-destructive biting and a choreo-athetoid movement disorder. There is no sensory deficit.
- If untreated, gouty tophi will develop.

FOLLOW-UP

Unfortunately control of the hyperuricaemia does not prevent abnormal neurological development in the Lesch-Nyhan syndrome[2].

[1] Lesch M et al. (1964) Am. J. Med., **36**, 561.
[2] Marks J F et al. (1968) Paediatrics, **42**, 357.

Porphyria

The porphyrias are a group of dominantly inherited disorders of haem metabolism resulting in excessive porphyrin production. The acute presentation is with colicky abdominal pain, vomiting, constipation or motor or sensory neuropathies[1]. There may also be psychiatric symptoms. In hereditary coproporphyria and variegate porphyria there is photosensitivity.

TREATMENT

1. The acute attack is treated with a high fluid intake and good analgesia with paracetamol, dihydrocodeine or morphine. When a neuropathy is present physiotherapy and splinting is helpful.
2. Avoidance of precipitating drugs including alcohol, barbiturates, chloramphenicol, chloroquine, theophylline and oestrogens is important.
3. When there is photosensitivity, the skin should be covered and a barrier cream used.
4. In congenital erythropoietic porphyria, splenectomy and chelation with cholestyramine may help.

PROGNOSIS

- Acute attacks vary considerably in severity. Occasionally they are so severe that assisted ventilation may be required.
- Photosensitivity may lead to hyperpigmentation and scarring.
- Congenital erythropoietic porphyria may lead to cirrhosis in adult life[2].

FOLLOW-UP

Relatives of patients should be screened and counselled about precipitating factors.

[1] Goldberg A (1959) Q. J. Med., **28**, 183.
[2] Magnus I A et al. (1961) Lancet, **ii**, 448.

Galactosaemia

Galactosaemia results from an autosomal recessive inherited deficiency of the enzyme galactose-1-phosphate uridyltransferase which enables galactose, derived from dietary lactose, to be turned into glucose. Thus the symptoms only develop after starting milk feeds. The higher the lactose content, the worse the symptoms so that breast-fed babies are severely affected. Symptoms include vomiting, diarrhoea, failure to thrive and prolonged jaundice. Often hepatosplenomegaly develops together with anaemia, clotting abnormalities, hypoglycaemic convulsions and cataracts.

TREATMENT

1. Treatment consists of a strict lactose and galactose free diet.
2. In the younger child soya-based feeds may be used, although some contain α-galactosides capable of releasing galactose[1].
3. Many foods, pills and medicines contain small amounts of unlabelled lactose so that a strictly lactose/galactose free diet needs expert dietary advice.

PROGNOSIS

- Untreated galactosaemia leads to mental retardation, behaviour problems, progressive cataracts and liver and renal damage[2].
- Less severe variants exist with cataracts as the chief manifestation of the disease[3].
- With good dietary control normal development should be possible.

- If the diet is relaxed during childhood, cataracts may develop and behaviour may deteriorate so the diet should probably be continued for life.
- Galactosaemic infants of heterozygote mothers may have cataracts at birth so that both homo- and heterozygous mothers should be on a diet during pregnancy until the status of the infant is known from prenatal diagnosis.

FOLLOW-UP

Maintenance of the diet requires close supervision and monitoring throughout childhood.

[1] Gitzelmann R et al. (1980) Galactose metabolism, hereditary defects and their significance. In Inherited Diseases of Carbohydrate Metabolism (Burman D et al. eds.). Lancaster: MTP Press.
[2] Buist N M R et al. (1984) Metabolic diseases. In Textbook of Paediatrics (Forfar J O, Arneil G C eds.). Edinburgh: Churchill Livingstone.
[3] Winder A R et al. (1983) Arch. Dis. Childh., 58, 362.

Fructose Intolerance

Hereditary fructose intolerance is caused by deficiency of fructose-1-phosphate aldolase (B) so that fructose-1-phosphate (which is very toxic) accumulates after ingestion of fructose[1]. This metabolite inhibits enzymes in the gluconeogenic and glycogenolytic pathways and so causes hypoglycaemia. Symptoms are those of hypoglycaemia, failure to thrive and disordered liver function – jaundice, hepatosplenomegaly, ascites and haemorrhage. Most patients develop an aversion to sweet food.

TREATMENT

Strict avoidance of fructose and sorbitol in the diet.

PROGNOSIS

- Provided an early diagnosis is made, normal development is possible.
- Liver damage may occur leading to cirrhosis.

FOLLOW-UP

Since fructose intolerance is an autosomal recessive trait, siblings should be screened before exposure to fructose. A liver biopsy may be needed to assess the patient's degree of hepatic damage.

[1] Woods H F (1980) Pathogenic mechanisms of disorders in fructose metabolism. In *Inherited Disorders of Carbohydrate Metabolism* (Burman D *et al.* eds.). Lancaster: MTP Press.

Glycogen Storage Disease

Glycogen storage disease (GSD) is characterised by an abnormal concentration or structure of glycogen in tissues. The type of tissue affected depends on which of 10 particular enzymes is affected but usually the liver is involved[1]. In most forms there is a deficiency in one of the enzymes involved in the breakdown of glycogen to glucose-6-phosphate (G-6-P). In the commonest form, type I or von Gierke's disease, glucose-6-phosphatase is deficient. While hypoglycaemia is the primary problem, there may also be lacticacidaemia, hyperlipidaemia, hyperuricaemia, bleeding and platelet dysfunction.

TREATMENT

1. *Type I GSD*

   a) Dietary management is the mainstay of treatment. The best results are obtained with continuous nocturnal direct intragastric feeding with glucose polymer solutions or Vivonex to provide 30% calories, the remainder being given by 2–4 hourly oral feeds by day[2].

   b) The aim should be to maintain blood glucose above 3.9 mmol/l (70 mg/dl). This helps to prevent formation of lactate, triglycerides and urate which result from the hypoglycaemic stimulus.

   c) Total parenteral nutrition may also be useful, especially in times of illness.

   d) Some children have received a portacaval shunt which also reduces the hepatic stimulation for glycogenolysis.

2. *Other GSDs*

   a) There is no effective treatment for Pompe's disease.

   b) Type III GSD may be treated in a similar way to type I.

PROGNOSIS

- Prognosis depends on the type.
- Type I (von Gierke's): glucose-6-phosphatase deficiency

  a) By one year of age, there is usually massive hepatomegaly, poor growth and recurrent episodes of hypoglycaemia which may affect intelligence.
  b) Bleeding and infections may also cause problems.
  c) Hepatic adenomas may develop during the second decade and may become malignant[3].
  d) Hyperuricaemia, gout and xanthomas become increasing problems.

- Type II (Pompe's): acid maltase deficiency

  a) Glycogen accumulates in the liver, muscle, heart, tongue and CNS. The cardiac problem leads to a severe dilated cardiomyopathy which may be fatal in the first year.
  b) Late infantile and adult forms are also known.

- Type III: Debrancher enzyme deficiency

  a) The clinical picture is similar to that of a mild form of type I GSD (von Gierke's).
  b) Presentation may be with just hepatomegaly in the childhood years. Lactic acidosis and hyperuricaemia do not occur.

  c) By puberty most patients are asymptomatic and adult height is not affected.

- Type V (McArdle's disease): muscle phosphorylase deficiency

  a) Muscle glycogen is unavailable for use as a fuel in vigorous exercise. Painful cramps may thus occur and myoglobinuria occasionally occurs; children are reluctant to climb hills[4].
  b) Lifespan is not affected.

FOLLOW-UP

After diagnosis, the feeding regimen will need to be established with frequent monitoring of blood glucose and lactate, insulin, glucagon, lipids, urate, liver function and clotting studies. Before hospital discharge, the parents will need to be able to learn to pass the nasogastric tube, operate the pump, mix the infusions and monitor blood and urine glucose. Hospital admission will often be needed at times of illness.

---

[1] Howell R R (1977) The glycogen storage diseases. In *The Metabolic Basis of Inherited Disease* (Stanbury J B, Wyngaarden J B, Fredrickson D eds.). New York: McGraw-Hill.
[2] Greene H L *et al.* (1979) *Adv. Pediatr.*, **26**, 63.
[3] Howell R R *et al.* (1976) *J. Am. Med. Assoc.*, **236**, 1481.
[4] Williams J *et al.* (1985) *Arch. Dis. Childh.*, **60**, 1184.

Hypoglycaemia

Many childhood conditions outside the neonatal period may present with hypoglycaemia. These include deficiencies of counter-regulatory hormones (e.g. growth hormone, ACTH, cortisol and catecholamines), liver disease (e.g. Reye's syndrome, fulminating hepatitis) and inborn errors of metabolism (e.g. galactosaemia, glycogen storage diseases, tyrosinaemia, maple syrup urine disease). It is important to exclude hyperinsulinism by measuring plasma insulin at the time of hypoglycaemia[1]; important causes of hyperinsulinism include nesidioblastosis, insulinomas, leucine sensitivity and the Beckwith–Wiedemann syndrome[2]. The presence of ketosis makes hyperinsulinism unlikely.

TREATMENT

1. The first priority is correction of the hypoglycaemia. This may require frequent or even continuous oral feeding, although in severe or symptomatic hypoglycaemia an intravenous bolus or infusion of 10–20% dextrose may be needed. Boluses of 0.5–1 g/kg of glucose (2–4 ml/kg of 25% dextrose) may be used in the acute emergency.
2. Infusion rates to maintain blood glucose are around 6–9 mg/kg/minute in the neonate falling to 2 mg/kg/minute in the adult. In the hyperinsulinaemic subject infusion rates up to twice these values may be required.
3. When hypoglycaemia persists despite a glucose infusion, hydrocortisone (2.5–5 mg/kg) or glucagon 0.5–1 mg may be tried.
4. Where there are hormonal deficiencies or inborn errors the next priority is the treatment of the underlying problem.
5. In hyperinsulinism steroids have only a transient effect. If the patient is leucine sensitive (as determined by a carefully controlled leucine tolerance test), a leucine restricted diet should be tried. The standard medical treatment for hyperinsulinism is diazoxide 5–20 mg/kg/day. Diazoxide is potentiated by a thiazide diuretic such as chlorothiazide.
6. Surgical treatment for hypoglycaemia consists of surgical resection of discrete insulinomas or partial pancreatectomy (75–80%) for nesidioblastosis.

PROGNOSIS

- The prognosis depends on the nature and early diagnosis of the underlying condition.
- Recurrent unrecognised hypoglycaemic episodes (particularly if nocturnal), may give rise to epilepsy, school failure, enuresis and even mental retardation.

FOLLOW-UP

Hypoglycaemic children should be stabilised in hospital initially and extreme care paid to their blood glucose control. Once they are discharged home, it is essential that the parents should have learned the techniques of blood glucose monitoring using chemical strips which may need to be performed several times daily, especially before meals. Glucagon should be provided for emergency treatment of hypoglycaemia at home and immediate telephone contact with the hospital should be available. The effect of surgical treatment needs to be carefully assessed as occasionally the pancreatectomy may be insufficient to control hypoglycaemia.

[1] Aynsley-Green A (1982) *Clin. Endocrinol. Metab.*, **11,** 159.
[2] Moncrieff M W *et al.* (1977) *Postgrad. Med. J.*, **53,** 159.

Mucopolysaccharidoses

The mucopolysaccharidoses (MPS) are a group of inherited lysosomal storage disorders with deficiencies of acid hydrolases which degrade the glycosaminoglycans (GAGs – one of the components of connective tissue). Mucopolysaccharidoses all have a progressive course after a period of apparent normality and have multisystem involvement. Mucopolysaccharide may be deposited in the cornea (corneal clouding), the skeleton (kyphoscoliosis), the skin (coarse facies), reticuloendothelial system (hepatosplenomegaly), CNS (mental retardation) and the heart.

TREATMENT

1. Treatment is mostly supportive rather than curative. Glaucoma, carpal tunnel syndrome, hernias and cardiac failure can all be treated in the usual ways.
2. The only attempt at cure which has met with any success is bone marrow transplantation. This has resulted in reduction in GAG concentrations and in some clinical improvement.

PROGNOSIS

● *MPS I (Hurler and Schie syndrome)*

  a) Hurler's syndrome becomes obvious in the first year of life and has all the features of an MPS.
  b) Mental development does not proceed much beyond mental age of 2–4 years.
  c) Corneal clouding is severe.
  d) Children develop heart failure and chest infections and usually die before the age of 10 years.
  e) The Schie variant has similar clinical features but a much slower rate of progression and patients survive into adult life.

● *MPS II (Hunter syndrome)*. All the MPS are autosomal recessive apart from Hunter's syndrome which is X-linked. The clinical features vary considerably in severity as with MPS I but are distinguished by the lack of corneal clouding.

● *MPS III (Sanfilippo's syndrome)*

  a) In Sanfilippo's syndrome the mental deterioration becomes apparent by the age of six

years, the corneal clouding is very slight and hepatosplenomegaly is not present.
  b) There are few contractures, the facies are only mildly affected and patients survive to adulthood.

● *MPS IV (Morquio syndrome)*

  a) Skeletal abnormalities predominate in MPS IV.
  b) The cornea is cloudy.
  c) There is severe shortening and a thoracic kyphosis and lumbar lordosis which come to affect respiratory function.
  d) Subluxation of the cervical spine may occur due to odontoid hypoplasia. The limb joints are also contracted.
  e) Intelligence is normal however and most survive until adult life.

● *MPS VI (Maroteaux-Lamy syndrome)*

  a) MPS IV is similar to MPS I and II but intelligence is not affected.
  b) Odontoid hypoplasia, optic atrophy, claw hand and hip dysplasia may develop.

● *MPS VII (β-glucuronidase deficiency)*. This form has a similar prognosis to Hurler's syndrome.

FOLLOW-UP

Families with children with MPS need the full range of supportive therapy; physiotherapy, occupational therapy and psychological support. All families should be offered genetic counselling as antenatal diagnosis is available.

Hyperlipoproteinaemia

Lipids are found in human plasma as esters of long-chain fatty acids in the form of triglycerides, phospholipids and cholesterol esters. Fatty acids and cholesterol also are present in the non-esterified form. Triglycerides may be absorbed from the diet as lymph chylomicrons or secreted by the liver as very low density lipoproteins (VLDL). Lipids are transported in plasma as lipoproteins being aggregates of lipids and apoproteins.

TREATMENT

1. Homozygous familial hypercholesterolaemia (FH) is treated with a low saturated fat diet supplemented with polyunsaturated fat, cholestyramine (0.15–0.6 g/kg/day), clofibrate 20–30 mg/kg/day and nicotinic acid. Folic acid and vitamins A and D may need to be given.
2. Heterozygous FH probably should be treated if cholesterol levels exceed 7.8 mmol/l (300 mg/dl). Diet alone may be tried but drugs may also have to be added.
3. Lipoprotein lipase deficiency may be treated with some fat restriction to about 10–20 g/day.

PROGNOSIS

● Familial hypercholesterolaemia

a) Familial hypercholesterolaemia (FH or type II hyperlipoproteinaemia) is an autosomal dominant single gene disorder with abnormal cell receptor binding for low density lipoproteins (LDL). Homozygous children develop xanthomas in skin and tendons in the first few years and cornus arcus and ischaemic heart disease (IHD) by the age of 10 years.
b) The prognosis for homozygous FH is very poor even with treatment and few patients survive beyond the age of 30 years.
c) Individuals with heterozygous FH are less likely to have signs but do have an increased risk of IHD.
d) 51% men and 12% women with heterozygous FH will have had a heart attack by the age of 50, which is three to four times more than normal controls.

● Familial lipoprotein lipase deficiency (type I hyperlipoproteinaemia) is a much rarer recessive disease in which there may be attacks of abdominal pain and pancreatitis but no increased risk of IHD.

FOLLOW-UP

Clinical and biochemical monitoring every 3–6 months throughout childhood and into adult life is needed.

Hypercalcaemia

Idiopathic hypercalcaemia may be present during the first year of life with vomiting, failure to thrive and constipation. The hypercalcaemia may be associated with hypercalciuria, nephrocalcinosis and impaired renal function. It is thought to arise from hypersensitivity to ingested vitamin D. Hypercalcaemia may be associated with a characteristic facies (the 'elfin face') with prominent lips, an upturned nose, prominent cheeks and low-set ears – William's syndrome. Other features include developmental delay, hypertension, supravalvular aortic or pulmonary stenosis and a bicuspid aortic valve[1]. William's syndrome may also exist without hypercalcaemia. Other causes of hypercalcaemia include vitamin D poisoning, primary hyperparathyroidism (usually from an adenoma), multiple endocrine neoplasia syndromes and extensive fat necrosis. Hypercalcaemia has also been described in low-birthweight infants[2].

TREATMENT

1. Acute hypercalcaemia over 3.5 mmol/l (14 mg/dl) is treated with frusemide 0.5–1 mg/kg combined with a high salt intake.
2. Frusemide should not be used for long-term treatment as it will lead to hypercalciuria and nephrocalcinosis.
3. Long-term treatment consists of reducing the intake of vitamin D and calcium in the diet and in infants a low calcium milk such as Locasol may be used.
4. Steroids reduce absorption of calcium from the gut and may be used in severe hypercalcaemia, e.g. prednisolone 5–10 mg/day. Steroids should not be used for more than 4 weeks because of the side-effects.
5. Primary hyperparathyroidism may need to be treated with a parathyroidectomy.

PROGNOSIS

- In idiopathic hypercalcaemia there is usually spontaneous resolution of the hypercalcaemia in the first two years of life even without treatment.
- William's syndrome is associated with signifi-cant long-term morbidity including hyperacusis (75%), obesity (50%), hypertension (29%) and kyphoscoliosis (19%)[3].
- Patients with William's syndrome have mild to moderate mental retardation (IQ 40–72), have better expressive than comprehensive language skills and have disturbed behaviour including hyperactivity[4].

FOLLOW-UP

Hypercalcaemic children should have at least weekly measurements of plasma calcium, urea and creatinine when starting treatment. Once the hypercalcaemia is controlled, these may be performed less frequently. Blood for serum calcium needs to be taken carefully as stasis will give rise to a falsely elevated value. Renal ultrasound may be used to look for nephrocalcinosis. Children with William's syndrome may need special schooling and psychological support.

[1] Garcia R E et al. (1964) New Eng. J. Med., **271**, 117.
[2] Lyon A J et al. (1984) Arch. Dis. Childh., **59**, 1141.
[3] Martin N D T et al. (1984) Arch. Dis. Childh., **59**, 605.
[4] Arnold R et al. (1985) Dev. Med. Child Neurol., **27**, 49.

Hypocalcaemia

The two major causes of hypocalcaemia outside the neonatal period are rickets and hypoparathyroidism. However, in rickets there is often secondary hyperparathyroidism, so that the calcium level may be only slightly lowered, while hypoparathyroidism is associated with severe hypocalcaemia. True hypoparathyroidism (low PTH levels) may be idiopathic, associated with other autoimmune diseases or following surgery.

Pseudohypoparathyroidism (PHP) is a dysmorphic syndrome associated with obesity, short stature, mental handicap and short fourth metacarpal bones. Parathormone (PTH) levels are normal but there is end-organ resistance to the effects of PTH leading to severe hypocalcaemia and hyperphosphataemia. The morphological features may also occur without the metabolic disturbances (pseudopseudohypoparathyroidism) (PPHP).

TREATMENT

1. Symptomatic hypocalcaemia can be treated with an infusion of 10% calcium gluconate (diluted to 2%) at a rate of 0.1 mmol/kg/hour (4 mg/kg/hour).
2. Oral treatment can then be started with 100 mg/kg/day of calcium given q.d.s.
3. The dose of vitamin D varies, depending on the condition. In hypoparathyroidism 2000 IU/day is usual.
4. Vitamin D metabolites (1α-hydroxyvitamin D and 1,25-dihydroxyvitamin D) are useful in renal rickets or where a short duration of treatment is needed, for example in neonates. The dose is 0.025–0.05 µg/kg/day.

PROGNOSIS

- Symptomatic hypocalcaemia may result in convulsions, tetany, laryngeal stridor and arrhythmias.
- Long-standing hypocalcaemia may cause mental disturbance, pseudotumour cerebri, enamel hypoplasia of the teeth and calcification of the basal ganglia.
- Hypocalcaemia due to idiopathic hypoparathyroidism responds well to treatment while hypoparathyroidism following thyroidectomy has a poorer prognosis. 5% subtotal thyroidectomies result in hypoparathyroidism[1].
- The hypocalcaemia of PHP responds well to treatment but the somatic and mental problems persist.

FOLLOW-UP

In idiopathic hypoparathyroidism, other autoimmune diseases may occur. These include Addison's disease, diabetes and chronic cutaneous candidiasis. During treatment, frequent monitoring of blood calcium is needed as hypercalcaemia may easily occur.

---

[1] Daneman D et al. (1982) Clin. Endocrinol. Metabol., **11**, 211.

10
Diseases of the Nervous System

R. O. Robinson

Neonatal Fits

The incidence of fits in the neonatal period is variously assessed at between 0.2–1.2% of all live births. Clonic fits are rare in the preterm infant, but may otherwise take the form of tonic or myoclonic fits or 'subtle' fits.

TREATMENT

1. Hypoglycaemic fits are treated with 0.5–1 g/kg as a bolus followed by an infusion of 10% glucose starting at about 75 ml/kg/day and continuing at a rate sufficient to maintain the blood glucose at more than 2.5 mmol/l.
2. Hypocalcaemic fits are treated with 0.2 ml/kg 10% calcium gluconate followed by 0.1 ml/kg 50% magnesium sulphate given slowly i.v.
3. Pyridoxine dependency responds to 100 mg pyridoxine i.v.
4. Status epilepticus is best treated with i.v. diazepam 0.4 mg/kg. If this is ineffective, paraldehyde 0.1 mg/kg by deep i.m. injection should be tried.
5. Frequent fits (as opposed to status) are best treated with phenobarbitone 15–20 mg/kg i.v. over 10 minutes or phenytoin 15–20 mg/kg over 45 minutes i.v. The latter is preferable since neither consciousness nor respirations are depressed, thereby allowing subsequent informative neurological assessment.
6. There is no convincing evidence that electrical fits without clinical concomitants, 'subtle' fits (respiratory irregularities, eye movements etc.) or myoclonic fits cause brain damage unless they are associated with hypoxia or hypoglycaemia. In these circumstances tempering therapeutic enthusiasm with discretion may avoid iatrogenic apnoea and hypotension (thereby causing decreased cerebral perfusion).

PROGNOSIS

- The prognosis depends largely on the cause.
- The outcome is usually excellent where hypocalcaemia or subarachnoid haemorrhage are the sole abnormalities.
- The rare child with pyridoxine dependency has a good prognosis if recognised and treated early.
- It is also better if no cause is found, with 60% being normal.
- The prognosis of fits following birth asphyxia, hypoglycaemia, intracerebral haemorrhage and meningoencephalitis is much worse with only some 10–20% surviving unscathed – the remainder being divided approximately equally into those who died and those who survived with handicap. About 20% of the survivors have epilepsy.
- The survival rate in term babies is much worse – about 30%[1,2].

FOLLOW-UP

Frequency of follow-up is determined by the response of fits to treatment. With lack of control, patients should be seen at least monthly to start with – more frequently if the family needs support.

[1] Rose A L et al. (1970) Paediatrics, **45**, 404.
[2] Holden K R et al. (1982) Paediatrics, **70**, 165.

Febrile Convulsions

Febrile convulsions are common, occurring in 2–3% all children.

TREATMENT

1. At the first febrile convulsion no child can be said to have more than a 50% chance of further fits – febrile or otherwise. Prophylaxis is rarely therefore considered until the child has had two or more.
2. Valproate or phenobarbitone reduce the likelihood of subsequent febrile convulsions. It is not known if they reduce the likelihood of subsequent epilepsy. Children with prior normal neurology and brief generalised febrile convulsions are a low risk group in terms of subsequent epilepsy or delayed development. The decision whether or not to treat these children after the second fit is determined as much by the parents' anxiety about fits and their attitude towards prophylactic medication as by the advice from their paediatrician.
3. Conversely, there is an obvious minority high risk group either for subsequent febrile convulsions or for epilepsy. In these children it would seem sensible to advise prophylaxis after the second fit. Dosage of either valproate or phenobarbitone must be continuous and such as to achieve at least minimum therapeutic levels. Giving either of these drugs only during a febrile episode is ineffective. Prophylaxis is continued until the child has been fit free for two years or until he is six years old – whichever is the shorter. Treatment is discontinued slowly over 4–6 weeks.
4. Equal consideration should be given to advising parents about temperature control during febrile convulsions. Since there is some recent evidence that the time-honoured practice of tepid sponging is ineffective at best, the most important measure is adequate dosage with paracetamol. There is an argument for giving regular 4-hourly 12 mg/kg doses while the fever lasts. Overheating the room or overwrapping the child should obviously be avoided – but the child should not be chilled sufficiently to provoke shivering.
5. It is also worth considering the use of prophylactic rectal diazepam (0.3 mg/kg) in a particularly susceptible child if the temperature is proving difficult to control.

PROGNOSIS

- 30–40% children in their first febrile convulsion will have one or more further febrile convulsions. About one-third will have only one more[1], but 10% will have multiple attacks. The two factors most closely related to recurrence are a history of afebrile seizures in the immediate family, and most powerfully, an early age of onset (in the first year of life)[2]. Half the children with an early first febrile seizure have one or more recurrences: the rate falling to 28% with onset after the first year.
- Complex seizures (see p. 174) are not predictive of recurrence of *febrile* convulsions.
- Overall 2% children who have experienced febrile seizures will have developed epilepsy by the age of seven[3]. The most important predictor for subsequent epilepsy is an abnormal neurological examination or delayed development before the onset of febrile convulsions. Other predictors include features of the first fit – more than 15 minutes, more than one a day, focal features, and a history of afebrile convulsions in a first degree relative.
- Rates of epilepsy per 1000 for children having febrile convulsions are as follows:

	Normal prior development	Suspect or abnormal prior development
No complex features	11	28
More than 15 minutes	14	91
More than one per day	14	111
Focal features	26	154

- 60% children developing epilepsy following a febrile convulsion will have no adverse features, 34% will have one adverse feature and 6% will have two or more.
- The risk of a child developing epilepsy by the age of seven if he has not had febrile seizures is 0.5%.
- If prior neurological status has been normal, the likelihood of subsequent epilepsy does not seem to be affected by how many febrile seizures the child has. However, if the prior status has been abnormal, the incidence of subsequent epilepsy rises with the numbers of febrile convulsions:

	1st fit	2nd fit	3rd fit	> 4 fits
Rates of epilepsy per 1000	28	28	74	100

- Prolonged febrile seizures do not seem to be associated with subsequent mental handicap if prior development is normal[4].

FOLLOW-UP

Follow-up should be at least monthly if fits are uncontrolled. Enquire for blunting of consciousness; and examine carefully for ataxia. If a child is on monotherapy checking anticonvulsant levels is only necessary if poor compliance or toxicity is suspected. If the child is on more than one drug and control is poor, anticonvulsant levels may determine therapeutic options. Liver function tests should be performed immediately in any patient on valproate if anorectic for more than 2–3 days. A repeat CT scan is justified if fits are focal and intractable. Repeat EEGs are rarely helpful.

[1] Freeman J (1980) *Paediatrics*, **65**, 1009.
[2] Nelson K D *et al.* (1978) *Paediatrics*, **61**, 720.
[3] Nelson K D *et al.* (1976) *New Eng. J. Med.*, **259**, 1029.
[4] Ellenburg J H *et al.* (1978) *Arch. Neurol.*, **35**, 17.

Afebrile Convulsions

The incidence of afebrile seizures by the age of seven following febrile seizures is about 2%. The incidence in children who have not developed febrile seizures is 0.5%. Seizures are a symptom of a brain disorder which may or may not be serious.

TREATMENT

1. The prophylaxis of the different seizure disorder types is treated separately. It remains here to deal with the management of status epilepticus.
2. Ensure that ventilation is unimpeded (turn the patient on his side and insert an airway).
3. Check for hypoglycaemia.
4. Give diazepam 0.3 mg/kg, i.v. if possible or rectally if not.
5. If this does not stop fits in 10 minutes, repeat the dose.
6. If this is ineffective give phenytoin 15–20 mg/kg i.v. over 45 minutes. Phenytoin is not absorbed adequately from an intramuscular injection. The intravenous preparation is unfortunately incompatible with dextrose – thus both the dead space of the giving set and the solution used to 'chase' the phenytoin through, must be either water for injection or saline not containing dextrose. Although this makes the procedure more complicated, it has the great advantage of allowing an informative neurological examination when the fit stops.
7. In the unlikely event of neither diazepam nor phenytoin being effective, set up a chlormethiozole infusion at 5–10 mg/kg/hour after an initial i.v. bolus of 5–10 mg/kg. An effective dose is usually one which causes drowsiness or a light sleep. If the seizures do not stop with the above, the infusion rate should be increased every 2 hours up to 20–30 mg/kg/hour until they do.
8. If all else fails, the patient should be paralysed

and ventilated under EEG control with continuing efforts with phenytoin or phenobarbitone to achieve electrical normality.

PROGNOSIS

- Estimates of recurrence after a single afebrile seizure vary widely between different series[1]. No very accurate figure can be given but it is of the order of 50%. However complete control with continuing afebrile seizures (i.e. epilepsy) can be achieved in at least 70%, with 50% of the total off medication after an interval[2].
- Many seizure disorders therefore represent a temporary disposition to fits. However, many

do not and a more accurate prognosis can be gained by considering the type of fit and the biological setting in which it occurs. This forms the basis for current classifications of epilepsy, one of which is adopted here[3].

FOLLOW-UP

Follow-up is as for febrile convulsions (p. 170).

[1] Robinson R J (1984) In *Recent Advances in Paediatrics no. 7* (Meadow R ed.), p. 155. Edinburgh: Churchill Livingstone.
[2] Annergers J F *et al.* (1979) *Epilepsia*, **20**, 729.
[3] Delgardo-Escueta A V *et al.* (1983) *New Eng. J. Med.*, **308**, 5108, 1576.

Grand Mal (Primary Generalised Convulsive Epilepsy)

Primary generalised fits occur when both EEG and the clinical features indicate simultaneous involvement of both cerebral hemispheres. This is a relatively uncommon form of childhood epilepsy occurring in a child who is both developmentally and neurologically normal and in whom there are no focal features to the attack nor other seizure types.

TREATMENT

1. Carbamazepine, phenobarbitone and phenytoin each achieve a seizure free remission rate of 60–70%. This, being the order of frequency of severe side-effects, is the order in which they should be used. Doses and therapeutic ranges are:

	Dose (mg/kg)	Therapeutic range (mg/l)
Carbamazepine	20–40	4–14
Phenobarbitone	3–10	20–50
Phenytoin	3–8	10–25

a) Start carbamazepine at 5 mg/kg/day for one week and then double on two successive weeks to achieve 20 mg/kg/day.

b) Phenobarbitone and phenytoin are usually given in two divided doses per day; carbamazepine in three divided doses.

2. As therapeutic ranges are wide and tolerance to side-effects is variable between patients, when only one drug is being used, the dose should be increased until toxic effects occur or fits stop whichever is soonest.

3. If none of the above three work alone combinations of any two should be tried.

PROGNOSIS

- With medication 60–70% children with such fits starting after infancy become seizure free[1].
- A population based study, which will not be so pure diagnostically, still gave a figure of 80% remission rate 15 years after diagnosis for generalised seizures starting under the age of 20[2].

Follow-up is as for febrile convulsions (see p. 170).

[1] Delgado-Escueta A V et al. (1983) New Eng. J. Med., **308,** 1508.
[2] Annegers J F et al. (1979) Epilepsia, **20,** 729.

Classical Petit Mal (Primary Generalised Non-Convulsive Epilepsy)

The diagnosis of classical petit mal requires a consistent clinical picture synchronous with a characteristic EEG (3/second synchronous spike and wave). It is not synonymous simply with absence attacks. It is a relatively uncommon form of childhood epilepsy.

TREATMENT

1. The two drugs of choice are:

   a) Sodium valproate (20–50 mg/kg/day in two or three divided doses, therapeutic range 40–100 mg/l).

   b) Ethosuximide (20–40 mg/kg/day in two divided doses, therapeutic range 50–100 mg/l).

   c) Livingstone et al.[1] in the pre-valproate era suggested that the subsequent development of grand mal could be suppressed by using phenobarbitone concurrently with ethosuximide. The effect of valproate in this regard is not clear but may give it a theoretical advantage over ethosuximide.

   d) Occasionally patients will respond to both drugs together when one alone fails.

2. For those patients refractory to these drugs the addition of acetazolamide (10–25 mg/kg/day in three divided doses) is worth trying, but the propensity for causing hypokalaemia should be checked.

3. In those patients refractory to drugs alone, a ketogenic diet may achieve control in some either alone or in combination with one of the two drugs of choice.

PROGNOSIS

- Classical petit mal is one of the more benign seizure disorders. 70–80% patients become seiz-ure free on treatment. Petit mal alone remits in early life.

- However, grand mal develops as well or subse-quently in about 40%. The likelihood of this is greater if the onset of petit mal is at an age of more than 8 years and is commoner in males. The grand mal is usually relatively easily con-trolled. The majority of those in whom the petit mal is relatively resistant to treatment, also develop grand mal.

FOLLOW-UP

Follow-up is as for febrile convulsions (see p. 170).

[1] Livingstone S et al. (1965) J. Am. Med. Assoc., **194,** 227.

Absence attacks

Absence attacks with accompanying myoclonus in children who also have tonic/clonic seizures have been described in children whose ictal EEG shows either 4–6 Hz multispike wave complexes or 8–12 Hz diffuse rhythms. These children are otherwise normal as is their interictal EEG. Their response to valproate is excellent but the spon-taneous remission rate of this type of seizure is unknown as yet. Absences with myoclonus also occur as part of secondary generalised epilepsy (see p. 173) when the prognosis and biological setting are very different.

Secondary Generalised Seizures

These are a common variety of seizure in childhood. They start as partial – either simple or complex seizures – which then progress to a generalised tonic and/or clonic seizure. This group also includes the myoclonic epilepsies (see p. 176). The first type are associated with lesions which may be developmental or acquired. Their prognosis is difficult to summarise since it depends on age of onset, aetiology and the coexistence of other neurological abnormalities. For this reason fits with these characteristics are rarely studied as a group and are included in childhood seizure disorders.

TREATMENT

Treatment of generalised tonic and/or clonic fits, complex partial or simple partial convulsive fits is with a major anticonvulsant (carbamazepine, phenobarbitone, phenytoin). If, as is frequently the case, there are associated myoclonic, absence or akinetic attacks, sodium valproate or a benzodiazepine may be necessary in addition.

PROGNOSIS

- Fits associated with demonstrable structural lesions are rarely fully controlled.

- Onset in the first year of life is usually associated with poor fit control and frequently delayed development.
- Accompanying mental handicap or focal neurological abnormality are usually associated with poor fit control.
- Association of several different seizure types in the same child is also a bad prognostic sign.

FOLLOW-UP

Follow-up is as for febrile convulsions (see p. 170).

Simple Partial Seizures

These start and remain as a focal discharge without impairment of consciousness. In children most types have a good prognosis. Several types are distinguished.

Rolandic epilepsy

Rolandic epilepsy accounts for 15% of all childhood seizures.

TREATMENT

It is easily controlled by a single anticonvulsant – usually carbamazepine as a single night time dose.

PROGNOSIS

- Attacks are typically nocturnal, usually occur in boys, and involve one side of the face and sometimes the arm.
- Prognosis is excellent since it self-remits during adolescence.

Benign epilepsy with occipital paroxysms

This type consists of visual ictal symptoms – usually either scotomata or simple visual hallucinations together with interictal occipital spike wave discharges which are aborted by eye opening. The children who are otherwise quite normal may experience other seizure types of which the commonest (43%) are hemiclonic.

TREATMENT

About 60% control is achieved with either carbamazepine, phenobarbitone, sodium valproate or a benzodiazepine.

PROGNOSIS

The prognosis of this type of seizure disorder is excellent, remitting completely during adolescence.

Benign psychomotor epilepsy

This is characterised by sudden fearful expression, usually with a scream, followed by salivation, oropharyngeal movements, often accompanied by autonomic expressions such as pallor, sweating or abdominal pain. The attack usually lasts 1–2 minutes. The EEG shows sharp waves in fronto-temporal or parietotemporal areas.

TREATMENT

Monotherapy with carbamazepine is nearly always completely effective.

PROGNOSIS

The prognosis is excellent with self-remission during adolescence.

FOLLOW-UP

Follow-up is as for febrile convulsions (see p. 170).

Complex Partial Seizures

Complex partial seizures start as a focal discharge following which consciousness becomes impaired. This is one of the commonest types of seizure in childhood.

Temporal lobe epilepsy

When the discharge starts in the anterior temporal lobe, there is a blank stare followed by automatisms such as lip smacking or forced searching. There may be accompanying autonomic phenomena or more complex subjective experiences. The attack usually lasts more than 10 seconds and therefore, if absence predominates, is not difficult to distinguish from primary generalised non-convulsive absences which last less than 10 seconds.

TREATMENT

1. Treatment is with one or more of the major anticonvulsants as with grand mal (see p. 171). In addition using acetazolamide as an adjunct to carbamazepine is worth trying.
2. Psychiatric disorders are particularly common in children with this type of epilepsy and may require expert help.
3. Children with continuing fits during adolescence should be considered as possible candidates for anterior temporal lobectomy. Indications include a disabling frequency of fits, despite adequate anticonvulsant therapy, not due to a gross space-occupying lesion, and a stable predominantly unilateral EEG focus. Results in such carefully selected cases are that about 50% patients are rendered fit free, with a worthwhile reduction of fits in a further 25%. Although there is no apparent relief from preoperative psychosis (which may indeed appear after surgery) uncontrolled aggression frequently improves. If subclinical seizure disorder has disabled the functioning of the resected lobe, cognitive functioning may also improve[1].

PROGNOSIS

- In one series[2] 33% became independent adults, off medication and fit free, 32% were independent but on treatment (mostly having some fits), 5% died during childhood and 30% were dependent and in institutions. The reasons for dependence were either mental handicap, psychosis, other behavioural disorders and/or continuing severe fits. Nearly all of the dependent group had had known brain insults, e.g. infections, or had suffered status epilepticus (more than 30 minutes).

- In general, those children with temporal lobe epilepsy who had a first or second degree relative with any kind of seizure had a better prognosis than those who did not (remission of fits occurred in 51% versus 9% respectively).
- Where there was no positive family history, the features associated with a poor outcome are early (aged less than 2 years 4 months) onset of fits, five or more grand mal attacks, more than one attack of temporal lobe epilepsy per day, and a left-sided focus. Additional features related to a poor outcome irrespective of family history are an IQ < 90, the hyperkinetic syndrome, catastrophic rage attacks and necessity for special schooling.
- Mental handicap and behavioural disorders were the strongest determinants of placement in adult life. Continuing fits through adolescence in males were associated in those less handicapped with sexual indifference and low likelihood of subsequent marriage or parenthood.
- Subsequent development of psychosis (9 of 87 child and adult survivors) is limited to those with a left-sided focus. Males with a left-sided focus had a 30% chance of developing psychosis. Continuing antisocial behaviour in adult life (12 of 87) was related to continuing fits and an EEG focus contralateral to the preferred hand (whether left or right).

Other complex partial seizures

Discharge from the orbital frontal cortex gives rise to olfactory hallucinations and autonomic phenomena. Discharge from the posterior temporal-parietal region gives rise to complex visual hallucinations and from the superior temporal gyrus, auditory hallucinations and vertigo. Spread of discharge from any of these areas may involve the temporal lobe or its medial structures including the amygdala. This is associated with impairment of consciousness (hence 'complex') and autonomic behaviour. They may thus closely resemble temporal lobe attacks (and hence the coinage of the catch-all phase 'psychomotor'), being distinguishable only by EEG analysis.

TREATMENT

1. Anticonvulsants as for grand mal are the drugs of choice.
2. As with temporal lobe epilepsy, patients refractory to treatment (the majority) should be considered for excision of the focus. Other criteria for selection include a stable focal EEG abnormality over a 3–5 year period. Results in suitable patients indicate 32% (frontal) or 45% (parietal) becoming fit free with overall improvement in two thirds[3].

PROGNOSIS

- Some 60% these disorders are refractory to anticonvulsant treatment.

FOLLOW-UP

Follow-up is as for myoclonic epilepsy (see p. 177).

[1] Polkey C E (1983) *J. Roy. Soc. Med.*, **76**, 354.
[2] Lindsay J et al. (1979) *Dev. Med. Child Neurol.*, **21**, 285, 433, 630.
[3] Rasmussen T (1969) *Clin. Neurosurg.*, **16**, 288.

Myoclonic Epilepsy

Myoclonus may be caused by a discharge arising from any level of the neuraxis. As such therefore, a number of syndromes with a widely differing prognosis have been described.

Benign myoclonic epilepsy of infancy

While the fits characteristic of this type of epilepsy present as generalised myoclonic fits mimicking infantile spasms, they do not occur in series, are usually brief (1–3 seconds) and are accompanied by a normal interictal EEG.

TREATMENT

Fits are easily controlled by valproate alone.

PROGNOSIS

● The prognosis is excellent.

Juvenile myoclonic epilepsy

This form of epilepsy presents with bilateral, single or repetitive jerks usually involving the arms. Fits mostly occur on awakening but can be precipitated by flashing lights. Most also have generalised tonic/clonic seizures. Brief generalised bursts of poly spike wave activity occur on a normal EEG background.

TREATMENT

There is an excellent response to valproate monotherapy.

PROGNOSIS

● The spontaneous remission rate is low (perhaps 10%).

Infantile spasms (West's syndrome)

This is the most familiar of the severe myoclonic encephalopathies of infancy with onset usually between 3 and 18 months of age. About 70% patients are either retarded or otherwise neurologically abnormal before the onset of spasms (the 'symptomatic' as opposed to the 'cryptogenic' group). Aetiology in the symptomatic group includes a wide variety of metabolic disorders, tuberous sclerosis, congenital malformations and chronic trauma. There is no evidence of association with pertussis vaccination.

TREATMENT

1. ACTH or prednisolone usually controls spasms and improves the hypsarrhythmic EEG. Conventional doses of the former start at 40 units i.m. daily and increase to 80 units by three weeks if there is no response. Prednisolone is usually started at 2 mg/kg/day; with the onset of response this is reduced to 20–30 mg on an alternate day schedule.
2. Steroids are usually continued for about three months. In the event of recurrence, a second course of steroids may be effective, failing which recourse may be had to valproate or one of the benzodiazepines.

PROGNOSIS

● Psychomotor regression occurs with the onset of spasms in 95% and is usually severe (88%).
● Spasms disappear before the age of 5 (about 50%) or evolve into the Lennox–Gastaut syndrome (see below).
● There is the impression that early and, if necessary, high dose steroids in the cryptogenic group may improve the prognosis for cognitive development.

Severe myoclonic epilepsy in infants

This term describes generalised or unilateral febrile clonic seizures starting at 5–6 months of age with subsequent appearance of generalised myoclonic attacks at about 18 months, sometimes' accompanied by partial complex seizures. The EEG shows generalised spike or polyspike waves, early photosensitivity, and multifocal spike wave abnormalities. Psychomotor development slows with onset of myoclonus, sometimes with ataxia and/or hyperreflexia.

TREATMENT

1. A combination of a major and a minor anticonvulsant (e.g. carbamazepine and valproate) may modify seizure frequency to some extent.
2. All children require special schooling.

PROGNOSIS

- The seizures do not remit and are extremely refractory to any anticonvulsants or a ketogenic diet.

The Lennox–Gastaut syndrome

The Lennox–Gastaut syndrome has three components: (1) a triad of seizure types – atypical absences, *axial* tonic seizures and drop attacks (either akinetic or myoclonic); (2) slow spike and waves on the awake EEG and 10 Hz bursts during sleep; and (3) psychomotor retardation.

TREATMENT

1. Seizures are relatively refractory. In some cases control may be gained with a combination of a major and a minor anticonvulsant (e.g. carbamazepine and valproate).
2. As in any chronic epileptic disorder the effect of or need for anticonvulsants requires regular review.

PROGNOSIS

- The condition is rarely (4–6%) self-remitting.
- After some years the epilepsy becomes less active in about 15–20%. Before this time the course is characterised by an apparently arbitrary waxing and waning of seizure activity.
- A minority became psychotic.

- The following features are predictive of a poor prognosis:

  a) Preceding developmental or neurological abnormality, particularly West's syndrome.
  b) Onset before the age of three years.
  c) Recurrent status and high seizure frequency.
  d) Slow background activity on EEG.

Myoclonic astatic epilepsy of early childhood

This term describes the onset in a previously normal child between the age of one and five years of symmetrical myoclonic jerks involving the arms and shoulders accompanied by akinetic drop attacks. About two-thirds cases start with generalised tonic/clonic or clonic, febrile or afebrile seizures. The EEG abnormalities are progressive from parietal theta activity to bilateral irregular 2–3 Hz spike wave and spike wave variants in a 4–7 Hz background with parietal accentuation.

TREATMENT

Treatment is with a combination of a major and a minor anticonvulsant (e.g. carbamazepine and valproate).

PROGNOSIS

- The prognosis is variable. Overall seizure control is achieved in 54% by the age of seven years[1].
- In some, spontaneous remission occurs. However, the following are predictive of a poor prognosis:

  a) Onset in infancy with febrile generalised seizures.
  b) Recurrence of minor motor status.
  c) Tonic nocturnal seizures.

- Those with poor prognosis develop slight ataxia, psychomotor retardation and continuing fits.

FOLLOW-UP

Follow-up should be at least monthly if fits are

uncontrolled. Enquire for blunting of consciousness; and examine carefully for ataxia. If a child is on monotherapy checking anticonvulsant levels is only necessary if poor compliance or toxicity is suspected. If the child is on more than one drug and control is poor, anticonvulsant levels may determine therapeutic options. Liver function tests should be performed immediately in any patient on valproate if anorectic for more than 2–3 days. A repeat CT scan is justified if fits are focal and intractable. Repeat EEGs are rarely helpful.

[1] Doose H (1985) In *Epileptic Syndromes in Infancy, Childhood and Adolescence* (Roger J, Dravet C, Bureau M, Dreifuss J E, Wolf P eds.), p. 78. London and Paris: John Libby Eurotext Ltd.

Migraine

Migraine is probably underdiagnosed in childhood since many adult sufferers can recall their first attacks, unrecognised at the time, occurring before puberty. One study has suggested a figure of 4% for school-age children[1].

TREATMENT

1. Treatment should be conducted on several fronts.
2. Reassurance of the essentially benign nature of the condition.
3. Assessment and as far as possible amelioration of stress and dietary provocations. Control of the stress should, if necessary in resistant cases, involve consideration of relaxation and biofeedback techniques.
4. The acute attack. Treatment is more likely to be successful if started with the onset of symptoms.

   a) A dose of paracetamol (e.g. 1 g in a seven year old) and lying down in the dark if preferred.
   b) If nausea and vomiting are prominent features, prochlorperazine suppositories (5 mg 1–2 years, 10 mg 3–5 years, 15 mg 6–12 years) may be used. Ergotamine preparations are useful in patients having attacks a month or so apart with well-defined auras and subsequent disabling headache. Ergotamine should not be used in 'complex' migraine – i.e. hemiplegic, basilar or ophthalmoplegic migraine—for fear of rendering a transient symptom permanent.

5. Prophylaxis should be recommended when attacks sufficiently severe to interrupt normal activity are occurring at least once a week. The list of possible effective agents is long, controlled trials are few, a placebo effect of at least 20% is to be expected and there is a known remission rate (see below). There is a definite – albeit fallible – clinical impression that some agents interrupt exacerbations.

   a) These agents include propranolol: in the prepubertal start at 10 mg t.d.s. and advance to 20–30 mg t.d.s.; in adolescence start at 20 mg t.d.s. and increase (if necessary) to 80 mg t.d.s.
   b) Phenytoin used in ordinary anticonvulsant doses (3–5 mg/kg/day) appears to be as effective as propranolol but is a drug of at least second choice in view of its known side-effects.
   c) Pizotifen up to 1.5 mg daily (maximum single dose at night 1 mg) or cyproheptadine (2–5 years 6–12 mg/day, 6–12 years 12–16 mg/day in three divided doses) are occasionally useful when propranolol or phenytoin have failed.
   d) Other drugs which also look promising but which are as yet relatively untested in children include:
      i) Naproxen sodium: an inhibitor of prostaglandin synthesis and platelet aggregation.
      ii) Calcium uptake blocking agents of

which nimodipine is said to be the most selective on cerebral vasculature.

iii) Methysergide is also effective but its propensity to cause retroperitoneal fibrosis prohibits its use in young children. If all else, including psychotherapy, fails in adolescents, it may be used to terminate an exacerbation but for no longer than three months (2 mg b.d. or t.d.s.).

e) In view of the common remission period in children, it is advisable to withdraw prophylaxis after 6–8 months at a time when stress is likely to be least, e.g. during the summer holidays.

PROGNOSIS

- Migraine tends to wax and wane in severity according to the level of stress (exacerbation) or equanimity (remission) in life. Exacerbation in children tends to last 6–8 months and may be

related to the school year. Exacerbations frequently present for 2–4 years followed by indefinite remission. Thus of 228 children followed for eight years, 29% had an eight-year remission[2].

- Perhaps 10% children have a clear dietary provocation (most commonly cheese and chocolate).

FOLLOW-UP

If the migraine is severe and uncontrolled 4–6 weekly follow-up is necessary to manage prophylaxis. If the child is on propranolol lying and standing arterial pressure must be checked. If the child is asymptomatic, 4-monthly follow-up is required to assess the overall situation and discuss stopping prophylaxis.

---

[1] Bille B (1962) *Acta Paediatr.*, **51** (suppl.), 136.
[2] Congdon P L *et al.* (1979) *Dev. Med. Child Neurol.*, **21**, 209.

Cerebral Tumours

Cerebral tumours are the most common solid tumour in childhood. There are probably 180–200 newly diagnosed cases each year in the UK.

Cerebellar astrocytoma

TREATMENT

1. As complete an excision as possible should be attempted. If this appears successful, prognosis is improved (15-year survival 75% in one series[1]).
2. Resection of recurrence should always be considered as this may also give further good quality survival.
3. The effect of radiotherapy on recurrence has not been demonstrated.

PROGNOSIS

- There is an overall recurrence rate of about

35%[2] with a median time to recurrence of one year.
- 32% require shunts for hydrocephalus.
- The mortality rate with recurrence is about 25%.

Medulloblastoma

TREATMENT

1. Surgery with neuraxial irradiation is the treatment of choice.
2. Chemotherapy (vincristine and lomustine) in addition to surgery and irradiation appears to be of benefit only in children under two years of age, with six-year survival rate of 57%.

179

PROGNOSIS

- With irradiation in addition to and following surgery there is an overall three-year survival rate of 70%.

Spinal tumour

PROGNOSIS AND TREATMENT

- The prognosis for spinal gliomas (without previous neurological deficit) has improved with the use of the Cavitron ultrasonic apparatus. These tumours grow slowly in children and some time will therefore elapse before meaningful figures for survival can be given.

Craniopharyngioma

TREATMENT

1. Surgical excision is the first line method of treatment.
2. These tumours are also radiosensitive. Since the surgical line of demarcation of the tumour is rarely clear, tissue from which recurrences can frequently arise remains after resection. Criteria for selection for postoperative radiotherapy on macroscopic, operative grounds therefore remain unclear.
3. Both surgery and radiotherapy can precipitate considerable neuroendocrinological disturbances with water and electrolyte imbalance which need close monitoring and treatment[3].

PROGNOSIS

- The overall recurrence risk after an attempted removal is about 10% but if there is evidence of tumour remaining on CT scan after operation, the recurrence risk rises to 60%[4].
- There is about a 10% postoperative mortality.

Optic glioma

TREATMENT

1. Resection is only indicated to control proptosis in a blind eye.

2. If there is neuroradiological evidence of continuing expansion or if there is diminishing visual acuity, it would appear that radiotherapy will halt further progression. However, as this is a self-limiting tumour the point can only be shown by a controlled trial which has not yet been carried out.

PROGNOSIS

- About 50% optic gliomas in childhood occur in the setting of neurofibromatosis. It has been suggested that in these cases, their growth characteristics are more aggressive. However, this has not been demonstrated satisfactorily.
- In both groups this seems to be an indolent tumour which may enlarge to cause symptoms early in life but remains static thereafter.

FOLLOW-UP

A CT scan should be performed three months after surgery or radiotherapy for baseline purposes in case of subsequent suspected tumour recurrence. If the child is asymptomatic after treatment, 6-monthly follow-up with careful neurological examinations is sufficient. If the hypothalamus has been irradiated, careful assessment of linear growth is mandatory with full hypothalamic–pituitary axis function testing after six months. For optic gliomas a 4-monthly assessment of the visual fields and acuity is required in addition to a yearly CT scan of the optic nerves.

[1] Bruno L et al. (1982) In Paediatric Neurosurgery (McLauran R L ed.), p. 307. New York: Grune and Stratton.
[2] Jerrias F (1978) Acta Neurol. Scand., 57, 31.
[3] Chapman S J et al. (1978) Dev. Med. Child Neurol., 20, 598.
[4] Raybaud C (1981) Proceedings of the XIIIth Meeting of Societie Internationale D'Oncologie Paediatrique (Paediatrique Oncologie Series 250). Amsterdam: Excerpta Medica.

Viral Encephalitis

Viral encephalitis usually presents with deterioration of consciousness, often associated with fits and sometimes with the acquisition of focal neurological signs. The differential diagnosis of this syndrome in paediatrics is wide, but when bacterial, traumatic, toxicological and other causes have been excluded, the remaining cases are nearly always associated with virus infections. These occur in 1–2:10 000 children under the age of 16 and are ten times more common in the first six months of life.

TREATMENT

1. The drug of choice for herpes encephalitis is acyclovir 10 mg/kg over 1 hour i.v., 8 hourly for 10 days[1].
2. Treatment otherwise devolves upon the maintenance of cerebral perfusion and the control of fits.

PROGNOSIS

- The prognosis depends upon the age of the child and the nature of the offending organism.
- Herpes simplex

  a) Neonatal herpes simplex encephalitis is fortunately uncommon. It may present either in isolation (local) or as part of a systemic infection (disseminated). The outcomes after treatment with vidarabine[2] are as follows (but see below):

	Mortality (%)	Morbidity in survivors (%)
Local infection	10	50
Disseminated infection	57	66

  After the neonatal period the outcome improves (until it declines again in patients over the age of 30).

  b) The prognosis for older age groups depends on the degree of consciousness at the start of treatment[1].

	Mortality (%)	Morbidity in survivors (%)
Lethargy	12	27
Semi coma/ coma	30	43

- Other viruses

  a) In a recent series[3] of children and infants with a wide range of viruses, the mortality was 10% with severe sequelae in only 7%.
  b) Features predictive of poor outcome were severe depression of conscious level, brainstem involvement, age less than one year and evidence of systemic involvement with renal failure.

FOLLOW-UP

Follow-up is unnecessary if full recovery is achieved, but otherwise should be as indicated for disabilities.

---

[1] Skoldenberg B et al. (1984) Lancet, ii, 77.
[2] Ch'ien L T et al. (1975) Paediatrics, 55, 678.
[3] Kennedy C R et al. Arch. Dis. Childh. (in press).

Meningoencephalitis

Meningoencephalitis is most commonly caused by viruses or bacteria. Bacterial infection of the meninges nearly always implies inflammation of the subjacent brain. The risk of meningitis occurring in a child by the age of five years (the commonest period) is between 1:400 and 1:2500.

TREATMENT

1. Antibiotics

   a) Organisms unknown: penicillin and chloramphenicol in the doses given below.

   b) *Haemophilus influenzae*: ampicillin 400 mg/kg/day in six divided doses i.v. and chloramphenicol 100 mg/kg/day in four divided doses i.v. until sensitivity is known.

   c) *Streptococcus pneumoniae*: penicillin G 250 000 units/kg/day (up to 20 000 000 units per day) given in six divided doses i.v. Chloramphenicol is an alternative in patients with penicillin sensitivity.

   d) *Neisseria meningitidis*: penicillin G. Half the calculated daily dose i.v. over 30–60 minutes at the start of treatment followed by 250 000 units/kg/day (not more than 20 mega U/day given in six divided doses i.v.). Chloramphenicol is an alternative in patients with penicillin sensitivity.

   e) Mycotuberculosis: isoniazid 20 mg/kg/day orally (up to 500 mg/day), streptomycin 20 mg/kg/day i.m. up to 1 g/day and rifampicin 15 mg/kg/day orally up to 600 mg/day. Streptomycin and rifampicin are continued for about two months after the onset of clinical improvement. Isoniazid alone is continued for a further additional 18–24 months.

2. Neonatal meningitis

   a) Group B streptococcus: penicillin G 300 000–400 000 units/kg/day given in four divided doses i.v.

   b) The treatment of meningitis caused by *Escherichia coli* in the neonate is unsatisfactory. Aminoglycosides penetrate poorly into the CSF. Chloramphenicol although penetrating well, has the disadvantage of being bacteriostatic only.

   c) *E. coli* or organism unknown: ampicillin 150–200 mg/kg/day given in four divided doses i.v. and chloramphenicol 25 mg/kg/day given in four divided doses i.v. in the first month in the preterm and in the first week in the term infant. (Only use when accurate and rapid chloramphenicol levels can be obtained. Therapeutic serum levels are 15–25 µg/ml. Levels more than 50 µg/ml are associated with the 'grey baby' syndrome.) Thereafter up to one month post-term 50 mg/kg/day in four divided doses i.v. or gentamicin 5 mg/kg/day in two divided doses i.m. in the first week or 7.5 mg/kg/day in three divided doses i.m. after the first week. (Dosage should be adjusted to achieve peak levels (30–60 minutes after injection) of 4–10 µg/ml.)

3. If organisms apparently sensitive to the antibiotics being used can still be cultured from lumbar CSF 72 hours after the onset of treatment, it is likely that ventriculitis is present and intraventricular antibiotics should be given daily – preferably by repeated ventricular puncture rather than by an indwelling ventricular catheter with subcutaneous reservoir which may itself be colonised. Close collaboration with the laboratory is strongly advised in order to establish that adequate antibiotic serum levels against the organism are being achieved. A week of intraventricular antibiotics usually suffices (as checked by daily ventricular CSF sampling). Systemic treatment should continue for about three weeks after the CSF has become sterile.

4. Initial reports[1] suggest that cefuroxime 60–75 mg/kg 8-hourly is as effective as ampicillin and chloramphenicol in the treatment of the three common organisms in older children.

5. Fits occur in 20–30% cases of bacterial meningitis and should be treated in the first instance with phenytoin.

6. In the acutely ill, intravenous fluids should be restricted to 50 mg/kg/day to minimise brain swelling. Raised intracranial pressure due to cerebral oedema should be treated as in Reye's syndrome. Subdural effusions causing pressure and/or focal signs, or hydrocephalus with accompanying clinical deterioration will require drainage.

PROGNOSIS

- Viral: aseptic viral meningoencephalitis is usually followed by rapid and complete recovery although ensuing sensorineural deafness has been described. In infants less than one year of age, enterovirus infection of the CNS may cause handicap, particularly depression of IQ and subsequent language delay[2].

- Bacterial: morbidity and mortality from bacterial meningitis depend upon the numbers and type of the infecting organism and the delay between onset of symptoms and start of adequate treatment. Approximate figures for the UK are:

	Mortality (%)	Major neurological sequelae in survivors (%)
H. influenzae type B	5–10	25
Strep. pneumoniae	17	25
N. meningitidis	5–10	18 (pre-chemo-therapeutic data)
Mycotuberculosis	20	23

- Neonatal meningitis is most commonly caused by *E. coli* and group B β-haemolytic streptococci. The *E. coli* organisms most likely to cause meningitis are those containing the K1 antigen, the figures for which are given below:

	Mortality (%)	Morbidity in survivors (%)
E. coli (K1)	31	29
Group B streptococcus (late onset)	15–20	12[3]
All organisms combined	50–70	30–55

FOLLOW-UP

If full recovery is achieved, follow-up is unnecessary, but otherwise is as indicated for disabilities.

---

[1] Swedish Study Group (1982) *Lancet*, **i**, 295.
[2] Sellers C J *et al.* (1975) *New Eng. J. Med.*, **293**, 1.
[3] Wald E R *et al.* (1986) *Paediatrics*, **77**, 217.

Brain Abscess

Brain abscesses are uncommon in children. The commonest association is with cyanotic congenital heart disease, but this is equalled by the number of children in whom there is no known cause. Other predisposing factors are suppurative middle ear and sinus infections.

TREATMENT

1. Treatment should be carried out in close consultation with neurosurgical colleagues. Abscesses may resolve with intensive antibiotic treatment alone, and this may be the method of choice when the abscess is surgically inaccessible or the child's general condition is very poor.
2. Abscesses are most commonly caused by staphylococci or a variety of anaerobic organisms. Initial treatment therefore may be started with methicillin 300 mg/kg/day in four divided doses i.v. and chloramphenicol 100 mg/kg/day in four divided doses i.v. If there is any particular reason to suspect anaerobic infection − such as gas in the abscess or if the abscess develops secondary to chronic otitis media, it would be reasonable to substitute penicillin 150 mg/kg/day in six divided doses i.v. for methicillin. Metronidazole 25 mg/kg/day in three divided doses i.v. as a third drug may be added in order to cover *Bacteroides* species not sensitive to chloramphenicol[1].
3. Aspiration or drainage by marsupialisation and total excision whenever possible have their neurological proponents.
4. Impending tentorial herniation is a strong indication for urgent surgery.
5. Dexamethasone 1–4 mg 6-hourly is efficient at reducing inflammatory oedema and consequent mass effect.

PROGNOSIS

- With the ready availability of CT scanning there has been a decline in mortality from 24% prior to CT scanning to 4% thereafter.
- The morbidity rate has similarly fallen from 74 to 46%[2].

FOLLOW-UP

Follow-up is unnecessary if recovery is assured, otherwise it should be as required for the management of disability or fits.

[1] Loovois J et al. (1977) *Br. Med. J.*, **2,** 981.
[2] Marshall W C (1983) In *Paediatric Neurology* (Brett E M ed.), p. 522. Edinburgh: Churchill Livingstone.

Hydrocephalus

The term hydrocephalus is used when there is ventricular enlargement due not to cortical atrophy, but to an imbalance between CSF production and flow.

TREATMENT

1. Intracerebral pressure is usually relieved with a ventriculoperitoneal shunt.
2. It has been suggested that when the hydrocephalus is not rapidly progressive and may be due to a self-limiting cause, isosorbide can be a successful temporising measure. The dose is 1.5–2.5 g/kg 6-hourly. Side-effects include diarrhoea and hypernatraemia (which should be looked for regularly).

PROGNOSIS

- The prognosis in hydrocephalus depends on the cause, the pressure effects and on the incidence of shunt complications.
- In one large series[1] there was a mortality of 7%. The IQ distribution was more than 110 in 7.7%, 90–109 in 5.2% with 10% mildly retarded, 13.4% moderately retarded and 17.1% severely retarded, the remainder (46.6%) having an IQ in the 70–89 range.
- Reported infection rates vary widely, but in the better centres are around 10%.

FOLLOW-UP

Serum electrolytes should be measured monthly if the child is on isosorbide. If the patient is stable or shunted, 6-monthly follow-up should be carried out with neurological examination to include careful ophthalmoscopy and monitoring of visual acuity. After shunting a CT scan is useful for baseline purposes in case of subsequent shunt malfunction.

---

[1] Hoffman H J et al. (1982) In Shunts and Problems in Shunts (Choux M ed.), p. 21. Basel: Karger.

Myelomeningocele

This is the most severe form of spina bifida where the abnormal neural plaque may or may not be covered by a thin membranous sac. While the incidence in the UK varies between 0.5 and 4:1000 live births, the overall incidence generally is on the decline possibly related to better maternal nutrition and health.

TREATMENT

1. Those who are likely to survive with severe or very severe handicap will have one or more of the following features at birth[1]:

   a) Thoracolumbar lesions.
   b) Severe paraplegia (paralysis below L3).
   c) Kyphosis or scoliosis.
   d) Hydrocephalus.
   e) Intracerebral birth injury.
   f) Other severe congenital defects.

2. Selective treatment usually means not immediately closing the sac in infants with one or more of these criteria. If they then subsequently develop hydrocephalus, ventriculoperitoneal shunting should be offered, not only on humanitarian grounds but also because the intelligence in survivors of deferred treatment may well be normal[2].

3. Walking during childhood can be achieved in the majority with the support of callipers and crutches. Orthopaedic intervention in the lower limbs is aimed at sufficient correction to allow the use of callipers and efficient weight bearing on a plantigrade foot. Where little flexion only of the hips is present, walking is usually abandoned in the teens for a wheelchair life.

4. The method of choice for urinary control is intermittent catheterisation, which the child can do for himself in due course[3]. Close attention to renal anatomy and function with the aim of preventing high pressure vesicoureteric reflux of infected urine is mandatory in order to prevent the onset of renal failure. Bowel control is usually possible with careful training and regular bowel stimulants.

5. Progressive instability of the spine may require operative fusion in due course, the timing of which may be deferred to some extent by supportive jacketing.

6. With close attention to detail, management decisions made in a multidisciplinary setting and appropriate support for the family and school an acceptable quality of life can be achieved for the more severely handicapped survivors[4].

PROGNOSIS

- Early mortality from ascending infection can be prevented by skin closure of the open lesions. Even when this is not done, 30–50% will survive some 25 years[5] since epithelialisation and spontaneous closure of the sac will occur. With active management, closing the defect in all, the overall mortality during childhood is about 30% with 90% of these dying in the first year, mostly of associated congenital defects and shunt complications.

- The grading of handicap in survivors of such a policy is approximately as follows[6]:

  1. Normal (normal IQ, walk without appliances, usually continent) 6%.
  2. Moderate (one third with low IQ, walk with callipers) 40%.
  3. Severe (walk not more than 20 yards if at all, many with severe kyphosis, some with severe mental handicap, nearly all incontinent) 39%.
  4. Very severe (not walking at all, severely mentally handicapped, some blind, all incontinent) 15%.

- 80% all cases develop hydrocephalus requiring treatment. 30–50% of these require shunt revision in the first year, 50–75% by the end of the second year and nearly all by the fourth year.

- If patients are selectively operated on at birth (see above) only 16% die by the age of seven years[7], 30% are normal and 70% are moderately handicapped.

FOLLOW-UP

Follow-up should be 6-monthly with examination to include fundoscopy, test of visual acuity, measurement of arterial pressure, fitting of orthoses and a wheelchair. Yearly x-ray of the spine, with measurement of serum electrolytes, creatinine and urea is required. An intravenous pyelogram should be performed every two years.

[1] Evans K *et al.* (1974) *Br. J. Prev. Soc. Med.*, **28**, 85.
[2] Hunt G *et al.* (1973) *Br. Med. J.*, **ii**, 197.
[3] Lorber J (1973) *Br. Med. J.*, **ii**, 201.
[4] Lorber J (1972) *Arch. Dis. Childh.*, **47**, 854.
[5] Menzies R G *et al.* (1985) *Lancet*, **ii**, 993.
[6] Borzyskowski M *et al.* (1982) *Br. J. Urol.*, **54**, 641.
[7] McCarthy G T (ed.) (1984) In *The Physically Handicapped Child*, p. 31. London: Faber and Faber.

Cerebral Palsy

This is a wide term embracing several patterns of motor handicap with different aetiologies and outcome. The overall incidence is 2–3:1000 live births. Each type will be considered separately.

Hemiplegia

The unilateral spasticity is frequently accompanied by sensory loss and hemianopia.

TREATMENT

1. Arm: the aim of physiotherapy, which should start by the age of 6 months, is to encourage symmetrical movement (two-handed activities), and promote awareness of the hand during washing, dressing, etc. Function may be promoted by ensuring propping during feeding, drawing, etc. and by adapting feeding utensils.
2. Leg: the initial aims are for efficient weight bearing and weight transfer. Equinus may be controlled in standing by bracing. Fixed deformities may be deferred or prevented by stretching once or twice a day. Handicapping equinus can be corrected by elongation of the Achilles tendon. Similarly persisting handicapping varus, valgus or foot instability is worth correcting surgically.
3. The use of baclofen to reduce spasm usually impedes function in this group.

PROGNOSIS

- About 30% have an IQ less than 70[2]. The CT scan may be helpful in this regard. If cortex or cortical association fibres are involved 55% have an IQ of less than 80.
- All walk eventually – most by the age of three.
- If hand function has not started by the age of three, it is unlikely that useful function will be gained.
- 30% have squint.
- About 40% have hemisensory loss.
- 10% have hemianopia.
- One-third to one-half has fits. This is particularly likely if fits have occurred in the neonatal period. There is a good correlation between paroxysmal EEG abnormalities and involvement of cortex on CT.

Diplegia

Here there is spastic involvement of both legs to a greater extent than in the arms. The borderline between diplegia and quadriplegia is ill defined, but the greater the degree of arm involvement, the higher is the rate of mental handicap, speech defects and fits.

TREATMENT

1. There is evidence that early treatment (less than 9 months) helps gait function[3]. These children

are best nursed prone. Sitting should be encouraged with the hips abducted and externally rotated. Standing balance may be, if necessary, promoted with standing apparatus but walking appliances are best avoided if possible since they tend to encourage the weight being taken through the arms rather than through the legs.

2. Orthopaedic involvement with surgical release of hip and knee contractures is indicated if useful weight bearing is feasible. Disabling foot equinus should be dealt with after correction of knee and hip flexion deformities. Disabling femoral anteversion may need an external rotation osteotomy.

PROGNOSIS

- Overall in this group 10% have mental handicap.
- 10% have fits; visual handicap due to refractive errors is relatively common.
- Speech delay is usually secondary to mental handicap.

Spastic quadriplegia

There is significant spasticity of the arms as well as of the legs.

TREATMENT

1. Movement is dominated by involuntary reflexes. Physiotherapy aims include the suppression of unwanted reflexes and the use of functional reflexes, e.g. the leg extensor thrust to facilitate standing. Acquisition of a functional gait is rare. Sitting posture to maximise head control and eye/hand coordination is central, usually involving individual prescription of an appropriate seating system. Powered mobility with an appropriate switch system should be considered.
2. Tongue thrust and exaggerated gag reflex thwart feeding and may be inhibited by desensitisation techniques.
3. Drooling can be helped in some by behavioural modification techniques and in others by posterior transposition of the submandibular ducts.

4. Regular changes in movement and posture with prone and sidelying boards may prevent 'windswept deformities' with secondary limb contractures, dislocated hips and scoliosis. Dislocating (if not dislocated) hips are painful and are less likely if the hip is maintained in external rotation and abduction. If necessary this can be facilitated by adductor tenotomy and obturator neurectomy. More extensive surgery is justified in established painful dislocations.
5. Baclofen is useful in this group of children in preventing painful flexor hip spasms.
6. A wide variety of alternative communication and educational aids is available.

PROGNOSIS

- Mental handicap is to some degree almost invariable.
- Major fits occur in 50%.
- Pseudobulbar palsy is common leading to additional difficulties with feeding, speech and middle ear disease.
- Squints occur in 50%.
- Visual handicap occurs in about 30%—half of whom have optic atrophy and half of whom are cortically blind.

Dyskinetic cerebral palsy

This refers to the combination of dystonia, chorea and athetosis, with the former usually predominating.

TREATMENT

The principles of treatment are broadly similar to those for spastic quadriplegia with inhibition of unwanted reflexes, acquisition of optimal sitting posture, prevention of secondary contractures and interfacing with appropriate aids. There is as yet no effective treatment for the suppression of unwanted movements.

PROGNOSIS

- During childhood the pattern of involuntary movements on the basis of disordered tone remains relatively static, although there have been isolated reports of further deterioration in motor function in early adult life.

- Approximately half have a normal IQ.
- 75% have speech defects of whom about one-third are non-verbal.
- Only a small proportion have fits or visual handicap.

FOLLOW-UP

Follow-up should be 6-monthly with attention to contractures, hip subluxation, spine scoliosis, visual acuity and hearing. There should also be 6-monthly developmental assessment with individual programme planning.

[1] Robinson R O *et al.* (1984) In *The Physically Handicapped Child* (McCarthy G T ed.), p. 115. London: Faber & Faber.
[2] Perlstein M *et al.* (1955) *Ann. J. Med.*, **34,** 391.
[3] Kanda T *et al.* (1984) *Dev. Med. Child Neurol.*, **26,** 438.

Guillain–Barré Syndrome

The Guillain–Barré syndrome or postinfectious polyneuritis is not rare in childhood. Clinical impressions suggest it is less severe than in adults. There is probably a male preponderance.

TREATMENT

1. Treatment is mainly supportive with physiotherapy to assist chest drainage and prevention of contractures (including ankle foot orthoses to prevent foot drop), with assisted ventilation if necessary.
2. The onset of cardiac arrhythmias may require insertion of a demand pacemaker.
3. Randomised trials suggest that plasma exchanges accelerate recovery. They may therefore have a place in the more severe cases. Steroids have not been shown to help.

PROGNOSIS

- The course of the illness is progressive weakness until a nadir is reached, followed by a plateau without further deterioration. There is then a period of recovery. The nadir is reached about 10.5 days after the onset of symptoms[1].
- Recovery starts usually within a week or two from the beginning of the period of maximum weakness. It is usually complete in 80–90%. When it is not, the duration of maximum weakness is predictive of incomplete recovery. Should 13 days elapse without improvement, there is a 56% probability of incomplete recovery: by 16 days this figure rises to 96%.
- A small proportion (less than 10%) cases also relapse (worsening before full recovery) or recur (worsening after full recovery).
- An even smaller proportion of cases (less than 5%) die either from autonomic involvement with cardiac arrhythmias, arterial pressure instability or from complications of assisted ventilation.

FOLLOW-UP

Follow-up is unnecessary after recovery but otherwise should be as required for management of disability.

[1] Eberte E *et al.* (1975) *J. Pediatr.*, **86,** 356.

Reye's Syndrome

Reye's syndrome is an acute complex disorder with hepatic dysfunction, cerebral oedema, disturbance of carbohydrate, protein and fat metabolism and clotting difficulties. The incidence is very variable. Epidemic cases in the USA follow varicella and influenza B infection. Sporadic cases appear to follow a variety of other viruses. Four case control studies have also shown an association with administration of aspirin in the prodromal period[1]. Although they inevitably suffer from the possible bias associated with voluntary case reporting, the evidence has been sufficiently suggestive for the DHSS to recommend avoiding aspirin in children less than 12 years of age. The syndrome may also be caused by organic acid, urea cycle and fatty acid oxidation disorders which contribute to the sporadic cases[2].

TREATMENT

1. Children with mild lethargy and vomiting with raised serum transaminases only require intravenous glucose with due attention to electrolyte concentrations.
2. Children with depression of consciousness sufficient to be unaware of their surroundings have several urgent and frequently simultaneous problems.

   a) Control of intracranial pressure is probably the most important problem. The advent of cerebral oedema produces life-threatening intracranial hypertension.
      i) Intracranial pressure monitoring should be instituted together with hyperventilation and boluses of mannitol for acute rises in pressure.
      ii) Barbiturate coma with EEG control may be necessary and even surgical decompression of the brain is a worthwhile consideration.
      iii) Control of intracranial pressure, while important in its own right, is only one of two determinants of cerebral perfusion – the mean arterial pressure being the other (which will also therefore require careful monitoring and management).
      iv) Cerebral oedema should be minimised by the restriction of i.v. fluids to 50 ml/kg/day.
      v) This whole complex exercise can only be carried out adequately in an intensive care setting with neurological experience.

   b) Hypoglycaemia may require correction with appropriate doses of intravenous glucose.
   c) Coagulation defects: thrombocytopenia may need correction with fresh platelet transfusions and prolonged prothrombin times may need correction with fresh frozen plasma.
   d) Hyperammonaemia: peritoneal dialysis and plasmapheresis have been advocated, but the evidence for their effect on outcome is less convincing than that for the successful control of intracranial pressure and maintenance of cerebral perfusion.

PROGNOSIS

- The prognosis depends on two factors – the clinical severity at presentation and the age of the patient (a worse outcome in the younger children).
- The overall mortality rate is quoted as around 45%.
- Figures for permanent sequelae vary widely from 10 to 50% survivors[3,4]. It seems that a relatively small proportion of survivors will be severely handicapped, but a significant proportion, depending on the length of coma, will have difficulty in one or more areas of learning. The degree of recovery over time in this latter group is not known.

FOLLOW-UP

Follow-up is unnecessary for the sporadic variety once there has been full recovery. However, if the attack was atypical (e.g. accompanied by acidosis and fits), recurrent, familial, or occurring in a young person, investigations for an underlying metabolic cause to be undertaken afterwards include blood ammonia, lactate, urinary organic acids, blood and urine amino acid chromatography.

[1] Hall S M (1986) *J. Roy. Soc. Med.*, **79,** 596.
[2] Robinson R O (1987) *Dev. Med. Child Neurol.* (in press).
[3] Crocker J (ed.) (1979) *Reye's Syndrome: Proceedings of a Symposium.* New York: Grune and Stratton.
[4] Brunner R L *et al.* (1979) *J. Pediatr.*, **99,** 706.

Von Recklinghausen's Neurofibromatosis

Von Recklinghausen's neurofibromatosis is one of the two commoner neurocutaneous syndromes with an estimated incidence of between 1:2500 and 1:3000 births. It is inherited as an autosomal dominant trait.

TREATMENT

1. Genetic counselling is based on accurate determination of the parents' status bearing in mind that at least 50% indexed cases are new mutations.
2. Many of the features of this disorder are remediable. For example morbidity from nerve tumours often arises from local pressure effects which can be relieved; optic gliomas are discussed on p. 180.
3. In view of the protean nature of this disorder and the major psychosocial burden it represents, management should ideally be concentrated in the hands of someone with a particular interest in this condition.

PROGNOSIS

- The prognosis is highly variable being determined by which of the many possible complications of this disorder are incurred by the individual patient.
- Learning disorders: attention deficits and/or specific learning disorders occur in 35% with an overall mental handicap rate of 2–5%. Speech impediments occur in 30–40%.
- CNS tumours: optic gliomas, astrocytomas, meningiomas and neurofibromas are the most common tumours. They account for a major proportion of the morbidity and are present in 5–10% patients.
- *Kyphoscoliosis* affects at least 2% with onset between 5 and 15 years of age.
- Growth disturbance

  a) Macrocephaly: the median head circumference lies on the 75th percentile.
  b) Short stature: the median height is on the 25th percentile.

- Constipation occurs in 10%.
- Neoplastic change is rare but occurs, with neurofibrosarcomas and malignant schwannomas being the two commonest types.
- In one group of clinic ascertained patients[1] 25% patients became moderately or severely affected – 30% of their life being in that state. Actuarial statistics are not available.

FOLLOW-UP

Follow-up should be 6-monthly, with investigations as indicated for symptoms. Careful examination of the spine for scoliosis and of visual acuity is mandatory.

[1] Riccardi V (1981) *New Eng. J. Med.*, **305,** 1617.

Friedreich's Ataxia

Friedreich's ataxia is the commonest of the primary neuronal degenerations. It is an autosomal recessive condition. It is diagnosed clinically by the combination of cerebellar ataxia, early loss of tendon reflexes in the legs and subsequent posterior column sensory loss.

TREATMENT

1. Pes cavus rather than neurological deterioration may be the initial predominant cause for walking difficulty. When this is the case an orthopaedic opinion should be sought for surgical stabilisation of the foot.
2. Cardiac symptoms are treated on their merits.
3. Usually parents have completed their family by the time symptoms appear. If not, they should be informed of the 1:4 recurrence risk. The risk of an affected person having an affected child is small if they marry non-consanguineously, i.e. half the carrier rate in the population (1:10).

PROGNOSIS

- The mean (± s.d.) age of onset is 10.5 ± 7.4 years[1].
- Ataxia tends to be the sole symptom for the first five years with subsequent development of dysarthria, pyramidal signs and posterior column sensory loss in all.
- The mean age of loss of walking ability is 25 years with 95% chairbound by the age of 44.
- Although optic atrophy develops in one-quarter of patients, about one-third of these have preserved visual acuity. It tends to be associated with diabetes mellitus (10% of all cases), mean age of onset 25 (± 10.6 years) and deafness (8% of all cases).

- Scoliosis develops in 80%. It is more common in those with symptoms before the age of 11 and can be rapidly progressive during growth spurts.
- Pes cavus develops in 55%.
- Cardiomyopathy: 75% develop an abnormal ECG and 40% of all cases have cardiac symptoms (dyspnoea, palpitations and angina).
- The presence of diabetes mellitus or cardiomyopathy has the strongest influence on the mode of death which usually occurs in the fourth or fifth decade. In the absence of cardiomyopathy, progressive weakness and scoliosis lead the patient to become bed-bound followed by death from infection and inanition.
- In general the outcome of pregnancy in women with Friedreich's ataxia is good[2]. Early investigation for diabetes mellitus as well as cardiovascular assessment by a cardiologist is clearly indicated.

FOLLOW-UP

Follow-up should be 6-monthly with attention paid to visual acuity, ophthalmoscopy, careful examination for scoliosis, ECG and fasting blood glucose. If scoliosis is already present, follow-up should be 3-monthly during growth spurts.

[1] Harding A E (1981) Brain, **104,** 589.
[2] MacKenzie W E (1986) Br. Med. J., **293,** 308.

Tuberous Sclerosis

Tuberous sclerosis is one of the two commonest neurocutaneous disorders. It is inherited as an autosomal dominant condition, penetrance of which may vary from an otherwise normal individual with one amelanotic naevus to a severely mentally handicapped child with intractable fits. There is an approximately 80% new mutation rate.

TREATMENT

1. Accurate genetic counselling can only be given after the status of the parents has been established. This should include careful examination (including Wood's light screening for amelanotic naevi, CT scan of the brain and ultrasound of the heart and kidneys). If neither parent has any evidence of tuberous sclerosis, their child is one of the majority with a new mutation, the recurrence risk for their future children therefore being negligible.
2. Treatment is symptomatic for the epilepsy and educational for the mental handicap.
3. Adenoma sebaceum can be disguised to some extent by suitable cosmetics, but dermabrasion or argon laser treatment are options to be considered.

PROGNOSIS

- Figures for the various manifestations of tuberous sclerosis, obtained largely from symptomatic populations, are as follows:

Epilepsy	80%
Infantile spasms	56%
Grand mal	43%
Myoclonic or	
psychomotor fits	67%
Mental handicap	60%
Adenoma sebaceum	53% by age 5
	100% by age 35[1]
Amelanotic naevi	
(present	
from infancy)	95%
Retinal phakoma	
(usually symptomless)	20%

- Hamartomas of the kidney, cardiac rhabdomyomas, lung cysts (causing pneumothorax), tubers blocking the foramen of Munro and neoplastic change in a brain tuber are all occasional complications.

FOLLOW-UP

Follow-up should be as necessary for the management of mental handicap or fits, otherwise if the child is asymptomatic, it is unnecessary.

[1] Bundey S et al. (1969) J. Neurol. Neurosurg. Psychiatr., **32,** 591.

Batten's Disease

Batten's disease is probably the most common neurodegenerative storage disorder in children in the UK. The biochemical defect has not yet been defined. The main features are blindness and dementia, often with myoclonic fits.

TREATMENT

1. On the supposition that intracellular membrane damage is due to free radical activity causing excessive lipid peroxidation[1] treatment of infantile Batten's disease with antioxidants has been proposed. This consists of:

   a) Vitamin E 0.5–1.5 g/day (to achieve serum levels of 30–45 mg/ml).
   b) Selenium 0.05–0.075 mg/kg (to achieve serum levels of 2–5 mmol/l).

2. The variability of the progress of this condition does not make assessment of the effects of drug therapy easy. This regimen seems at best to retard the rate of decline but does not defer it indefinitely.

PROGNOSIS

● The outlook is poor (see below).

	Age at onset of signs	Morbidity	Mortality
Infantile years	8–18 months	Simultaneous dementia, visual failure, ataxia and myoclonus	Vegetative by 3 years, death 3–9 years
Late infantile	1–2 years	General delay followed by visual failure	6–7 years
Juvenile	5–8 years	Visual failure followed by general delay	Late teens

FOLLOW-UP

Follow-up frequency is dictated by rapidity of decline and parents' counselling needs. Selenium levels should be monitored 6-monthly if the child is on antioxidant therapy.

[1] Santavuori P (1984) Personal communication.

Metachromatic Leukodystrophy

Metachromatic leukodystrophy is probably the second commonest neurodegenerative storage disorder of childhood in the UK. It is an autosomal recessive condition due to arylsulphatase deficiency.

TREATMENT

One isolated report[1] of a successful recipient of a bone marrow transplant who, suffering from the late infantile disorder, had not regressed by 44 months suggests a possible method of treatment.

FOLLOW-UP

Follow-up frequency is dictated by rapidity of decline and counselling needs but should be at least 4–6 monthly.

PROGNOSIS

- The prognosis is poor (see below).

---

[1] MacFaul R *et al.* (1982) *Arch. Dis. Childh.*, **57,** 168.
[2] Bayever G *et al.* (1985) *Lancet*, **ii,** 471.

	Age at onset of symptoms	Symptoms	Age at death
Late infantile	6–25 months (mean 17)	Gait disorder followed by global decline	5 months – 8 years from onset
Intermediate	4–6 years (mean 5)	Gait disorder with simultaneous educational and behavioural problems	$3\frac{1}{2}$ – more than 17 years from onset
Juvenile	6–10 years	Educational and behavioural problems followed 6 months to 4 years later by gait disorder	5–11 years from onset

Intracranial Arteriovenous Malformation

While large arteriovenous malformations may occur in infancy presenting with high output cardiac failure, the commonest presentation is somewhat later with intracranial haemorrhage.

TREATMENT

1. If the malformation is accessible and resectable (41% in one series[1]) this should be attempted for the prognosis is then excellent.
2. Selective catheterisation of feeding vessels is sometimes feasible with embolisation of the malformation.
3. Stereotactic radiosurgery is available in a few centres. Currently, it is limited to lesions less than 2.5 cm in diameter but is nevertheless an alternative when neither of the first two options is possible.
4. Finally, proton beam therapy (currently available in only two centres in the USA) appears effective in surgically unresectable lesions of more than 5 cm in diameter[2].

PROGNOSIS

- Over two-thirds of cases present with subarachnoid haemorrhage.
- The total mortality rate for 33 patients aged between 7 and 20 years was 21%[3]. 12% died as a result of the first haemorrhage. Recurrent bleeding occurred in 41% cases with a mortality rate of 25%. The remainder present with focal fits or focal headaches.
- Ischaemia of the cortex from a steal phenomenon may occasionally cause progressive cognitive deficits.

FOLLOW-UP

Follow-up should be 6-monthly if the patient is asymptomatic, with careful neurological examination, otherwise as indicated for management of disability or fits.

[1] Matson D (1969) Neurosurgery of Infancy and Childhood, 2nd edn. Springfield, Ill.: C C Thomas.
[2] Kjellberg R N et al. (1983) New Eng. J. Med., **309**, 269.
[3] Sedzimer C B et al. (1973) J. Neurosurg., **38**, 269.

11
Diseases of the Bone, Joint and Muscle

J. P. Osborne and A. E. Fryer

Systemic Onset Juvenile Chronic Arthritis

Juvenile chronic arthritis (JCA) affects 1 in 1000 children before the age of 16. Symptoms should persist for more than three months and other causes must be excluded before the diagnosis is made. Systemic onset disease is the rarest type of JCA.

TREATMENT

1. Activity and exercise should be maintained whenever possible. Bed rest, if essential because of systemic illness, severe pain or surgery, should be brief and accompanied by passive physiotherapy and splints.
2. Splints to preserve the joint in position of optimum function or serial splints to correct deformity are often essential.
3. Physiotherapy and hydrotherapy increase muscle strength and maintain joint mobility.
4. Aspirin 80 mg/kg/day is the drug treatment of choice.
5. Indomethacin 2.5 mg/kg/day can be added to aspirin if symptoms continue.
6. Ibuprofen 20 mg/kg/day can be increased to 60 mg/kg/day in severe cases intolerant of aspirin or indomethacin.
7. Steroids are only used when the above treatments fail to control the disease. Alternate day single dose treatment is best, although it takes longer to control the disease initially: it must be used for maintenance treatment. Suggested dose of prednisolone 40 mg/m²/single dose initially.
8. Gold, penicillamine and chloroquine – see *Polyarticular juvenile chronic arthritis* (p. 200). These drugs are frequently required to control joint disease[1], but do not help the systemic manifestations.
9. Surgery should be considered where appropriate.

PROGNOSIS

- The younger the child, the worse the prognosis.
- High platelet levels and high IgA levels at onset are a poor prognostic sign.
- By 3 months from onset, 50% have developed arthritis.
- Loss of systemic features and mild arthritis only after one year is a good sign.
- 50% are in complete remission 5 years after the start of symptoms.
- 40% still have active arthritis at 5 years.
- 10% experience a remitting/relapsing course at 5 years.
- Infection can be lethal early in the disease.
- Amyloidosis can be lethal when active disease persists.

FOLLOW-UP

Children should be supervised daily by parents who have been taught the appropriate exercises. In addition to medical assessment there should be frequent reassessment of the family and social background, including arrangements for schooling and psychological support if necessary. Every child, but especially those with a positive antinuclear factor (ANF), should have regular eye assessments including slit-lamp examination.

[1] Manners P J et al. (1986) Paediatrics, **77,** 99.
[2] Ansell B M (1980) Rheumatic Disorders in Childhood. London: Butterworths.

Pauciarticular Juvenile Chronic Arthritis

Juvenile chronic arthritis (JCA) affects 1 in 1000 children before the age of 16. Symptoms must have lasted for at least three months and other causes must be excluded before the diagnosis is made. Two-thirds are pauciarticular, i.e. affecting up to four joints, usually medium sized ones – particularly the knees[1].

TREATMENT

1. A full range of joint movement should be maintained if at all possible.
2. Exercise to maintain muscle strength: swimming and bicycle riding have the lowest risk of trauma.
3. Splints are used to regain a full range of movement, especially at night. Wrist splints maintain the position of optimum function. Prone-lying is useful to maintain hip extension.
4. Non-steroidal anti-inflammatory drugs prevent pain and encourage mobility: naproxen 10–15 mg/kg/day given b.d., aspirin 80 mg/kg/day given q.d.s. or benorylate 200 mg/kg/day given b.d. Indomethacin 1–1.5 mg/kg is useful as a single night dose for refractory morning stiffness.
5. Intra-articular steroid injections are reserved for persistently troublesome joints, often with large effusions which should be drained first.

PROGNOSIS

- Knees, ankles and elbows are most often affected.
- Up to 50% those with antinuclear antibodies (ANA) develop chronic iridocyclitis: especially those aged less than five years (and never after 10 years of age)[2]. Less than 10% ANA negative patients will be affected. Chronic iridocyclitis develops within 5 years in 90% those who will be affected.
- Up to 50% will be free of disease within five years.
- Long-term joint disease is rare provided contractures are prevented.
- A few patients, especially girls, gradually develop a true polyarthritis.
- A few patients have more than four joints affected but not usually all at the same time.

FOLLOW-UP

Follow-up should be regular while the disease is active with self-referral for increasing loss of range of movement and for relapses. Slit-lamp examination of the eyes should be performed every six months for five years for those who are ANA positive to exclude iridocyclitis.

[1] Ansell B M (1980) *Rheumatic Disorders in Childhood.* London: Butterworths.
[2] Leak A M *et al.* (1986) *Arch. Dis. Childh.*, **61,** 168.

Polyarticular Juvenile Chronic Arthritis[1]

Juvenile chronic arthritis (JCA) affects 1 in 1000 children before the age of sixteen. Symptoms must have lasted more than three months and other causes must be excluded before the diagnosis is made. 15% are polyarticular at onset, i.e. affect five or more joints. All joints can be affected. More girls are affected than boys.

TREATMENT

1. Activity and exercise should be maintained whenever possible. Bed rest, if essential because of systemic illness, severe pain or surgery, should be brief and accompanied by passive physiotherapy and splints.
2. Splints to preserve the joint in the position of optimum function or serial splints to correct deformity are often essential.
3. Physiotherapy and hydrotherapy increase muscle strength and maintain joint mobility.
4. Aspirin 80 mg/kg/day is the drug treatment of choice.
5. Indomethacin 2.5 mg/kg/day can be added to aspirin if symptoms continue.
6. Ibuprofen 20 mg/kg/day can be increased to 60 mg/kg/day in severe cases intolerant of aspirin or indomethacin.
7. Gold: sodium aurothiomalate 1 mg/kg/week for a minimum of six months unless severe side-effects occur (rash, proteinuria, haematuria, blood dyscrasia, jaundice or DIC) in severe persistent disease with functional or radiological deterioration, especially erosions. As rheumatoid factor negative patients have a better prognosis consider gold only if significant disease continues for some years. If treatment is effective, reduce the frequency of injections gradually, but continue for some years as relapse is not infrequent after short (six months) courses.
8. Penicillamine is probably as effective as gold but there is less experience of this drug in children. The maximum dose is 20 mg/kg/day. Proteinuria, haematuria, blood dyscrasia and nausea can occur.
9. Chloroquine phosphate 4 mg/kg/day or hydroxychloroquine 6 mg/kg/day for a maximum of two years if side-effects occur with gold or penicillamine. The eyes must be examined for retinopathy: if large doses are used this is essential. After six months continue if necessary, but reduce to alternate day dose if possible.
10. Azathioprine, chlorambucil or even cyclophosphamide may be required if amyloidosis develops or other drugs are contraindicated.

PROGNOSIS

- Older children (peak age 8–10) are usually girls. If IgM rheumatoid factor positive, the prognosis is worse – this is true juvenile rheumatoid arthritis.
- *Rheumatoid factor negative patients* can get progressive bony changes, usually symmetrical, in hands, knees and tarsus and, in 30%, the cervical spine within five years. The lower jaw may fail to grow. Persistent activity can occur into adult life with involvement of elbows, hips and shoulders, despite which function can be maintained. In general the prognosis is good. This is the commonest variety of polyarticular disease.
- In *rheumatoid factor positive patients* nodules, erosions and progressive disease occur. Tendon rupture and atlantoaxial subluxation are serious complications and hip destruction more common. Disease activity may continue throughout life: by age 15 years up to one-third have severe limitation of function.
- Amyloidosis is rare.

FOLLOW-UP

Depends on disease activity and the drugs in use. If on gold or penicillamine, check for bleeding, rashes, haematuria, proteinuria and do a full blood count every 1–2 weeks until established on treatment when monthly will suffice.

[1] Ansell B M (1980) *Rheumatic Disorders in Childhood*. London: Butterworths.

Juvenile Ankylosing Spondylitis[1]

Juvenile ankylosing spondylitis (JAS) affects 15% children with juvenile chronic arthritis. Around 80% present with peripheral joint disease before spondylitis. Enthesopathy and hip disease are suggestive of the diagnosis, especially in boys who account for 90% those affected. HLA B27 is carried by 90%; a family history of ankylosing spondylitis or acute iritis is therefore not unusual.

TREATMENT

1. Naproxen 15 mg/kg/day given b.d. or indomethacin 2.5 mg/kg/day are better than aspirin.
2. Mobility and maintenance of a full range of movement, especially of the hip and back are important.
3. Physiotherapy is essential as a means to encourage exercises, especially swimming.
4. Gold and penicillamine are not helpful.

PROGNOSIS

- Atlantoaxial subluxation can occur as the presenting feature.
- Knees and ankles usually recover fully.
- Sacroiliac x-ray changes are present in the majority after 5 years, but are difficult to interpret until after puberty.
- 25% have had acute iridocyclitis 15 years from onset.
- 60% are functioning normally 15 years from onset.
- 33% have serious hip disease 15 years from onset. Hip replacement may be required; it works best for those with loss of joint space and erosions.
- Aortic incompetence, bowel disease and amyloidosis are uncommon at 15 years.
- Long-term outlook is not known, but is thought to be no worse than that for adult-onset disease.

FOLLOW-UP

It is arguable that these patients should never be discharged from follow-up because of the potential for insidious spondylitis.

[1] Ansell B M (1980) *Rheumatic Disorders in Childhood*. London: Butterworths.

Congenital Dislocation of the Hip[1,2]

The prevalence of congenital dislocation of the hip (CDH) in unscreened populations is 1 in 1000. The prevalence of clinical instability on neonatal screening is 1 in 100. Predisposing factors include female sex (70%), breech presentation, positive family history, twins, caucasians and muscle weakness.

TREATMENT

1. Hips clearly unstable at birth should be splinted for 6 weeks, usually in an Aberdeen splint. Consideration should be given to a longer period of splinting (up to 12 weeks) and the use of the Von Rosen splint in the most unstable hips.
2. Reduction is usually obtained in late diagnosed cases under 6 months by serial splinting, abduction traction or Pavlik sling.
3. Adductor tenotomy open reduction, femoral osteotomy and acetabular reconstruction become increasingly necessary the later the diagnosis, or following failure of conservative methods of treatment.

PROGNOSIS

- Nine out of 10 hips unstable on neonatal screening become stable without treatment.
- Splinting from birth rarely causes avascular necrosis: only 1 in 100 of those splinted remains unstable, requiring surgery.
- The incidence of late CDH in those clinically stable at birth is 1 in 2000.
- Late diagnosis (outside the neonatal period) carries a good prognosis provided it is not left beyond six months.
- Cases diagnosed after six months show an increased incidence of premature osteoarthritis, avascular necrosis and pseudoarthrosis.
- Progressive deterioration continues in severe cases, usually those requiring open surgery.

FOLLOW-UP

Patients splinted from birth should be followed-up until independent stable walking is observed. X-rays should be obtained if there is any doubt at any stage. A check at six months is crucial.

[1] Dunn P M *et al.* (1985) *Arch. Dis. Childh.*, **60**, 407.
[2] Leck I (1986) *J. R. Coll. Phys. (Lond.)*, **20**, 56.

Perthes' Disease

Perthes' is a disease of unknown aetiology characterised by avascular necrosis of the femoral head. This results in a pathological subchondral fracture, which being painful, heralds the clinical onset[1]. Its prevalence is 1 in 2000, mainly affecting 4–9 year olds. It is four times commoner in boys and bilateral in up to 15% cases.

TREATMENT

1. There is no consensus view apart from the need to prevent subluxation of the femoral head[2,3].
2. Early treatment to prevent femoral head deformity is sometimes recommended in those more than six years old at onset and those with more than 50% femoral head involved as well as those with subluxation of the femoral head when weight bearing. Some form of osteotomy is the most frequent treatment.
3. Non-surgical symptomatic treatment includes traction, abduction casts or orthoses and crutches.
4. Late surgery to correct femoral neck deformity and limb length discrepancy is usually undertaken following resolution of the disease of the femoral head.
5. Hip replacement in adult life can be performed if necessary.

PROGNOSIS

- In the long term 40% have symptomatically normal hips, 40% have minor symptoms and 20% have pain or stiffness. Less than 10% require hip replacement.
- The age at onset affects outcome. No child less than five years old at onset develops significant arthritis even in the presence of significant femoral head deformity. 40% patients aged 6–9 years developed significant arthritis as did 100% of those 10 years old or more.
- Girls have more severe disease than boys.
- Femoral head deformity of more than 3 mm deviation from sphericity is a poor prognostic sign. Loss of more than 2 mm (compared to the opposite side) of head height (from base of femoral head to roof of the acetabulum) is a very poor sign[4].
- Subluxation of the femoral head is a poor sign leading to pain and loss of movement.
- It has been suggested that the extent of the femoral head involvement may be predicted from the extent of the subchondral fracture in the earliest phase of the disease.
- 50% patients have a good prognosis and require intermittent symptomatic therapy only.

FOLLOW-UP

Regular x-ray monitoring is necessary to ensure that the femoral head is not subluxing.

[1] Salter R B (1984) *J. Bone Jnt. Surg.*, **66**, 961.
[2] Lloyd–Roberts *et al.* (1976) *J. Bone Jnt. Surg.*, **58**, 31.
[3] Leader (1986) *Lancet*, **i**, 895.
[4] Hall G Personal communication.

Transient Synovitis of the Hip

Transient synovitis of the hip (irritable hip, observation hip) refers to the child presenting with pain causing restricted movement in the hip joint where other causes have been excluded. The peak age incidence is between 4 and 10 years and the aetiology is unknown. It is the commonest cause of hip pain in childhood accounting for 90% children with hip pain presenting with a limp[1]. Boys are more commonly affected than girls.

TREATMENT

1. It is essential to exclude other causes of hip pain. An x-ray of both hips (for comparison) in anteroposterior view should be normal but may occasionally show an increased joint space. In the older child frog's view should be obtained to exclude a slipped epiphysis. In all children the ipsilateral femur should be x-rayed to exclude a tumour.
2. Bed rest in order to avoid weight bearing is the mainstay of management. Traction is of little benefit except in keeping the hyperactive child in bed. Most children can therefore be managed at home.
3. When a *full* range of pain free movement is obtained, gentle mobilisation can be started.
4. Trauma, and therefore physically competitive sport, should be avoided for a few weeks following mobilisation.

PROGNOSIS

- 90% cases settle within seven days.
- Recurrence occurs in 15% cases, 40% within six months, the majority within a year. Late occurrences several years later are well recognised[2].
- The long-term prognosis in those accurately diagnosed as having transient synovitis is unknown.
- Medium term follow-up suggests there is no complication after the initial first decade[3].

FOLLOW-UP

Follow-up is unnecessary in those with a rapid and complete resolution of symptoms and signs where the initial x-ray was normal[4]. The child should be reviewed if pain or a limp recurs. Caution should be exercised in those with an insidious onset. Some patients with recurrent symptoms on repeat x-ray will be found to have Perthes' disease, where it is known that up to 30% patients may have an initial normal x-ray.

[1] Illingworth C M (1978) *Clin. Paediatr.*, **17,** 139.
[2] Illingworth C M (1983) *Arch. Dis. Childh.*, **58,** 620.
[3] Sharwood P F (1981) *Acta Orthop. Scand.*, **52,** 633.
[4] Jacobs B W (1971) *Paediatrics*, **47,** 558.

Acute Septic Arthritis

80% episodes of septic arthritis occur in the weight-bearing joints (hips, knees and ankles). 50% cases affect children aged three and younger. *Staphylococcus aureus* is the commonest pathogen at all ages but *Haemophilus influenzae* is common in children under the age of four years[1]. Beware of coincidental osteomyelitis, especially with infections of the hip joint.

TREATMENT

1. Intravenous antibiotic therapy alone is acceptable for cases presenting within 48 hours of onset except for infections of the hip. Joint aspiration for diagnostic purposes with removal of as much pus as feasible should be part of initial management.
2. Blood cultures should always be taken.
3. There is a good case for aspiration as a minimum, and preferably open surgical drainage as a primary procedure in septic arthritis of the hip[2].
4. If necessary aspiration should be repeated every 24–48 hours. If there is no improvement after 4–5 days consider open surgical drainage.
5. Antibiotic therapy should consist of ampicillin and flucloxacillin in those under four years of age and penicillin with flucloxacillin with or without fusidic acid in older children. Antibiotics should be changed when the results of cultures are known.
6. Intravenous treatment for a minimum of 48 hours or until there is clinical improvement followed by a minimum of three weeks' oral therapy is usually recommended. In refractory cases and where *Staphylococcus* is the cause, consider treatment for 6 weeks.

PROGNOSIS

- If appropriate antibiotic treatment is begun within 48 hours of onset, the outlook is excellent.
- The prognosis is not related to the causative organism except for *Gonococcus* where the outlook is good. Involvement of the hip joint has the worst prognosis: 40% hip joints are permanently affected[3].
- 30% ankle joints are permanently affected, but only 10% knee joints.

FOLLOW-UP

Regular follow-up is essential until independent walking in young children.

---

[1] Nade S (1977) *Arch. Dis. Childh.*, **52,** 679.
[2] Scoles P V *et al.* (1984) *J. Bone Jnt. Surg.*, **66,** 1487.
[3] Howard J B *et al.* (1976) *J. Am. Med. Assoc.*, **236,** 932.

Acute Osteomyelitis

Most cases (70%) occur in weight-bearing bones, predominantly the femur and tibia. It is most common in the first year of life with no age predominance thereafter. Three-quarters of all cases are due to *Staphylococcus aureus*. Boys tend to outnumber girls.

TREATMENT

1. Antibiotics to cover the most common pathogens should be started and treatment modified if necessary when the results of cultures are known.
2. In the newborn, flucloxacillin and an aminoglycoside to treat staphylococci and enterococci are usually recommended.
3. Six weeks' treatment is required with intravenous treatment for 5–7 days minimum. Group B streptococci and gonococci only need 14 days' treatment if surgical drainage has been performed.
4. In older children flucloxacillin and penicillin (100–200 mg/kg/day of each) will cover staphylococcal and streptococcal infection. If *Staphylococcus* is confirmed add fusidic acid (20 mg/kg/day i.v. or oral) in place of the penicillin. In penicillin-sensitive patients use fusidic acid and erythromycin as alternatives.
5. In patients with sickle cell disease use ampicillin to treat *Salmonella* infections.
6. Infection following penetrating trauma can be due to *Pseudomonas*. An aminoglycoside with piperacillin or ticarcillin is usually recommended, but ceftazidime is also effective.
7. In older children intravenous therapy is often only needed for 2–3 days.
8. Pain is relieved by immobilisation. Physiotherapy should begin once the pain has settled.
9. Surgery is usually indicated if symptoms have been present for more than 48–72 hours or if symptoms continue for more than 48 hours despite antibiotic therapy. Aspiration for diagnosis is important in immunocompromised patients. Vertebral osteitis is usually cured without surgery.

PROGNOSIS

- The prognosis is worse in the newborn where damage to the epiphyseal growth plate is most likely. Subsequent leg length discrepancy is common and destruction of the whole epiphyseal growth centre can occur. In infancy the growth plate is still at risk, but in older children the metaphysis is the primary site of infection.
- The primary success rate is 95% whether or not early surgical decompression is performed[1].
- Treatment within 48 hours of the onset results in complete cure without surgery in 90% cases[2].
- Treatment delayed until after three days is associated with a marked increase in the incidence of chronic osteomyelitis[3].
- Chronic osteomyelitis occurs in less than 5% cases. Presentation is often some years after the initial episode.

FOLLOW-UP

In young children follow-up is required to confirm adequate growth of the affected bone.

---

[1] Anderson J R et al. (1981) *J. Antimicrob. Chemother.*, **7**, 43.
[2] Neligan G A et al. (1965) *Br. Med. J.*, **1**, 1347.
[3] Nade S (1977) *Arch. Dis. Childh.*, **52**, 679.

Reiter's Disease

Reiter's disease is a predominantly lower limb seronegative arthropathy in association with one or more of the following: urethritis, conjunctivitis, oral ulceration or keratoderma blennorrhagica. It is rare in childhood where it usually follows acute infective bowel disease[1]. 90% carry HLA B27.

TREATMENT

1. Reiter's disease responds best to indomethacin (2.5 mg/kg/day) but mild cases may only need naproxen (10–15 mg/kg/day).
2. Steroid injections into non-responsive joints and areas of enthesopathy can be very helpful.

PROGNOSIS

- Symptoms usually develop within about 10 days and settle within one month to one year.
- Mucocutaneous symptoms settle quickly.
- Iritis is usually acute but can be persistent, requiring treatment.
- Urethritis is often mild and transient.

- Arthritis varies from a mild form affecting two or three joints to severe widespread disease.
- Recurrent attacks usually follow a further acute bowel infection.
- The long-term outlook is unknown. In adults approximately 10% will be sufficiently incapacitated in the long term to be unable to work[2].

FOLLOW-UP

Open access for recurrent attacks following recovery from the initial episode is recommended.

[1] Rosenberg A M *et al.* (1979) *Am. J. Dis. Childh.*, **133**, 394.
[2] Fisk P (1982) *Br. Med. J.*, **284**, 3.

Systemic Lupus Erythematosus

One-fifth of cases of systemic lupus erythematosus (SLE) begin in childhood. Before puberty, it is three times more common in girls; after puberty it is eight times more common. If SLE presents in very young children complement defects should be sought. Blacks are affected more frequently than whites. Drug-induced SLE can occur in childhood[1].

TREATMENT[2,3]

1. Treatment should be designed to suppress disease activity and once this has been achieved reduced to the minimum to restore normal growth and development.
2. Steroids are the mainstay of treatment. Large doses of prednisone (2 mg/kg/day) can be reduced when the disease is under control. First change to alternate day therapy using $2\frac{1}{2}$ times the previous daily dose every 48 hours in a single dose.
3. Immunosuppression with other agents is required if the disease remains uncontrolled or steroid dependence develops. Azathioprine (2.5–3.0 mg/kg/day) is the drug of choice. Cyclophosphamide can also be used but has more side-effects.
4. Plasmapheresis can be used in severe disease particularly that affecting the kidney, the CNS and for severe arteritis.
5. Antimalarial drugs can have a steroid sparing effect. Skin disease can respond rapidly (within a week) and arthritis and arthralgia may also improve. Hydroxychloroquine (6 mg/kg/day)

is usually recommended as retinal toxicity is rare at this dose[3].

6. Hypertension should be treated conventionally.

7. Infection can be difficult to diagnose and should be treated vigorously with the emphasis on microscopy and culture as unusual organisms are common. Sometimes helpful are levels of the C reactive protein which are often low in acute SLE but rise during episodes of infection.

8. Exposure to ultraviolet light exacerbates disease in up to 50% cases. Barrier creams are not always effective.

9. Patients should be strongly advised against smoking.

PROGNOSIS

- Before the use of steroids SLE in children under 12 was generally fatal.
- There is now a 90% 5-year survival. Few survivors (15%) go into complete remission, most require constant management.
- Renal involvement occurs in 80% and is closely linked with prognosis. There is a 75% 10-year survival. Proliferative glomerulonephritis and membranous nephritis are the most aggressive forms of disease.
- CNS lupus occurs in up to 50%. If due to arteritis it rapidly responds to steroids. If, however, it is due to a direct effect on neurons the prognosis is poor in the short term.
- Arthritis is common but rarely causes significant sequelae.
- Pulmonary lupus is not often troublesome in children.

- Cardiac lupus and myocardial infarction can occur in patients under 20 years of age.
- Raynaud's disease occurs in 10% cases but is not usually severe.
- Haematological abnormalities (leucopenia, thrombocytopenia and Coombs'-positive haemolytic anaemia) are common but only occasionally troublesome.
- Severe infection occurs in 20% patients at some time in their lives. All fevers should be carefully monitored for infection before it is assumed they are due to the disease process.
- Death and serious complications are frequently due to the side-effects of treatment.
- Neonatal SLE occurs following a background of high risk pregnancy with a high risk of abortion and hypertension causing growth retardation. Discoid skin lesions can occur in isolation. Haematological abnormalities occur and the most serious defect is complete heart block. This may be present antenatally and is more common in those with anti-Ro antibodies. The outlook is good but heart block is occasionally permanent.

FOLLOW-UP

Regular follow-up should be prolonged as relapses are frequent before the menopause. DNA antibody titres and complement levels as well as circulating immune complexes can herald exacerbations before clinical signs are apparent.

[1] Schaller J (1982) *Clin. Rheumatic Dis.*, **8,** 219.
[2] Kornreich H K (1976) *Clin. Rheumatic Dis.*, **2,** 429.
[3] Fleck B W *et al.* (1985) *Br. Med. J.*, **291,** 782.

Dermatomyositis

Dermatomyositis is a chronic inflammatory disease predominantly affecting muscle and skin. Arthralgia and carditis can occur and gastrointestinal vasculitis can be troublesome. Onset is usually with insidious weakness, but acute weakness can occur. Rarely the skin rash is the presenting feature: the characteristic violaceous hue is almost diagnostic. One-third of cases present in childhood when dermatomyositis is not associated with an underlying malignancy.

TREATMENT

1. Steroids are the treatment of choice. Children frequently respond to 'low dose' steroids (1–1.5 mg/kg) given daily[1]. It is often possible to reduce doses by 2.5 mg per day each week until a dose of 10 mg/day is achieved. Each week thereafter it should be possible to reduce the dose by 1 mg per day.
2. It is better to achieve adequate control of the disease initially than to continue with prolonged steroid treatment.
3. Those patients who are steroid dependent should be tried on alternate day steroids and if necessary immunosuppression with azathioprine 2.5–3.0 mg/kg given once daily.
4. Vigorous physiotherapy is essential to minimise contractures. Swimming is an excellent activity.

PROGNOSIS

- Untreated, one-third of patients die, one-third are left severely crippled and one-third survive functionally normal[2].
- With careful use of steroids, mortality is 5–10%, 10% are left severely crippled and approximately 10% remain functionally impaired.
- Death usually results from progressive weakness, gastrointestinal vasculitis or from complications of treatment, usually sepsis.
- Severe vasculitis on muscle biopsy, or when affecting the skin or in the gut is a poor prognostic sign.

- Calcinosis, when it develops, is usually evident within three years of onset. Deposits can continue to occur for some years until the disease is controlled. Although subcutaneous calcinosis can cause troublesome ulceration with extrudation of deposits, calcification within muscles is more likely to lead to permanent damage. Fascial calcification also occurs. Early use of steroids in treatment with early reduction in dose is thought to reduce the incidence of calcinosis.
- Some patients have only one attack, but 50% relapse within the first two years. Of those relapsing some respond to steroids and some have persistent disease despite steroids. The latter group has a worse prognosis[3].
- Muscle enzyme levels and the ESR are unreliable indicators of disease activity. Levels are frequently normal despite active disease and conversely may remain raised despite adequate control of disease.
- Sunlight exacerbates the skin disease and may provoke muscle relapse. However, continuing skin disease is not always associated with continuing muscle disease.

FOLLOW-UP

Follow-up is required with clinical assessment of severity until quiescent.

[1] Miller G et al. (1983) Arch. Dis. Childh., 58, 445.
[2] Malleson P (1982) J. Roy. Soc. Med., 75, 33.
[3] Spencer C H et al. (1984) J. Pediatr., 105, 399.

Myasthenia Gravis

Myasthenia gravis is rare in children who account for less than 10% cases. Three types are recognised: a) transient neonatal; b) congenital (not due to maternal antibodies: mothers are unaffected); and c) juvenile: the juvenile group includes generalised myasthenia and the purely ocular form.

TREATMENT

1. Transient neonatal

   a) Observe and monitor babies at risk on the special care unit for a minimum of three days. Edrophonium and neostigmine must be available.
   b) If symptoms develop give edrophonium 1 mg i.v. Repeat test dose if necessary; a saline control injection is often useful.
   c) Treatment can usually be continued orally (neostigmine bromide 1 mg initially increasing to 5 mg according to response). Neostigmine methylsulphate 0.1–0.25 mg i.m. may occasionally be required.
   d) Maintain adequate ventilation throughout and keep the airway clear of secretions; i.v. feeding may be required.
   e) Exchange transfusion should be considered in refractory cases and those requiring ventilation.

2. Congenital

   a) Anticholinesterase drugs as for juvenile myasthenia gravis are the mainstay of treatment. Other forms of treatment are usually of no value.
   b) Some cases are recessively inherited; genetic counselling should be sought.

3. Juvenile

   a) Admit children to hospital to start treatment, during significant illness and for all surgery.
   b) Pyridostigmine (1 mg/kg) 4-hourly or neostigmine (0.25 mg/kg) 3-hourly are the drugs of choice. Toxicity includes colic, diarrhoea, excessive salivation and respiratory difficulty. Increase the dose slowly until maximum benefit is achieved. When dysphagia is a problem, neostigmine should be used half an hour before meals (it has a more rapid onset of action than pyridostigmine). Crises due to under treatment (myasthenic) or over treatment (cholinergic) occur. When in doubt try effect of edrophonium 1 mg i.v. If doubt persists, stop all drugs and give respiratory support for 48–72 hours before restarting treatment.
   c) Cholinergic crises are treated by stopping all drugs and giving supportive treatment. Atropine (0.02–0.04 mg/kg) 4-hourly controls some side-effects.
   d) Myasthenic crises are treated by increasing anticholinesterase treatment.
   e) Steroids are indicated for seriously ill patients before thymectomy, for those responding poorly to thymectomy, those with pure ocular disease and those with a poor response to anticholinesterase treatment. Since steroids can exacerbate symptoms for 24–48 hours, patients should be admitted to hospital for the commencement of treatment. Potassium supplements *must* be given simultaneously. Improvement takes 1–6 weeks to be evident. Prednisolone 60 mg/m^2 is the usual single dose on alternate days, but i.v. methylprednisolone (2 g over 12 hours every five days for a maximum of three doses) is said to cause less exacerbation of the symptoms[1].
   f) Plasmapheresis can buy time during a crisis.
   g) Gammaglobulin (0.4 g/kg i.v. daily for five days) has been recommended in the seriously ill ventilated patient[2].
   h) Thymectomy is indicated in patients with poor control regardless of length of disease. Postoperatively patients are more sensitive to anticholinesterase drugs which should be given with care.

i) Avoid drugs which exacerbate myasthenia. These include bulk laxatives (which reduce drug absorption), quinine, propranolol, anti-arrhythmics, aminoglycosides. Diuretics causing hypokalaemia will increase muscle weakness. CNS depressants can exacerbate respiratory difficulty.

4. Ocular myasthenia

a) Pure ocular disease is treated with anticholinesterase drugs.
b) Steroids are the second line of treatment and are usually very effective.
c) Thymectomy is not indicated.

PROGNOSIS

- Transient neonatal: this occurs in 10% babies born to myasthenic mothers. Symptoms (mainly respiratory and marked hypotonia) usually start within 2–3 days (rarely up to 7 days) and last for 2–4 weeks. Prognosis for neuromuscular function is normal. Contractures are rare.
- Congenital: predominant symptoms are ocular. Generalised weakness, bulbar involvement and respiratory difficulty are usually mild. Death is uncommon, although spontaneous improvement is unusual and response to treatment frequently poor and unreliable.
- Juvenile: this runs a fluctuating course with symptoms frequently worse later in the day, after exercise and just prior to menstruation. Exacerbations are precipitated by infections, surgery and some drugs.

a) 40% patients develop respiratory compromise at some stage.
b) Overall 80% children survive to 40 years of age.
c) Spontaneous remission or improvement occurs in 30–60% patients who have not undergone thymectomy.
d) Thymectomy results in remission or improvement in 80% cases. Most remissions occur in the first year after thymectomy but several years may pass before the maximal effect is seen. Bulbar symptoms, other autoimmune disease, and thymectomy within 12 months of onset of symptoms all favourably affect the response to thymectomy[3].
e) There is an increased incidence of other autoimmune diseases, seizures and neoplasia.

FOLLOW-UP

Regular follow-up is required over many years for congenital and juvenile myasthenia gravis.

[1] Arsura E et al. (1985) Arch. Neurol., **42,** 1149.
[2] Ippoliti G et al. (1984) Lancet, **ii,** 809.
[3] Rodriquez M et al. (1983) Ann. Neurol., **13,** 504.

Osteogenesis Imperfecta

Osteogenesis imperfecta or brittle bone disease is a heterogeneous group of disorders of collagen, resulting in a high risk of fractures. It occurs overall in 1:10 000 live births. The prognosis and treatment is related to the type of disease and hence the severity[1].

TREATMENT

1. There is no effective drug treatment.
2. Physiotherapy is important. Exercise should be encouraged since the resulting increase in muscle mass decreases the number of fractures. The most severe cases can only undertake light exercise, but swimming is helpful for all patients. Immobilisation for any reason should be kept to a minimum.
3. Braces and splints should be used to aid ambulation both regularly in those with severe disease and to reduce the time a limb requires immobilisation following a fracture. As soon as adequate callus has formed mobilisation should be encouraged with the use of a splint.
4. Surgery may be required to straighten deformities resulting from fractures. In addition, intramedullary rod fixation can be used for internal splinting to reduce recurrent fracturing. This is most often required in the lower limbs and deformity from previous fractures can be corrected at the same time. In the upper limb surgery is rarely indicated because great deformity is compatible with good function[2].
5. Deafness is frequently conductive and ossicular reconstruction and stapedectomy can help. Hearing aids should also be considered.
6. Attention should be given to appropriate dental care because of coincident dentigenosis imperfecta.
7. Stool softeners with or without stimulant laxatives may be needed to combat the frequently seen constipation.
8. Genetic counselling is complicated and important. It is important to look for signs of mild disease in other members of the family who should have skull x-rays to look for wormian bones. In at-risk pregnancies, prenatal diagnosis by ultrasound is possible from 16 weeks. DNA collagen gene probes are now available and may help diagnose some types of osteogenesis imperfecta. The lethal variety (type II) is usually sporadic but occasional recessive cases occur.

PROGNOSIS

- The majority (80%) cases are type I. Inheritance is autosomal dominant with occasional new mutations. The disease is relatively mild with fractures occurring more frequently in childhood. Scoliosis occurs in 20% and can be significant. Ultimate stature is nearly normal. Deafness increases with age from 7% in childhood to more than 50% by 50 years.
- Lethal disease (type II) has at least two subgroups (broad boned and thin boned). The patients have grossly deformed skeletons and die at or near birth.
- Type III disease is a heterogeneous group of patients with severe disease who survive the neonatal period. Deformity is progressive and most never walk unaided. Growth is severely limited and death may occur in early childhood often from respiratory infections.
- Type IV disease is rare. It is dominantly inherited but the bone disease is more severe than type I and also stature is considerably reduced. The sclerae are of normal colour in this type.
- If a child is born with fractures (this can occur with all types) the chances of survival are poor if the fractures are numerous, affect the ribs and if there is defective skull ossification.

FOLLOW-UP

Long-term survivors with moderate or severe disease require a multidisciplinary approach with regular physiotherapy and braces, splints and surgery as indicated.

[1] Smith R (1984) Br. Med. J., **289**, 394.
[2] Root L (1984) In Orthopaedics: Metabolic Bone Disease (Lane J M ed.), p. 775. Philadelphia: Saunders.

Familial Periodic Paralysis

This is a rare group of diseases, usually autosomal dominant in inheritance but occasionally sporadic in adults. Brief self-limiting episodes of muscle paralysis occur.

TREATMENT

1. Hypokalaemic patients are treated with oral potassium chloride (3–10 g). Prophylaxis with Slow K and/or acetazolamide is usually effective.
2. Hyperkalaemic attacks usually require no treatment. If required calcium gluconate 10% is safer than glucose and insulin. An inhalation with salbutamol is rapidly effective[1]. Thiazides are also effective.
3. Normokalaemic patients respond to sodium chloride. Prevention with acetazolamide and fludrocortisone is effective.

PROGNOSIS

- Hypokalaemic periodic paralysis[2]

    a) Attacks last several hours.
    b) Speech and breathing are maintained.
    c) A heavy carbohydrate meal or rest following exercise precipitates attacks.
    d) A progressive myopathy after repeated attacks is preventable by good control.

- Hyperkalaemic periodic paralysis[3]

    a) Attacks begin by 5 years in 50% and by 10 years in 100%.
    b) Carbohydrate meals are protective.
    c) Rest after exercise precipitates attacks.
    d) Initially attacks last only a few minutes but become longer in adolescence and improve in adult life.
    e) Myotonia occurs on exposure to cold.

- Normokalaemic periodic paralysis[4] is rare and severe with attacks lasting several days.

FOLLOW-UP

Follow-up should be aimed at preventing attacks. Mild cases can be seen when necessary.

[1] Wang P et al. (1976) Lancet, i, 221.
[2] Johnson T (1981) Dan. Med. Bull., 28, 1.
[3] Gamstorp H et al. (1957) Am. J. Med., 23, 385.
[4] Poskanzer D C et al. (1961) Am. J. Med., 31, 328.

Duchenne Muscular Dystrophy

Duchenne muscular dystrophy affects 1 in 3000 boys. It is X-linked but new mutations are frequent. Serum creatinine phosphokinase levels are grossly elevated[1].

TREATMENT

1. The muscle disease is progressive and untreatable.
2. Prevention of deformities is best achieved by maintaining walking for as long as possible. Leg callipers can prolong walking for 2–3 years and rolators may help further.
3. Once walking is lost spinal bracing, usually with a lightweight jacket, is important. The prevention of foot deformity maintains comfort. Attention to detail of posture in a wheelchair is essential. Surgery to the spine is not usually recommended in the UK[2] but is used in the USA[3].
4. Avoid immobility: muscle power is rapidly lost never to be regained following even brief periods of immobility.
5. The families should be referred to a genetic clinic for evaluation of recurrence risks. DNA probes can help to quantify risks in the extended family.

PROGNOSIS

- Mild mental retardation is common; the average IQ is 80%.
- Delayed motor milestones occur in one-third of cases.
- Gower's sign (using the hands to climb up the legs and therefore extend the back) occurs by 4–6 years of age.
- Most patients are unable to walk by 8–11 years. If still walking at 12–13 years Becker dystrophy is a more likely diagnosis.
- Inability to self propel a wheelchair occurs by 13–14 years.
- Scoliosis occurs rapidly once walking is lost, as do contractures of the hip flexors, Achilles tendon, knee flexors and feet (equinovarus deformity).
- Swallowing, facial and ocular muscles and continence are preserved.
- Respiratory disease is the commonest cause of death: cardiac disease may also be a terminal event, due to arrhythmias because of the underlying cardiomyopathy.
- Death occurs between 14 and 20 years in most cases.

FOLLOW-UP

Regular follow-up by a multidisciplinary team is essential.

---

[1] Gardner–Medwin D (1977) *Br. J. Hosp. Med.*, **17,** 314.
[2] Gardner–Medwin D (1979) *Dev. Med. Child Neurol.*, **21,** 659.
[3] Shapiro F *et al.* (1982) *J. Bone Jnt. Surg.*, **64,** 1102.

Spinal Muscular Atrophy

Spinal muscular atrophy (SMA) is a group of disorders, genetically determined, characterised by death of the anterior horn cell with consequent denervation of the muscle motor spindle. It affects both sexes with a frequency of 1 in 10 000[1].

TREATMENT

1. Respiratory disease must be treated energetically, with antibiotics and physiotherapy.
2. Independent walking should be maintained as long as possible. This helps prevent development of scoliosis.
3. Wheelchairs must then be provided; at this stage spinal jackets are frequently required.
4. Scoliosis develops early – average age of seven years, but later in those who maintain walking. It causes considerable discomfort and significantly reduces lung function.
5. Scoliosis surgery prevents the lordotic posture required for independent walking and is usually delayed until walking is lost. It may reduce wheelchair mobility slightly[2].
6. Spinal fusion should be considered before respiratory function is less than 30% of normal in order to prevent further deterioration.
7. Anterior spinal fusions risk reducing the effectiveness of the diaphragm and should be avoided[3].
8. Posterior spinal fusion usually requires simultaneous Harrington rod instrumentation to provide stability.
9. The disease is usually inherited recessively with rare dominant cases. Affected siblings usually follow the same clinical course but not necessarily so. Type I and type III disease have occurred in the same family.

PROGNOSIS

- Type I (Werdnig–Hoffmann disease) presents in the first year, is inexorably progressive and death occurs within three years, often in the first year.
- Type II (intermediate) can present in the first year. Symptoms usually develop within two years and run a more protracted, intermittently downhill course with survival beyond four years, usually to adolescence, occasionally later.
- Type III (Kugelberg–Welander disease) presents with delayed motor milestones or later with an abnormal gait. Progression is mild, often intermittent, with loss of independent walking after prolonged immobilisation, often at puberty and usually by the end of the third decade. Postural deformity of the spine and feet are frequent, increasing with age.
- Death is usually due to respiratory disease. The intercostal muscles deteriorate early, the diaphragm late.
- Swallowing is maintained until late except in Fazio-Londe disease. This is a rare type of SMA which affects the motor nuclei of the brain stem.

FOLLOW-UP

Regular follow-up every 6–12 months should include lung function studies and assessment of scoliosis.

[1] Gardner-Medwin D (1977) Br. J. Hosp. Med., **17,** 314.
[2] Aprin H et al. (1982) J. Bone Jnt. Surg., **64,** 1179.
[3] Shapiro F et al. (1982) J. Bone Jnt. Surg., **64,** 785.

Ewing's Sarcoma[1]

Ewing's sarcoma is a primary malignant bone tumour, with peak incidence in the second decade. Metastatic disease, usually in the lungs or bones, is present in 15–20% cases at diagnosis.

TREATMENT

1. Treatment is usually in specialist centres involved in multicentre trials.
2. Treatment of the primary tumour is by radiotherapy or surgery (amputation or excision of entire bone). Surgery is frequently used for expendable bones (e.g. fibula or ribs), lesions of the feet or hands which may be functionally impaired by radiotherapy, resectable pelvic lesions and in young children where radiotherapy would involve the epiphyseal plate of a long bone causing an excessive leg length discrepancy.
3. Radiotherapy (often 5000–5500 cGy over 5–6 weeks) with adjuvant chemotherapy controls local disease in more than 90% cases affecting the leg. Complications include unequal growth, joint deformity, fractures, soft tissue changes and secondary neoplasia.
4. Late recurrences do occur and chemotherapy is primarily aimed at preventing this. Effective drugs in combination include vincristine, actinomycin D, cyclophosphamide, doxorubicin (adriamycin), VP 16 and cisplatin. Prophylactic pulmonary radiation is occasionally recommended.
5. Complete remission in relapsed unresponsive patients has been achieved with cyclophosphamide, melphalan and autologous bone marrow transplantation.

PROGNOSIS

- Before the advent of radiotherapy there was a 20% five-year survival.
- The most important prognostic feature is the site of the primary tumour: the three-year survival rate for tumours of the distal extremity is 68%, the ribs 50%, and pelvis 40%.
- Other factors said to be of prognostic significance include the lymphocyte count (a high count is favourable), the neutrophil count (a high count is unfavourable) and the time from onset of symptoms to diagnosis (less than one month is favourable). A raised serum lactate dehydrogenase is thought by some to be unfavourable.

FOLLOW-UP

Initial monthly chest x-rays are required.

[1] Jaffe N (1985) *Pediatr. Clin. North Am.*, **32**, 801.

Osteosarcoma

This is a primary malignant bone tumour with a peak incidence in the second decade. It is commoner in boys. There are 200 cases per year in the UK[1]. It is a rapidly growing tumour and gross metastatic disease in lung and/or bone is present in 10–20% at diagnosis. 80% are thought to have micrometastases at presentation. It is often seen as a second tumour in cases of familial retinoblastoma.

TREATMENT

1. Treatment is usually in specialist centres involved in multicentre trials.
2. Amputation was the treatment of choice for the primary tumour. Now limb-sparing operations are advocated where possible.
3. A current European study includes chemotherapy both preoperatively and postoperatively and where possible conservative surgery. Cisplatin, doxorubicin and high dose methotrexate are the most commonly used agents. Where one or two pulmonary metastases are present or develop, local resection and chemotherapy is usually advocated. Occasionally multiple metastases can be removed.
4. In patients with advanced disease at presentation, palliative amputation will prevent painful local recurrence.

PROGNOSIS

- Prognosis has improved dramatically in the last 15 years, although optimum therapy has not necessarily been found.
- Before 1972, five-year survival was 20%[2].
- During the 1970s, five-year survival improved to 50–60% whether or not patients received chemotherapy.
- Adjuvant chemotherapy has increased survival further[3].

- Adverse prognostic factors include:

  a) Age less than 10 years.
  b) Male sex.
  c) Tumour diameter more than 15 cm.
  d) Duration of symptoms less than 2 months.
  e) Involvement of femur or humerus.
  f) Cell type – osteoblastic or chondroblastic.

- Gross metastatic disease at initial diagnosis carries a long-term survival rate of 10–20%. Patients with bony metastases do less well.
- Where relapses occur, 80% are in the lung only. 90% occur within two years of diagnosis.
- First relapses after five years are unusual. Aggressive treatment of pulmonary relapse has resulted in a 40% survival in this group. 90% survivors received chemotherapy as well as resection of the pulmonary metastases.

FOLLOW-UP

Initially monthly chest x-rays are required to look for metastases.

[1] Editorial (1985) *Lancet*, **ii**, 131.
[2] Goorin A M *et al.* (1985) *New Eng. J. Med.*, **313,** 1637.
[3] Link M P *et al.* (1986) *New Eng. J. Med.*, **314,** 1600.

12

Diseases of the Eye

J. O'Day and G. W. Harley

Refractive Disorders in Childhood[1-6]

Myopia

20% children will become shortsighted by late adolescence. Myopia is often first detected at school when a child has difficulty seeing writing on the blackboard. Onset of myopia is commonly after the age of six years. Occasionally it is present at birth when the error is usually quite high and is non-progressive. Myopia is often bilateral and is not usually associated with degenerative changes in the eye.

Pathological myopia

TREATMENT

1. Spectacle correction is usually necessary to improve distance vision.
2. Contact lenses are not usually prescribed for young children because of the difficulties in lens maintenance and the changing refractive error.

PROGNOSIS

- It is not possible to predict which myopic child will develop pathological myopia. However, it is more common with high myopic errors.
- A small number of children who develop myopia will go on to progressive enlargement of the globe with thinning of the retina and choroid. Focal areas of atrophy may develop in the choroid and retina particularly around the optic nerve head and the macula. There is often associated degeneration of the vitreous and peripheral retina with increased risk of retinal detachment. Premature macular degeneration may lead to loss of central vision. These complications tend to occur in adult life.
- There is no evidence that constant wearing of spectacles or eye exercises will reduce the final myopic refractive error.

Unilateral myopia

TREATMENT

1. Spectacles are prescribed to correct the refractive error.

2. The normal eye is patched to improve the vision in the amblyopic eye.
3. Once the vision is improved the spectacles are worn with periodic vision checks until the vision remains stable.

PROGNOSIS

- When one eye is significantly myopic and the other has normal vision within the first six years of life, then amblyopia (lazy eye) may occur.

Hypermetropia

75% all newborns are long sighted (hypermetropic) at birth. This refractive error diminishes, although 50% adults still remain a little hypermetropic.

TREATMENT

Prescribe spectacles to correct moderate to severe hypermetropia which will give clear vision and permit single binocular fusion reflexes to develop.

PROGNOSIS

- Infants have great powers of accommodation and may overcome up to 10 dioptres of hypermetropia. However, this rapidly diminishes over the next few years and significant degrees of hypermetropia will require spectacle correction in childhood.
- Minor degrees of hypermetropia will lead to the patient requiring spectacle correction for reading at an earlier age.
- The condition is usually bilateral, however, if the error is greater in one eye, then amblyopia will develop if spectacle correction is not worn.

Astigmatism

Astigmatism causes an image to be blurred both in the distance and near. This may arise from an abnormality in any of the refracting elements.

However, nearly all cases arise from an alteration in the curvature of the cornea, being steeper in one meridian than another. The eye is shaped more like a lemon than an orange. There may be hypermetropia or myopia present as well.

TREATMENT

1. Prescribe spectacles.
2. The major factor is to make sure the axis of the cylindrical correction is accurate.

PROGNOSIS

- The condition is usually bilateral. However, if astigmatism is present in one eye then amblyopia will develop if spectacle correction is not instituted.

- Minor degrees of bilateral astigmatism require no treatment.
- Astigmatism is present from birth and in many children will disappear in the first six years of life. In other children with astigmatism the axis and degree will remain constant unless modified by disease, trauma or surgery.

[1] Harley R D (1983) *Pediatric Ophthalmology*, 2nd edn, ch. 10, p. 11. Philadelphia: Saunders.
[2] Duke-Elder S *et al.* (1978) *Practice of Refraction*, 9th edn, p. 67. Edinburgh: Churchill Livingstone.
[3] Curtain B J (1985) *The Myopias: Basic Science and Clinical Management*. Philadelphia: Lippincott.
[4] Stewart-Brown S (1985) *Br. J. Ophthalmol.*, **69,** 847.
[5] Ingram R M *et al.* (1986) *Br. J. Ophthalmol.*, **70,** 16.
[6] Gwiazda J *et al.* (1984) *Invest. Ophthalmol. Vis. Sci.*, **25,** 88.

Strabismus[1-5]

Strabismus (squint) is present when the axis of alignment of the eyes is not parallel and there is a deviation either inwards (esotropia), or outwards (exotropia) from the line of visual fixation. Vertical deviations also occur. Many children with straight eyes appear to have a convergent squint due to prominent epicanthic folds. 3% children have strabismus. The most common type is non-paralytic, where there is a full range of ocular movements with deviation present in all directions of gaze. Diplopia does not occur in young children since there is suppression of the image from the deviating eye. Strabismus may be latent and only revealed when the stimulus of binocular vision is suppressed such as in the alternate cover test. Alternatively, it may be present constantly or intermittently. Infants develop coordinated eye muscle movement at 3–5 months.

TREATMENT (principles)

1. Regardless of age, all children in whom strabismus is suspected should be examined carefully to exclude:

   a) An underlying disease, e.g. retinoblastoma.
   b) Refractive error.
   c) Amblyopia.

2. The establishment of good visual acuity in both eyes and binocular vision.
3. The realignment of the eyes in a good position for cosmetic purposes.

Congenital convergent squint (esotropia)

Congenital esotropia presents in the first six

months of life and is occasionally associated with weakness of the lateral rectus muscle.

TREATMENT

1. Refractive error and eye disease must be excluded; an examination of the child is performed using atropine to dilate the pupil and paralyse accommodation (cycloplegia). Under 12 months of age atropine 0.5% drops are put in both eyes three times a day for three days prior to the examination. In older children, particularly with dark irides atropine 1% is used. The reduced dosage of atropine in young children lowers the risk of systemic toxicity.
2. Surgical correction of the squint. This involves either recessing both medial recti or operating on one eye and recessing the medial rectus and resecting the lateral rectus.
3. Best results are obtained if the eyes are aligned before the age of 18 months. More than one operation may be necessary.

PROGNOSIS

- There is usually a large angle of deviation.
- The likelihood of a full binocular fusion reflex developing is small, even when surgery is performed at a very early age.

Acquired convergent squint

An acquired convergent squint usually commences between the ages of two and four years. The angle of deviation is often greater for near than far distance. There is often associated hypermetropia and amblyopia.

TREATMENT

1. Refraction under cycloplegia – atropine is used as above.
2. If the child is hypermetropic, spectacles are prescribed. This may control the squint.
3. If one eye is amblyopic then patching or some other form of fogging of the vision of the other eye is performed until the vision is equal in both eyes, or the squint becomes alternating in children too young to test.

4. Strabismus surgery may be required (same as for *Congenital convergent squint*) when the refractive error and amblyopia have been corrected.

PROGNOSIS

- Without treatment the condition will remain unchanged.

Divergent squint (exotropia)

TREATMENT

1. Cycloplegic refraction (see above) is performed and any necessary spectacles prescribed.
2. Amblyopia is less common in exotropia than esotropia. However if present, the eye with the better vision is patched until vision is equal in both eyes.
3. Surgical correction with recession of the lateral recti or resection of the medial recti is performed depending on the size of the squint and whether the squint is larger for near or far distance.

PROGNOSIS

- Exotropia is less common than esotropia in childhood.
- Exotropia may be latent or manifest, and present predominantly for near or for distance vision. When exotropia is present in far distant vision the child will often close one eye when outside and this is a common presenting symptom. The squint may not be revealed unless the child fixates on an object well beyond six metres.
- Condition tends to worsen with time.

Vertical deviation

TREATMENT

1. A small vertical deviation without diplopia will require no treatment.
2. Children with complicated vertical deviations due to oculomotor palsies with diplopia or abnormal head posture, require careful assessment and appropriate surgery.

PROGNOSIS

- Particularly in patients with congenital convergent squint whose eyes have been horizontally aligned, vertical deviation may become apparent when the eyes are dissociated. Most of these do not require surgical treatment.
- If there is inferior oblique muscle overaction the adducting eye will deviate upwards. If the condition is bilateral a 'v' pattern will be present with the eyes turned in maximally in downgaze.

[1] von Noorden G K, Burian H M (1980) *Binocular Vision and Ocular Motility: Theory and Management of Strabismus*, 2nd edn. St Louis: Mosby.
[2] Publications Committee (1971) *Symposium of Strabismus*. New Orleans Academy of Ophthalmology. St Louis: Mosby.
[3] Parks M M (1975) *Ocular Motility and Strabismus*. Hagerstown, Md: Harper and Row.
[4] Crawford J S et al. (1983) *The Eye in Childhood*. New York: Grune and Stratton.
[5] Reinecke R D (1982) *Strabismus 11*. New York: Grune and Stratton.

Blepharitis[1]

Blepharitis is a condition characterised by hypertrophy and desquamation of the epidermis near the lid margin leading to erythema and scaling of the lids. This lesion is subject to infection and ulceration and to closure of the glands supplying the hair follicles causing a stye, or to closure of the meibomian glands leading to a meibomian cyst.

TREATMENT

1. Thoroughly clean the scale away from the eyelashes. This is best done with a moist cotton bud and if there is any difficulty in removing the scale, baby shampoo or similar astringent can be used on the tip of a cotton bud and then washed away. This needs to be done as often as the scale recurs and it may be necessary in the early stages to do it three times a day.
2. Topical antibiotic drops or ointment. The most usual commensal organism is *Staphylococcus aureus* which is sensitive to a wide variety of antibiotics including chloramphenicol and neomycin.
3. Topical steroid preparations (e.g. prednisolone acetate eye drops) are used if there is an allergic or inflammatory response. These can be used three times a day.

PROGNOSIS

- There are two main types of blepharitis. Ulcerative blepharitis often begins in childhood, is due to a staphylococcal infection and there may be an associated low-grade conjunctivitis. Squamous blepharitis occurs from adolescence onwards and is associated with dandruff and seborrhoeic dermatitis. Occasionally there is a combination of the two. In both cases symptoms are likely to recur and treatment will control rather than eradicate the disease. Intense treatment is needed during exacerbations.
- Occasionally a third cause of blepharitis are chemical irritants such as eye drops or cosmetics. This allergic response will be prevented by banning the offending irritant.

FOLLOW-UP

No routine follow-up is necessary.

[1] Dougherty J M et al. (1984) *Br. J. Ophthalmol.*, **68**, 524.

Chalazion

A chalazion (meibomian cyst) is a lipogranuloma of the meibomian gland. It produces a swelling in the eyelid which tends to point inwards.

TREATMENT

1. Topical antibiotics (e.g. neomycin, chloramphenicol or sulphafurazole) are often used to prevent secondary infection.
2. Surgical incision (with curettage) through the tarsal plate from the conjunctival surface may be necessary.

PROGNOSIS

- A chalazion usually begins as a small nodule and enlarges slowly without acute pain or inflammation.
- It may rupture, or persist leaving a lump requiring curettage. In children, slow resolution without intervention is common.
- There is a tendency to recurrence in other meibomian glands.

FOLLOW-UP

Follow-up to check for recurrence.

Hordeolum (Stye)

A stye is an acute infection of the gland of Zeis which is related to the lash follicle and appears on the anterior surface of the eyelid.

TREATMENT

1. Topical antibiotics (e.g. chloramphenicol or neomycin ointment) combined with hot compresses.
2. If this fails, surgical incision with drainage may be necessary.

PROGNOSIS

- A stye appears over a matter of hours or days with pain and inflammation. It usually ruptures spontaneously leaving no residual lump.

FOLLOW-UP

No follow-up is required.

Nasolacrimal Duct Obstruction[1]

Nasolacrimal duct obstruction is commonly caused by a failure of canalisation of the duct and the most common site of blockage is at the lower end of the duct. The condition is characterised by persistent or recurrent discharge from the affected eye.

TREATMENT

1. During exacerbations treatment with antibiotic drops such as neomycin, framycetin or chloramphenicol is used empirically.
2. Frequent massage over the lacrimal sac to express retained secretions.
3. Probing of nasolacrimal duct under general anaesthesia. This will need to be carried out if there is no spontaneous resolution after the infant is four months old, particularly if there is a copious discharge.
4. Rarely, probing the nasolacrimal duct is not sufficient and a more complicated procedure such as dacrocystorhinostomy is performed in which an opening is made between the lacrimal sac and the nose directly. Intubation of the lacrimal passages is sometimes a feasible alternative.

PROGNOSIS

- Approximately 6% fullterm infants are affected. There is often a membrane across the opening which may spontaneously open in the first six months of life.

FOLLOW-UP

Routine surveillance of the infant.

[1] Ernest J T (1985) *The Year Book of Ophthalmology*, ch. 1, p. 15. Chicago: Year Book Medical Publishers Inc.

Conjunctivitis

Conjunctivitis is usually a benign self-limiting condition characterised by a watery or purulent discharge with conjunctival injection requiring no specific treatment beyond topical antibiotics. Neonatal conjunctivitis should be considered separately since there are two causes of conjunctivitis requiring specific treatment, i.e. gonorrhoea or chlamydial infection.

Gonococcal conjunctivitis

Gonococcal conjunctivitis is caused by neonatal infection within the mother's birth canal and presents in the first two to five days after birth as a profuse mucopurulent discharge.

TREATMENT

1. Conjunctival swab with Gram stain and culture to detect the Gram-negative diplococci.
2. Penicillin 50 000 U/kg/day intravenously. Cefuroxin or spectinomycin may be necessary for β-lactamase-producing organisms.
3. Sulphacetamide eye drops hourly as soon as the diagnosis of gonococcal conjunctivitis is suspected.
4. Treat in isolation.

PROGNOSIS

- Corneal involvement may rapidly cause corneal ulceration, perforation and blindness unless adequate treatment is commenced immediately.

FOLLOW-UP

Must include treatment of parents.

Chlamydial conjunctivitis

Chlamydial conjunctivitis causes approximately 20% cases of neonatal conjunctivitis. It often starts two or three weeks after birth and may be associated with infection of the respiratory tract and other sites.

TREATMENT

Erythromycin 50 mg/kg/day for 14 days, and sulphacetamide drops (20%) 2-hourly, or tetracycline ointment four times a day.

FOLLOW-UP

Must include treatment of parents.

Acute bacterial conjunctivitis

Bacterial conjunctivitis should be suspected when there is production of a mucopurulent discharge in association with conjunctival injection. *Pneumococcus* and *Staphylococcus* are the most likely infecting organisms. Visual acuity is normal and any age group may be affected. Both eyes are normally involved.

TREATMENT

1. In severe cases take adequate conjunctival swabs before commencement of treatment.
2. There is no common consensus regarding the best eye drop preparations to use before the results of culture and sensitivity are known. Broad spectrum cover is suggested.

FOLLOW-UP

Epidemic spread must be prevented especially in institutions. Particular care must be taken with dirty cotton swabs, towelling, bedclothes and the tip of the antibiotic dropper.

Adenovirus conjunctivitis

Viral conjunctivitis may commence in one eye but usually becomes bilateral and is associated with ocular irritation and watery discharge. The conjunctiva is injected and follicles are seen in the conjunctiva particularly beneath the tarsal plate. Conjunctivitis may occur in association with an upper respiratory tract infection.

TREATMENT

Antibiotic drugs are often prescribed but are not essential since the risk of secondary bacterial infection is small.

PROGNOSIS

- The disease is usually benign and self-limiting.
- There can be secondary involvement of the cornea with punctate epithelial opacities. These may remain for months to years.

Trachoma

Trachoma is conjunctival infection with an organism of the genus *Chlamydia*. It is the world's most prevalent eye disease.

TREATMENT

1. Improved living standards and hygiene are the greatest factors in eradication of the disease or prevention of repeated attacks, together with eradication of the fly which is the vector for spread of the disease.
2. Local: terramycin ointment three times a day for 3–4 weeks.
3. Systemic sulphonamides.
4. Surgical treatment of lid deformities is necessary to prevent further corneal ulceration, to relieve pain and discomfort and to make the eye less watery and therefore less attractive to flies.

PROGNOSIS

- Worldwide about 500 million people are affected, of whom 100 million suffer some visual handicap and at least 2 million become totally blind. It vanished from Europe after the arrival of better housing and hygiene.

- Children frequently have attacks. Loss of vision is due to primary corneal involvement followed by secondary corneal damage caused by scarred upper eyelids with inturned lashes traumatising the cornea with each blink. Secondary bacterial infection is common causing further damage to the eye.

FOLLOW-UP

Since recurrence is so common, regular follow-up is important.

Herpes simplex

Herpes simplex may produce a follicular form of conjunctivitis indistinguishable from other forms of viral conjunctivitis. Look for small skin vesicles around the eyes. Following secondary infection dendritic corneal ulcers may occur. It usually only affects one eye.

TREATMENT AND PROGNOSIS

See *Corneal ulceration* (p. 229).

Herpes zoster ophthalmicus

If the ophthalmic division of the fifth nerve is infected by herpes zoster ocular involvement may occur. This is rarely seen in children unless they have compromised immune function, e.g. in leukaemia.

TREATMENT

1. Uveitis

    a) Steroid eye drops (e.g. prednisolone) up to hourly depending on the severity of the inflammation. Be certain of the diagnosis before starting this treatment because other viral diseases of the cornea are aggravated by steroids.
    b) Consider topical acyclovir ointment five times a day as an alternative to topical steroids.
    c) Pupil dilatation, e.g. homatropine 2% drops four times a day.

2. Glaucoma

    a) Acetazolamide (Diamox) 15 mg/kg/day in divided dosage.
    b) Timolol maleate (Timoptol) 0.5% twice daily eyes drops.

3. Consider topical acyclovir ointment five times a day as an alternative to the topical steroids in the management of iritis.

PROGNOSIS

- Herpes zoster may cause a punctate keratitis, iritis, glaucoma, optic neuritis and cranial nerve palsies.
- Fortunately, only a small proportion of those patients with herpes zoster involving the first division of the ophthalmic nerve develop eye inflammation.

FOLLOW-UP

Post-herpetic neuralgia should be treated with carbamazepine orally.

Allergic Keratoconjunctivitis (Vernal, Atopic)[1-3]

Allergic keratoconjunctivitis is a reaction involving the conjunctiva particularly beneath the tarsal plate and in more severe cases with an oval corneal ulcer which is typically in the upper half of the cornea. Patients with this condition often complain of itching of the eyes, watering, photophobia and have an allergic diathesis. Mild cases of allergic conjunctivitis associated with slight itching and soreness of the eyes are often misdiagnosed as having minor refractive errors and given spectacles which are of no help.

TREATMENT

1. Mild: eyedrops containing antihistamines and a decongestant four times a day may be sufficient to control the mild cases.
2. Moderate: if symptoms are more severe sodium cromoglycate eye drops are used four times a day producing symptomatic relief. The drops prevent mast cell degranulation and consequent histamine release.
3. Severe

   a) Combine above treatment with corticosteroid eye drops which need to be given frequently.
   b) Often there is an increased production of sticky mucus which can be hydrolysed with acetylcysteine eye drops 5% or 10% used every hour.
   c) The mucus plaque associated with the corneal ulcer will usually settle down when the corneal disease is improving. Occasionally a superficial keratectomy will be required to remove the plaque.

PROGNOSIS

- For the mild cases the prognosis is excellent. In the more severe cases the condition is likely to be recurrent. Large corneal plaques may lead to permanent corneal scarring.

[1] Sandstrom K I et al. (1984) J. Pediatr., **105,** 707.
[2] Darougar S et al. (1986) Br. J. Ophthalmol., **69,** 2.
[3] Wishart P K et al. (1984) Br. J. Ophthalmol., **68,** 653.

Orbital Cellulitis[1,2]

Infection of the paranasal sinus in children will often lead to orbital cellulitis because of the free communication between the sinuses and the orbit. This produces a tender swelling of the eyelids with associated proptosis and restriction of eye movements.

TREATMENT

1. Systemic antibiotics will need to be given once the diagnosis is made to reduce the risk of visual loss and prevent the spread of infection intracranially. It is important to include cover for anaerobe infection during antibiotic treatment; metronidazole should also be given.
2. Adequate surgical drainage including fronto-ethmoidectomy may be necessary.
3. Management in children is usually a team effort with physicians monitoring antibiotic therapy, the ophthalmologist monitoring vision and the ENT surgeon performing the necessary surgery on the paranasal sinuses.

PROGNOSIS

- Vision may be lost in patients inadequately treated.

FOLLOW-UP

Follow-up within a week of stopping antibiotics. And then dependent on ENT findings.

[1] Barkin R M (1978) *Paediatrics*, **62**, 390.
[2] Lawless M *et al.* (1986) *Aust. J. Ophthalmol.*, **14**, 211.

Corneal Ulcers[1-3]

Viral ulcers

Many viral diseases involving the conjunctiva may cause a secondary keratitis with small punctate epithelial opacities. In the acute state these are on the surface and may stain with fluorescein. Gradually they become subepithelial and may last for up to one year. The viral infection which produces the most serious corneal disease is herpes simplex causing characteristic corneal dendritic ulcers. They may spontaneously improve or go on to ulceration involving the corneal stroma.

Adenovirus

TREATMENT

1. Specific antiviral drugs have no effect on adenovirus conjunctivitis.
2. Topical antibiotics, e.g. neomycin and chloramphenicol are used to reduce the risk of secondary bacterial infection which fortunately is small.

PROGNOSIS

- Adenovirus will produce an acute follicular conjunctivitis which may be unilateral or bilateral and can be associated with superficial punctate epithelial opacities. The conjunctivitis will commonly heal spontaneously within three weeks while the opacities may persist for one year or longer.

Herpes simplex

TREATMENT

1. Idoxuridine ointment five times a day or hourly as drops.
2. Either idoxuridine or vidarabine ointment are continued until the corneal ulcer has disappeared. Corneal toxicity is likely to occur when the treatment has been given for longer than one week. This is characterised by the development of punctate epithelial staining of the corneal and conjunctiva.
3. If the ulcer is unresponsive to idoxuridine or vidarabine, acyclovir ointment five times a day is commenced.
4. Avoid steroid eye drops with dendritic ulcers as the steroids may potentiate virus replication leading to a more severe corneal infection and can even result in corneal perforation.
5. Disciform keratitis: as an exception, disciform keratitis is sometimes treated with low-dose steroid eye drops. However, there is always a risk of potentiating the epithelial disease if it recurs and the stromal disease will often recur unless the steroid eye drops are reduced very slowly.

PROGNOSIS

- Primary herpes simplex causes a follicular conjunctivitis indistinguishable from adenovirus but may go on to develop dendritic corneal ulcers.
- Correctly treated most dendritic ulcers heal within seven days.
- Recurrences of the dendritic ulcers are common and characteristically involve the same eye.
- A small proportion of patients may develop large corneal ulcers involving the epithelium and stroma or purely stromal disease with ulceration (disciform keratitis).
- Some patients may also develop a severe iritis.

Bacterial ulcers

TREATMENT

1. Take conjunctival scrapings and swabs for microscopy and culture and sensitivity.
2. Topical antibiotics are the mode of treatment for corneal ulcers. The choice of topical antibiotic therapy should be determined by the results of the microbiological assessment. However, until this is known, broad spectrum cover such as tobramycin eye drops and neomycin eye drops can be applied quarter hourly.
3. Subconjunctival antibiotics are given if the infection is more severe.
4. Systemic antibiotics are rarely indicated since effective local tissue levels are reached with topical and subconjunctival injections without the risk of systemic side-effects.

PROGNOSIS

- Most bacterial corneal ulcers are secondary to damage to the corneal epithelium, disease of other ocular structures or occur in debilitated or immunocompromised children.
- Certain virulent organisms such as *Neisseria gonorrhoeae* may attack an intact corneal epithelium leading to ulceration and loss of the eye unless appropriate treatment is instituted quickly.
- Even with the right antibiotic treatment, the outlook for recovery of sight is poor if this organism is virulent, e.g. *Pseudomonas aeruginosa* or *Staphylococcus aureus*.

---

[1] Symposium on Bacterial Infection and the Eye (1986) *Trans. Ophthalmol. Soc. UK*, **105,** 18.
[2] Leibowitz H (1984) *Corneal Disorders: Clinical Diagnosis and Management*, ch. VII, p. 16. Philadelphia: Saunders.
[3] Coster D *et al.* (1983) *Aust. J. Ophthalmol.*, **11,** 1.

Iritis[1-3]

Iritis is inflammation in the anterior chamber of the eye characterised by pain, photophobia and blurred vision. Clinical examination reveals an inflamed eye with a constricted pupil. Examination with a slit lamp will reveal flare and cells in the anterior chamber of the affected eye. This is commonly a unilateral condition but may be bilateral. There are occasional indolent forms of uveitis in which there is little pain or photophobia, characteristically found in juvenile arthritis. There may be little clinical evidence of inflammation but later band keratopathy (calcium deposition in the exposed central zone), vitreous opacification and cataract formation develop.

TREATMENT

1. Search for and treat an underlying disease such as toxoplasmosis, herpes simplex, sarcoidosis, Behçet's disease, syphilis, arthritis and chronic bowel disease. In many patients no cause will be found.
2. Moderate iritis: corticosteroid eye drops as frequently as hourly depending on the severity of the inflammation. Mydriatics drops, for example homatropine 2% four times a day, or atropine 1% three times daily.
3. Severe iritis: addition of systemic prednisolone (2 mg/kg/day maximum) or subconjunctival injection of steroids depending on the age of the patient.

PROGNOSIS

• The prognosis is good for an acute attack of iritis since it will usually settle down with treatment. Subsequent attacks may occur.
• Indolent iritis will often flare up again when treatment has ceased.

FOLLOW-UP

Regular slit lamp examination of patients who have arthritis associated with uveitis is necessary to avoid the complications mentioned above.

[1] Kanski J J et al. (1984) Ophthalmology (Rochester), **91**, 1247.
[2] Perkins E S et al. (1984) Ophthalmologica, **189**, 36.
[3] Geraint D et al. (1976) Trans. Ophthalmol. Soc. UK, **96**, 108.

Cataracts[1,2]

Opacities in the lens causing significant visual impairment are uncommon in childhood. They may be congenital or acquired. A young child with a cataract will often present with a squint or white pupil reflex. If the child is over three months of age nystagmus may be the presenting feature. Maternal infection with rubella or cytomegalovirus during the first trimester is a significant cause of cataract at birth. Systemic diseases associated with cataract include diabetes mellitus, toxoplasmosis, hypoparathyroidism, homocystinuria, atopic dermatitis, Marfan's syndrome and Down's syndrome. One systemic abnormality which is often not clinically obvious at presentation is galactosaemia. Patients and siblings should be reviewed to exclude an hereditary cataract. The common form is autosomal dominant.

TREATMENT

1. *Cataract surgery*

   a) Early cataract surgery and appropriate correction with extended wear contact lenses in neonates and young infants is important to allow for a clear retinal image and visual development before nystagmus resulting from visual deprivation develops at about the age of three months. In these patients, the lens is removed with a suction cutter so that there is no framework on which any residual lens fibres can proliferate and obstruct the pupil.

   b) In older children who have developed cataracts because of systemic disease or trauma, there is not the same urgency to obtain a clear pupil and the current techniques of extracapsular surgery used in adults can be employed, with the advantage that the surgery can usually be performed through an incision only large enough to admit the infusion–aspiration system. The nucleus of a child's cataract is not solid and can be sucked out. Any thickening of the remaining posterior capsule which may occur later can readily be treated by the YAG laser without admission to hospital.

2. It is generally accepted that intraocular lenses (IOL) are contraindicated in children for four reasons:

   a) The infant eye is developing in size and is soft.

   b) The long-term complications of posterior chamber IOLs and their supporting polypropylene loops have not been fully evaluated.

   c) The final refractive error of the developing eye cannot be predicted.

   d) The size of the corneal incision necessary for the insertion compromises the integrity of the eye itself.

PROGNOSIS

- If the cataract is unilateral and present from birth the chance of improving vision significantly with surgery is extremely low, because the associated amblyopia is difficult to treat and secondly, the eye with the cataract has often other associated defects which preclude a successful visual result.

- Bilateral cataracts will need to be assessed carefully and if it is thought that there is significant visual impairment then surgery is recommended to allow normal visual development.

[1] Taylor D (1981) *Trans. Ophthalmol. Soc. UK*, **101**, 114.
[2] Hoyt C (1984) Treatment of congenital cataracts. In *Cataract Surgery* (Steele A D McG, Drews R C eds.). London: Butterworths.

Retinoblastoma[1-3]

Retinoblastoma occurs in approximately one in 20 000 live births and, although a potentially fatal tumour, the prognosis is extremely good if diagnosed early. 60% cases of retinoblastoma are sporadic. The remaining 40% are hereditary transmitted by an autosomal dominant gene. Deletion of part of the long arm of chromosome 13 has been found in some cases of hereditary retinoblastoma. All bilateral cases of retinoblastoma are hereditary and 8% unilateral cases of retinoblastoma are hereditary. This is a tumour which arises from photoreceptor elements and may grow into the vitreous (endophytic) or grow outwards under the retina causing a retinal detachment (exophytic). Rarely it produces a diffuse infiltrating tumour in the retina. Secondary dissemination of the tumour may result from invasion of the optic nerve and dissemination through the subarachnoid space or from invasion into the choroid and to the systemic circulation. Most patients with retinoblastoma present before the age of two years with the hereditary retinoblastoma presenting on average nine months earlier than the sporadic case. The common mode of presentation is strabismus, a cat's eye, a white reflex, reduced vision or a red painful eye.

TREATMENT

1. In the sporadic cases diagnosis may sometimes be difficult and retinoblastoma needs to be carefully differentiated from:

   a) Persistent hyperplastic primary vitreous.
   b) Retrolental fibroplasia.
   c) Posterior cataract.
   d) Coloboma of the choroid.
   e) Toxocara endophthalmitis.
   f) Coat's disease.

2. The patient with suspected retinoblastoma should be examined under general anaesthesia to confirm the diagnosis and assess the size of the lesion.
3. The aim of initial treatment is to preserve life and hopefully also preserve sight in the affected eye, particularly in the bilateral cases.
4. Unilateral tumours

   a) If the lesion is small a number of options are available including cryotherapy, laser coagulation and cobalt-60 plaque. When the lesion is large, a megavoltage irradiation through a lateral portal to avoid the lens may be used.
   b) In practice since most unilateral tumours present when the tumour is large with no chance of preservation of sight, enucleation is performed.

5. Bilateral tumours

   a) In bilateral cases either cobalt-60 plaque or megavoltage radiation is commonly used. If there are small tumours less than 2 disc diameters in size, cryotherapy or photocoagulation are often effective.
   b) All bilateral retinoblastoma patients have hereditary disease and this group has a higher incidence of osteogenic sarcoma and other second tumours, primarily at the site of radiotherapy but also at distant sites. Therefore the dosage of radiotherapy given is kept to a minimum to reduce the risk of late onset osteogenic sarcoma in the field of irradiation.
   c) If metastatic spread has occurred or if the risk of this is high then prophylactic chemotherapy has been advocated.

PROGNOSIS

- Prognosis depends on the speed at which diagnosis is made. If diagnosis is delayed until there is secondary spread, mortality approaches 100%.
- A cure should be possible in over 95% patients who have a tumour occupying less than half the volume of the eye and not extending out into the choroid or into the subarachnoid space around the optic nerve.
- There is a 1% incidence of spontaneous disappearance of retinoblastoma, hence the parents of a child with retinoblastoma need to be

reviewed to see if they have evidence of a lesion that may have undergone spontaneous resolution.

- It is important to differentiate between hereditary and sporadic cases of retinoblastoma for genetic counselling.
- Patients with a family history of retinoblastoma have about a 50% chance of transmitting the disease to their offspring. Those with an affected child but no previous family history have a 1% chance of transmitting the tumour to their second child.

[1] Ellsworth R M (1985) Retinoblastoma. In *Clinical Ophthalmology* (Duane T D ed.), pp. 3:35 (1–18). Philadelphia: Harper & Row.
[2] Cavenee W K *et al.* (1986) *New Eng. J. Med.*, **314**, 1201.
[3] Abramson D H *et al.* (1984) *Ophthalmology (Rochester)*, **91**, 1351.

FOLLOW-UP

Regular examination required throughout childhood.

Glaucoma[1-3]

Glaucoma in childhood is an uncommon disease and the symptoms and signs of childhood glaucoma are quite different from those in the adult, particularly if the disease is manifested in the first year of life. During this time, the affected eye will often partly compensate for the rise in intraocular pressure with progressive enlargement (buphthalmos). This leads to photophobia in sunlight, and on clinical examination, an enlargement of the cornea and sometimes clouding of the cornea in more severe cases. Visual field defects may be detected in older children. Glaucoma in children may be primary or associated with systemic disease such as neurofibromatosis and Sturge–Weber syndrome or with developmental abnormalities of the anterior segment of the eye.

TREATMENT

1. Topical medication

   a) Eye drops pilocarpine 2%, four times a day.
   b) Eye drops timolol maleate (Timoptol) 0.25–0.5% twice daily.
   c) Eye drops dipivefrin HCl (Propine) 0.1% twice daily.
   d) Acetazolamide (Diamox) 10–15 mg/kg/day, usually given in four divided doses.

2. Surgery will be necessary for severe cases and those not responding quickly to medical treatment.

   a) *Goniotomy*: in primary open angle glaucoma there is a membrane over the trabecular meshwork from the iris. Under gonioscopic control, a knife can be inserted across the iris to cut this membrane through one quadrant or more. The operation may need to be repeated.
   b) *Trabeculotomy*: if clouding of the cornea will not permit an adequate view for a goniotomy procedure, a trabeculotomy will produce a similar lowering of intraocular pressure. The canal of Schlemm is opened and a probe is passed in breaking through into the anterior chamber creating a track for drainage.
   c) *Trabeculectomy*: for most other forms of glaucoma, a draining procedure is indicated such as a trabeculectomy in which a piece of trabecular meshwork is removed under a small scleral trapdoor. The operation probably works by allowing fluid to escape from the anterior chamber through the scleral trapdoor to beneath the conjunctival space (a filtration procedure). The results are often unsatisfactory in children due to healing of the fistula.

d) *Cyclocryotherapy* and molten tubes are other procedures resorted to in desperate cases.

PROGNOSIS

- Without satisfactory management of the intraocular pressure, irreversible blindness due to damage to the optic nerve and retinal elements will occur.
- If the pressure is very high, damage to the cornea may lead to clouding of the cornea and reduced vision.
- In arrested cases of glaucoma in the first year of life, the progressive enlargement of the eye may result in this eye being short sighted (myopic).

FOLLOW-UP

Regular follow-up throughout childhood is essential.

[1] Anthony C B *et al.* (1984) *Arch. Ophthalmol.*, **102,** 51.
[2] Shaffer R N *et al.* (1970) *Congenital and Pediatric Glaucoma.* St Louis: Mosby.
[3] Walton D (1983) Glaucoma in infants and children. In *Pediatric Ophthalmology* (Harley E D ed.). Philadelphia: Saunders.

Ocular Injury[1-3]

The history is important in ocular injury in children since the cause of the injury will alter the management. Children are likely to give misleading information where air gun or explosives are involved in order to protect their friends who may have been responsible.

Non-penetrating eye injury
Corneal foreign body

TREATMENT

1. Apply topical anaesthesia, e.g. benoxinate, amethocaine.
2. Remove the foreign body with a cotton bud, or if more deeply imbedded, the tip of a 25-gauge needle.
3. If there is a rust ring remaining, this can be removed with either a dental burr or the tip of the 25-gauge needle. If the rust ring is difficult to remove, wait 24 hours and then try again as material will often soften in that time and be easier to remove.
4. Leave the rust ring if the trauma of its removal could lead to excessive scarring or perforation of the cornea.
5. Instil topical antibiotics, e.g. chloromycetin, neomycin and cycloplegic agents and drops to dilate the pupil, e.g. Mydriacyl and homatropine. Both are used until the epithelium is healed and the stromal reaction settled.

PROGNOSIS

- Corneal foreign bodies will cause ocular irritation with watering.
- Instillation of local anaesthetic will relieve symptoms and facilitate examination.
- Staining of the cornea with fluorescein will reveal scratch marks if the foreign body is beneath the tarsal plate.

FOLLOW-UP

Review daily until healed.

Alkali burn

TREATMENT

1. Immediate copious water lavage.
2. Topical steroids and antibiotics four times a day for the first five days.
3. With more severe burns, admit the child to hospital and add collagenase inhibitors topically, such as 20% acetylcysteine.
4. Corneal grafting is often unsuccessful due to the associated lid scarring and reduced tear film.

PROGNOSIS

- Chemical burns from materials splashed in the eye may lead to blindness particularly with alkali agents.
- The likelihood of serious visual loss increases in alkaline burns if, at presentation, there is conjunctival ischaemia and clouding of the cornea over one-third of the surface.
- The long-term problems relate to loss of the tear film and persistence of corneal epithelial defects and activation of collagenase with lysis of the corneal stroma and subsequent perforation.

Traumatic hyphema

Blunt trauma from a flying object or involvement in any trauma may lead to rupture of blood vessels in the anterior segment of the eye causing a hyphema.

TREATMENT

1. Rest the child in bed, preferably in hospital.
2. Pad and shield the affected eye.
3. Give light sedation if necessary.
4. If the intraocular pressure is elevated, then use acetazolamide (Diamox) 15 mg/kg in divided dosage orally, topical timolol maleate (Timoptol) 0.25% twice daily or dipivefrine hydrochloride (Propine) 0.1% twice daily.
5. Keep the patient under close observation for five days. The risk of re-bleed is maximal in the first three days and drops rapidly thereafter.
6. Make sure aspirin or aspirin-related compounds are not given for analgesia as this will increase the risk of re-bleeding due to its effect of platelet function.
7. *Surgery*

    a) If there is a total hyphema with very high rise in intraocular pressure which does not settle within 24 hours, the clot will need to be evacuated surgically.
    b) Surgery may consist of aspiration of part of the blood clot in the anterior chamber with the remainder spontaneously resorbing.
    c) If there are repeated re-bleeds with organising clots in the anterior chamber, sodium

hyaluronate or similar viscostatic substance can be injected through a small hole at the limbus inferiorly. An incision can be made superiorly through which the clot can be expressed. The major problem with the removal of a hyphema surgically is that there is poor visualisation of the anterior segment structures which may be damaged by surgical manipulation.

PROGNOSIS

- Most hyphemas clear spontaneously. The danger is of a re-bleed with formation of a total hyphema, raised intraocular pressure and subsequent permanent damage to the eye.
- Persistence of blood in the anterior chamber under pressure can cause blood staining of the cornea and there may be fibrous ingrowth obliterating the anterior segment.
- The risk of re-bleed is higher in children than in adults and is not related to the extent of the original bleed.

FOLLOW-UP

Assessment at six weeks is made to exclude the development of glaucoma, to examine the posterior segment of the eye for associated retinal haemorrhages and tears in either the choroid or retina, and to look carefully at the periphery to exclude a retinal detachment.

Penetrating eye injuries
TREATMENT

1. Carefully suture the corneal and scleral wounds directly under microscope control.
2. If the lens has been damaged, this may require removal.
3. A retained intraocular foreign body in the posterior segment of the eye, if it is magnetic, may be removed with a magnet applied to the outside of the eye or an intraocular magnet introduced through a small entrance site at the pars plana. A similar incision would be needed to remove an intraocular foreign body through the pars plana with a magnet used on the outside of the eye.

4. If iris is incarcerated in the wound, it often becomes adherent to the wound and will need to be excised.

PROGNOSIS

- The prognosis is worsened in penetrating eye injuries where there is both an entrance and an exit wound, where there is disruption of the lens or damage to the posterior segment of the eye.
- If there is a history of hammering metal against metal, even if a penetration of the eye cannot be seen, take an x-ray to exclude an intraocular foreign body. Intraocular foreign bodies composed of iron almost always need to be removed since if left in the eye they lead to siderosis with progressive nerve cell death and blindness.
- Copper intraocular foreign bodies can produce a massive inflammatory response, 'chalcosis', and need to be removed also.

- Late complications of penetrating eye injuries include retinal detachment often as a result of contraction of fibrous adhesions between the vitreous and retina, which may develop rapidly in children.

FOLLOW-UP

Following penetrating eye injuries, there may rarely develop inflammation in the other eye 'sympathetic ophthalmitis' which will threaten sight in the eye. Therefore, check the non-injured eye carefully, particularly if the patient complains of glare or photophobia – symptoms that might suggest the development of iritis.

---

[1] Romano P E (1986) *J. Pediatr. Ophthalmol.*, **23**, 92.
[2] Crouch E R (1986) *J. Pediatr. Ophthalmol.*, **23**, 95.
[3] Paton D *et al.* (1976) *Management of Ocular Injuries*. Philadelphia: Saunders.

13

Diseases of the Ear

M. H. Bellman and S. C. Bellman

External Ear (Pinna and Auditory Meatus)

Accessory auricles

TREATMENT

Plastic surgery is possible. The lobule is the most important abnormality to correct cosmetically.

PROGNOSIS

- Accessory auricles are of cosmetic importance provided the external auditory meatus is patent.

Malformed auditory meatus (stenosis, atresia)

TREATMENT

If hearing loss is present and is:

1. Unilateral – no treatment is necessary.
2. Bilateral – hearing aids and reconstructive surgery starting at the age of 5–7 years may help, although results are questionable.

PROGNOSIS

- There is complete conductive hearing loss (60 dB) if the auditory meatus is atretic. Sensorineural hearing loss is present in 20% these cases.

Pre-auricular pits

TREATMENT

If infection is persistent treatment is by complete surgical excision of the track.

PROGNOSIS

Recurrent infection is likely if the pits are deep.

Furunculosis

TREATMENT

1. Systemic antibiotics, e.g. ampicillin/flucloxacillin, for five days.
2. Use of an astringent wick – a small piece of ribbon gauze soaked in 13% aluminium acetate, inserted into the meatus.
3. Analgesia as appropriate.

PROGNOSIS

- These boils are very painful, and may recur.

Otitis externa

Predisposing factors include otitis media, moist ear, allergy and trauma.

TREATMENT

1. Prevention
   a) Treatment of predisposing factors, e.g. chronic otitis media.
   b) Keep ears dry at all times – ear plugs or cotton wool with vaseline for baths or showers, avoid swimming.
   c) Stop scratching.
   d) Treat allergy (steroid drops).

2. Take swab and culture to identify bacterial (or fungal) infection with antibiotic sensitivities.
3. Regular aural toilet. Using a head mirror for direct vision, clean out all discharge with sterile cotton wool. Gentle suction or syringing can be used in cooperative children.

4. Astringent (aluminium acetate) drops.
5. Antibiotic/steroid drops or wick, e.g. dexamethasone plus framycetin plus gramicidin (Sofradex) drops, either 2–3 drops 3–4 times daily into the meatus or soaked on to ribbon gauze placed in meatus and changed daily for five days. Avoid longer use of antibiotic drops because of the risk of local hypersensitivity aggravating the condition. If allergy is a major problem use steroid drops, e.g. betamethasone (Betnesol).
6. Oral antibiotics are of no value for otitis externa except when it occurs as a complication of otitis media.

PROGNOSIS

- The condition tends to recur, especially if the primary cause is not identified.

Wax impaction

Wax impaction in children is usually due to attempts to clean out the ears with cotton wool/ matchsticks, etc. Occasionally it is due to pressure from hearing aid moulds.

TREATMENT

1. Prevention: ban cotton 'buds' for cleaning ears.
2. Most wax does not need removal. If necessary use olive oil or sodium bicarbonate drops followed by syringing/manual removal under direct vision. Do not syringe if there is a history of recent or persistent perforation. Ensure water is at body temperature. Direct a continuous flow of water at the posterior–superior wall of the meatus. Mop dry thoroughly afterwards.

PROGNOSIS

May recur if the cause is not identified and stopped.

Foreign bodies

TREATMENT

1. Removal by ENT surgeon. Other doctors should only attempt to remove objects clearly visible and extruding from the meatus with an obvious point to grasp with forceps (NB not round objects). Always remove under direct vision.
2. If in doubt – don't! Incorrect removal can cause trauma and infection and even damage to the tympanic membrane and ossicles, which may have medico-legal consequences.
3. Insects can be syringed out.

PROGNOSIS

- If impacted, foreign bodies cause conductive hearing loss and infection.

Middle Ear[1-4]

Congenital abnormalities

Congenital abnormalities range from minor deformation of the ossicular chain to absent middle ear cavity (e.g. in Treacher Collins' syndrome). They can be associated with atresia of the external and/or dysplasia of the inner ear.

TREATMENT

1. If the abnormality is unilateral, no treatment is necessary.
2. For bilateral abnormalities hearing aids will be necessary.
3. X-rays may reveal an abnormality theoretically correctable by surgery at the age of 5–7 years. Surgery may be impossible in some abnormalities, e.g. Treacher Collins' syndrome, otopalatodigital syndrome.

PROGNOSIS

- There is often complete conductive hearing loss in the abnormal ear. If the abnormality is unilateral there is no functional problem. If the abnormality is bilateral there may be 60 dB hearing loss (see *Deafness* p. 244).

Acute otitis media

Acute otitis media is the commonest infective disorder of children (occurs in 50% children by school age). Bacterial infection is often secondary to primary viral infection (e.g. respiratory syncytial virus, measles).

TREATMENT

1. Analgesia as appropriate.
2. Aural toilet.
3. Many cases are of viral aetiology and settle spontaneously with analgesia alone.
4. Systemic antibodies should only be used if there is no spontaneous resolution, i.e. persistent pyrexia and severe otalgia, after 48 hours, or if other complications (e.g. mastoiditis) are suspected. Use a broad spectrum antibiotic (amoxycillin, cephalexin, co-trimoxazole) unless the organism is known to be penicillin sensitive. Recent evidence suggests that a short course (3 days) is sufficient.
5. If there is severe pain or the ear drum is acutely red and bulging consider myringotomy.
6. If there are recurrent infections look for the source of infection, e.g. infected adenoids may need adenoidectomy, secretory otitis media will need grommets.
7. Antibiotic prophylaxis (co-trimoxazole) can be useful in some cases, e.g. those with medical disorders which increase the liability to persistent infections.
8. Polyvalent pneumococcal vaccine may become available in future.
9. Hearing loss due to a scarred drum (tympanosclerosis) may be improved surgically (tympanoplasty).

PROGNOSIS

- 90% cases resolve spontaneously with or without perforation leaving no sequelae.
- The ear drum may rupture and heal with scarring causing minor conductive hearing loss.
- Spread of infection from the middle ear cavity on occasion results in mastoiditis with the danger of cerebral abscess.
- Recurrent attacks may occur in immuno-compromised children or those with persistent secretory otitis media.

Otitis media with effusion (secretory otitis media, glue ear)

Glue ear is the presence of fluid, usually thick, within the middle ear, due to a variety of causes. It is very common affecting up to 30% school-age children. In pre-school children it especially affects those in day nurseries. Predisposing factors include partially treated or recurrent acute otitis media, recurrent upper respiratory tract infections, barotrauma caused by air travel or diving, abnormal anatomy (e.g. cleft palate), syndromes such as Down's, mucopolysaccharidoses and allergy, particularly for cow's milk.

TREATMENT

1. *Prevention.* Recurrent episodes may be reduced by long-term antibiotics, e.g. co-trimoxazole, insertion of ventilation tubes (grommets), and adenoidectomy.
2. Medication has not been found helpful in controlled trials. Decongestant and antihistamine drugs are commonly used but have no scientific justification. It has been claimed that mucolytics (Mucodyne) are helpful postoperatively.
3. Antibiotics are indicated only when acute otitis media is present or if the presence of infection elsewhere (e.g. tonsils, sinuses) is relevant.
4. Steroids should not be used.
5. Surgical myringotomy and aspiration of middle ear fluid relieve symptoms.
6. Ventilation of the middle ears by insertion of grommets should prevent reaccumulation of fluid. These stay in place for 6–24 months before being extruded spontaneously. Up to 20% children have occasional otorrhoea while grommets are *in situ*. Treatment is with antibiotic/steroid drops (as above).
7. Tympanostomy tubes stay in longer and are better in susceptible cases (e.g. children with cleft palate or Down's syndrome). The ear drum heals quickly. Scarring (tympanosclerosis and atrophy) occur in up to 40% cases but does not usually affect hearing. Persistent perforation is present in 4% and may require treatment by myringoplasty.

PROGNOSIS

- It may resolve spontaneously.
- It may cause conductive hearing loss while fluid is in the middle ear.
- Longstanding secretory otitis media may cause adhesions and fibrosis in the middle ear causing a degree of permanent conductive hearing loss.

- When episodes are frequent or persistent, the hearing loss may inhibit optimal language development.

Chronic suppurative otitis media

Chronic suppurative otitis media is divided into two main types.

Tubo-tympanic disease (safe)

The middle ear is infected and there is central perforation of the para tensa. Mastoid x-rays demonstrate the extent of disease.

TREATMENT

1. Aural toilet is essential including a swab to identify the organism and sensitivity.
2. Keep ear dry to prevent reinfection (vaseline on cotton wool).
3. Topical medication is usually an antibiotic-steroid combination. Drops should preferably not contain ototoxic drugs, e.g. gentamicin, neomycin, kanamycin, framycetin. If such drugs are essential following antibiotic sensitivity tests, the length of course should be short (5–7 days). This has the added advantage that it will prevent sensitisation leading to otitis externa.
4. Treatment of factors predisposing to chronicity (e.g. maxillary sinusitis, infected tonsils and/or adenoids) is important.
5. Tympanoplasty is indicated when the ear is dry and the child is older (10–12 years plus) so that infections are less likely. (Some surgeons will operate on younger children with wet ears.) Successful operation prevents re-infection by repairing the tympanic membrane and also restores hearing by reconstruction of the eardrum and ossicular chain if necessary. Results are good if eustachian tube function is adequate (with more than 95% achieving a dry ear).

PROGNOSIS

- Long-term prognosis is good if the condition is treated adequately.
- Chronic central perforations in children sometimes heal spontaneously if the ear remains dry.

Attic disease (unsafe)

Attic perforation/retraction pockets are associated with cholesteatoma. It can be seen following long-term glue ear, e.g. in Down's syndrome and children with cleft palates. Otorrhoea is not always present at first.

TREATMENT

1. Safety is the primary aim of treatment.
2. Very early lesions are treated by regular removal of debris and examination under microscope by an experienced ENT surgeon.
3. Surgery ranges from tympanotomy to modified radical mastoidectomy, with possible later reconstruction, depending on the extent of the disease.

4. Bilateral disease may cause conductive hearing loss sufficiently severe to require the patient to use hearing aids.

PROGNOSIS

- This is a progressive, destructive disease. It is unsafe and can lead to local damage, e.g. VII nerve palsy or vestibular symptoms, and ultimately cerebral complications, e.g. abscess or venous sinus thrombosis.

[1] Bluestone C D *et al.* (1983) *Paediatrics*, **71**, 639.
[2] Diamant M *et al.* (1974) *Arch. Otolaryngol.*, **100**, 226.
[3] Paradise J L (1980) *Paediatrics*, **65**, 917.
[4] Shurin P *et al.* (1980) *J. Pediatr.*, **96**, 1081.

Deafness[1-3]

Hearing impairment in childhood, particularly during early language development, may permanently compromise communication abilities. It is extremely important to detect and treat affected children and this requires a systematic policy for population screening using appropriate hearing tests. In general, the prognosis for communication depends on: degree of hearing loss; duration of hearing loss; age of onset; associated developmental handicaps; intelligence; family and social support; audiological rehabilitation services; and special educational facilities.

Conductive deafness

Conductive deafness is the most common type of hearing loss in children. It can be due to secretory otitis media, acute otitis media or congenital abnormality of the middle or external ear.

TREATMENT

1. Early detection and appropriate treatment will minimise the problems.
2. In severe conductive loss due to congenital abnormalities primary treatment is with hearing aids (bone conduction if no external auditory meatus), audiological rehabilitation, special educational help and speech therapy. Reconstructive surgery may be possible at 5–7 years of age.

3. For intermittent conductive deafness provided speech and language development is not delayed, do not intervene but review ears (otoscopy, audiogram and tympanometry) and speech/language every 3–4 months. Deterioration or onset of behavioural/educational symptoms indicate a need for referral to an ENT surgeon.
4. Persistent hearing loss is an indication for referral to an ENT surgeon for consideration of myringotomy, aspiration of middle ear fluid, insertion of grommets and adenoidectomy. Hearing aids should be considered as a temporary solution.
5. In all cases advice should be given to the child, parents and teachers on facing the child directly, reducing distance (e.g. sitting at front of class) and cutting out background noise.

PROGNOSIS

- Untreated, the hearing loss range is 20–60 dB.
- Deafness worse than 40 dB

  a) If the deafness is of this degree normal (conversational) speech can barely be heard and language development is thus severely impaired.
  b) If the problem is continuous (congenital abnormality or chronic middle ear disease) the prognosis for speech and language is poor and the consequences for educational progress, emotional development and social integration far reaching.

- Deafness 30–40 dB

  a) With deafness of this degree loud speech is audible but word discrimination poor. It may be missed by early screening hearing tests.
  b) If hearing loss is intermittent prognosis for language is relatively good.
  c) Continuous moderate deafness causes delayed language development (verbal comprehension and expression) and impaired phonation with poor intelligibility. This often results in frustrated communication and behaviour problems, e.g. withdrawal, aggression, temper tantrums and sleep disturbance.

- Deafness 20–30 dB

  a) The normal voice can be heard but low energy speech sounds (some consonants, e.g. t, p, v) are missed. It is detectable only by formal speech or pure tone audiometry.
  b) Language impairment is subtle or mild, but may cause failure of optimal school progress especially if persistent.

Sensorineural deafness

The incidence of congenital hearing loss (greater than 50 dB) in western Europe is approximately 1:1000 live births. 2% school children have special educational needs due to hearing loss. Aetiology includes genetic causes, e.g. Down's syndrome, intrauterine infection, e.g. rubella or cytomegalo-virus (CMV), perinatal causes, e.g. anoxia or hyperbilirubinaemia, ototoxic drugs, e.g. aminoglycosides, antibiotics or antineoplastic agents, post-meningitis, e.g. there is a 6–10% incidence following influenza/meningococcal meningitis, or 40–50% incidence following pneumococcal meningitis, or as a sequel of exanthem, e.g. measles or mumps.

TREATMENT

1. Well-organised screening programmes for detection of infants with sensorineural deafness are essential. Neonatal screening is possible using the auditory response cradle. Screening of high risk cases with brainstem evoked responses would identify 50–70% children with congenital hearing impairment. Accurate screening at 7–9 months of age by distraction testing should identify all affected children. Check lists of normal hearing responses can alert parents and professionals to the child at a younger age. Children who fail these tests must be quickly referred to an audiological unit for assessment and treatment.

2. Hearing aids

   a) A wide range of electronic hearing aids is now available and these should be fitted at the youngest age possible. They are worn in both ears and switched on for the maximum time during waking hours.
   b) Aids are prescribed according to the specific pattern of hearing loss and should be managed by appropriately trained and experienced audiologists.
   c) Most children can wear two ear level aids but a bodyworn aid is still better for a few.
   d) Adaptations available:
      i) Limitation of maximum output.
      ii) Selective frequency transmission.
   e) Special aids
      i) Radio aids. This eliminates distance effect and enables the child wearing receivers to be active while the speaker wears a microphone and transmitter.
      ii) Induction loop system (partly superseded by radio aid). The speaker wears a microphone which magnetically activates a wire loop laid round a building

—aids are functional within the loop. Still used in many schools and partial hearing units.

f) Even with highly sophisticated hearing aids, a deaf patient cannot hear normally.

3. Audiological rehabilitation includes:

   a) Teacher of the deaf (peripatetic) counselling of family and carers, management of hearing aids and coordination with school.

   b) Speech therapy to promote speech and language development.

4. Education

   a) Moderately affected children may manage in a normal school with special help.

   b) Severely deaf children are often better placed in a partial hearing unit with appropriate staff and facilities. The emphasis is on communication which may include oral and manual language techniques and lip reading.

   c) Health education: hearing impaired patients still suffer social stigma which must be removed prior to their acceptance and integration.

5. Associated audiological problems such as tinnitus and vestibular disorders may occur with sensorineural deafness and should be investigated if there are symptoms.

6. Genetic counselling. Aetiological diagnosis should be attempted in all cases. In at least 50% cases the cause is genetic and advice on recurrence risks should be offered.

PROGNOSIS

- Apart from temporary shifts in sound level thresholds due to brief acoustic trauma or some ototoxic drugs (e.g. aspirin or frusemide), sensorineural hearing loss is invariably permanent.

- Eventual outcome is determined by communication abilities. The type of hearing loss is important — high frequency sounds (consonants) are more essential for understanding speech than low frequency sounds (vowels).

- Infants with congenital sensorineural deafness must be identified in their first six months of life for optimal results.

- In acquired deafness the prognosis becomes better the later the age of onset after acquisition of language.

- Severe deafness with prelingual onset can cause almost total isolation with profound social, educational and emotional handicaps.

- The deafness resulting from some causes (such as rubella, CMV, or some genetic conditions) may deteriorate with increasing age.

- When associated with other handicaps (e.g. cerebral palsy, complex syndromes), problems are multiplied disproportionately. Evolving disorders (e.g. Usher's syndrome) can cause catastrophic physical and emotional disablement especially if not anticipated.

[1] Bellman S (1986) *Arch. Dis. Childh.*, **61,** 42.
[2] Newton V (1985) *J. Laryngol. Otol.*, Suppl. 10.
[3] Riko K *et al.* (1985) *Laryngoscope*, **95,** 137.

Cleft Lip and Palate

The extent of cleft lip and palate varies from a notch in the lip vermilion or submucous cleft of the palate to a complete bilateral cleft of the lip and palate. Prognosis depends on the size and complexity of the lesion and care should be carried out by a multidisciplinary team including plastic, orthodontic, ENT surgeons, speech therapist and audiologist[1].

Cleft lip[2]

TREATMENT

1. Plastic surgery at 2–3 months old. Muscle realignment is important for good appearance and function.
2. Cosmetic surgery on the nose is required when growth is complete (in the late teens) to correct abnormal shape due to misaligned muscle insertions.

PROGNOSIS

- The major complication is the cosmetic appearance.

Cleft palate[2-4]

TREATMENT

1. Oral surgery. Palate repair should be undertaken at 5–10 months of age. In order to achieve good function palatal muscles, submucous and mucous layers must be carefully dissected and realigned.
2. Orthodontics. Suitable appliances should be used when secondary dentition is established. Bone defects may need repair by grafting.
3. ENT surgery. Ventilation of middle ears with grommets or T tubes helps to prevent persistent effusions.
4. Speech therapy. Help with speech therapy should be offered from approximately 2 years of age onwards.

PROGNOSIS

- Prognosis depends on the extent of abnormality.
- Cosmetic: external appearance is normal in isolated cleft palate.
- Feeding: regurgitation of oral contents into nose occurs.
- Orthodontic: the defect in the alveolus often leads to an abnormal number or position of teeth.
- Audiological: there is a very high incidence of secretory otitis media and consequent conductive hearing loss in young children. This may resolve spontaneously but can be followed by persistent middle ear disease and deafness in adult life.
- Speech: the voice is hypernasal due to nasal escape of air.

[1] Holve L M (1982) *J. Craniofacial Genet. Dev. Biol.*, **2**, 201.
[2] Bardach J *et al.* (1984) *Ann. Plastic Surg.*, **12**, 235.
[3] Ainoda N *et al.* (1985) *Ann. Plastic Surg.*, **15**, 415.
[4] Egyedi P (1985) *J. Maxillofacial Surg.*, **13**, 177.

14

Diseases of the Skin

J. I. Harper

Birthmarks[1,2]

Strawberry naevus (capillary haemangioma)

Strawberry naevus is a common abnormality which appears as a protuberant vascular nodule, during the first few weeks of life. It slowly increases in size reaching a maximum during the first year. Multiple lesions are sometimes seen.

TREATMENT

1. In spite of parental pressure, management must be conservative and surgical intervention avoided.
2. Indications for active treatment are those lesions which, by virtue of their size and site, compromise vital structures, such as the airway or the eyes. In this emergency situation, the treatment of choice is a short course of oral prednisolone (2 mg/kg body weight/day, initially).
3. A rare complication of one or more large haemangiomas is thrombocytopenia due to platelet trapping (Kasabach-Merritt syndrome).

PROGNOSIS

- Over 90% will resolve spontaneously by school age, usually with no residual scarring. If any blemishes remain, these can be removed by plastic surgery at a later date.

FOLLOW-UP

Regular follow-up is essential to give reassurance and to note any changes or complications.

Port wine stain (naevus flammeus)

Port wine stain is present at birth as a large, irregular, deep, red/purple, flat area of skin which is usually unilateral, often on the face.

TREATMENT

1. As the child grows older and becomes more self-conscious, camouflage make-up is useful (Covermark).
2. Recently, argon laser therapy has been shown to have some beneficial effect, although these results are preliminary.
3. Rare complications include meningeal involvement (Sturge-Weber syndrome), and gross hypertrophy of a limb (Klippel-Trenaunay-Weber syndrome).

PROGNOSIS

- This birthmark persists; there is no tendency to fade or spread.

FOLLOW-UP

Regular follow-up is required to monitor developments and advise parents and patients on treatment possibilities.

Pigmented naevi

Although pigmented naevi may be present at birth, most appear during childhood and adolescence. In childhood, they are usually flat or only slightly elevated.

TREATMENT

The larger congenital melanocytic naevi should be excised, the sooner the better. Some specialist centres are now encouraging surgery (dermabrasion) as early as the first few weeks of life.

PROGNOSIS

- With maturation the majority become intradermal in adult life and are completely benign.
- Congenital melanocytic naevi, especially the giant pigmented hairy lesions, have a significant predisposition to malignant melanoma.

For the larger congenital melanocytic naevi, regular follow-up is important.

[1] Alper J C et al. (1983) Pediatr. Dermatol., **1**, 58.
[2] Atherton D J et al. (1986) In Textbook of Dermatology (Rook A, Wilkinson D S, Ebling F J G, Champion R H, Burton J L eds) 4th edn, vol 1, p. 167. Oxford: Blackwell Scientific Publications.

Infantile Seborrhoeic Eczema

Infantile seborrhoeic eczema[1,2] is an acute erythematous scaly eruption of unknown cause. It starts soon after birth as cradle cap and/or nappy rash which spreads rapidly and may become extensive in an otherwise healthy baby.

TREATMENT

1. Often no treatment at all is necessary, apart from a bland emollient, such as aqueous cream.
2. For the more severely affected use 0.5% or 1% hydrocortisone alone or in combination, for example, with clioquinol (Vioform-Hydrocortisone), clotrimazole (Canesten HC) or miconazole (Daktocort), applied sparingly once or twice daily.
3. The thick scaling of cradle cap can be removed by the use of arachis oil massaged into the scalp prior to washing with a mild baby shampoo.

PROGNOSIS

- This condition is self-limiting and usually clears spontaneously within a few weeks.

- There is no evidence that these children are more likely to develop atopic eczema.

FOLLOW-UP

Routine follow-up as necessary. Reassurance is essential.

[1] Atherton D J et al. (1986) In Textbook of Dermatology (Rook A, Wilkinson D S, Ebling F J G, Champion R H, Burton J L eds), 4th edn, vol. 1, p. 246. Oxford: Blackwell Scientific Publications.
[2] Yates V M et al. (1983) Br. J. Dermatol., **108**, 633.

Nappy Rash

Nappy rash[1,2] affects almost all infants to some extent. The main causes are chemical irritation and infantile seborrhoeic eczema. Chemical irritation (primary irritant dermatitis) of the nappy area is due to occlusive contact of urine and faeces with the perineal skin. The rash is bounded by the margins of the nappy with sparing of the skin folds. Prolonged contact can lead to erosions of the skin. Infantile seborrhoeic eczema involves the flexures and the nappy area is usually affected as part of a more widespread eruption. Skin colonisation with *Candida albicans* is common.

TREATMENT

1. A prophylactic protective covering of zinc and castor oil cream applied after each nappy change is usually all that is required. Metanium (titanium in a silicone base) is another useful protective preparation that is widely used.
2. Advise parents to avoid the use of plastic pants or disposable nappies, leave off the nappy when possible and change the nappy frequently.
3. Treatment of established nappy rash comprises an anti-candida/hydrocortisone application, for example, clotrimazole and hydrocortisone (Canesten HC), nystatin and hydrocortisone (Nystaform HC) or miconazole and hydrocortisone (Daktacort).
4. Strong fluorinated topical steroids are contraindicated.

PROGNOSIS

- Primary irritant nappy rash may be seen at any time until the infant is continent.
- Infantile seborrhoeic eczema is seen as a problem mainly during the first three months of life.

FOLLOW-UP

Follow-up is not usually necessary.

[1] Kozinn P J et al. (1961) *J. Pediatr.*, **59**, 75.
[2] Swift S (1956) *Pediatr. Clin. North Am.*, **3**, 759.

Atopic Eczema

Atopic eczema[1-4] affects 1–3% all infants. The onset is usually between 3 and 18 months of age. About 70% have a positive family history of atopy (eczema, asthma, hayfever). Itching is prominent and often the baby is fretful because of this. The disease typically waxes and wanes. Although skin prick tests for specific allergens are often positive, they provide little guide to clinical management as multiple factors are usually involved.

TREATMENT

1. Bland emollients (such as emulsifying ointment or aqueous cream): these should be used frequently both as a soap substitute and as a bath additive.
2. Topical steroids: the minimum potency topical steroid should be used. Application of 1% hydrocortisone ointment is usually sufficient, although occasionally a stronger topical steroid may be required for a short period to treat an acute exacerbation. Steroid ointments should be applied sparingly once or twice daily to the affected areas only. All topical steroids are best avoided on the face, except when it is obviously necessary.
3. Antibiotics: a flare-up of eczema is often associated with secondary infection and these children require frequent courses of a broad spectrum oral antibiotic (flucloxacillin and penicillin V, or erythromycin for seven days). Skin swabs for microbiology should be taken prior to therapy. It is important to check the antibiotic sensitivities. Staphylococcal resistant strains on the skin surface are common in this group of children.
4. Antihistamines: an antihistamine elixir, such as trimeprazine (Vallergan) or promethazine (Phenergan), is helpful at night.
5. Diet: it has been suggested that avoidance of cow's milk protein in the first few months of life may be beneficial. However, exclusion diets appear to benefit only a few and should be reserved for young children with severe eczema who have not responded to conventional therapy or where there is a clear history of specific food intolerance.
6. General measures: the most important part of management is supportive care emphasising the good prognosis. Excessive heat should be avoided and the child should be dressed in cool, loose, cotton clothing. Other factors which are known to aggravate eczema include synthetic fabrics, clothing washed in biological detergents, irritant foods (for example, citrus fruits or tomatoes) causing perioral eczema, cigarette smoke, dander from pets and housedust.
7. It is important that the school-leaver with atopic eczema is given career guidance to avoid contact with chemical irritants which would aggravate and possibly potentiate the eczema, as for example in hairdressing, catering, nursing and engineering.

PROGNOSIS

- There is a general tendency towards improvement throughout childhood and over 90% will clear by the age of 15.

Eczema herpeticum

Eczema herpeticum is a serious complication of atopic eczema which occurs as a result of an increased susceptibility to herpes simplex. Exposure to the virus may result in widespread dissemination of herpes simplex lesions. Prompt treatment with intravenous acyclovir (Zovirax) is indicated if the herpetic lesions are spreading and the child unwell.

FOLLOW-UP

Regular follow-up is important. It is helpful to give the family an 'open appointment' to attend the clinic when necessary.

Contd.

[1] Atherton D J (1986) *Prescribers' J*,: **26,** 140.
[2] Champion R H *et al.* (1986) In *Textbook of Dermatology* (Rook A, Wilkinson D S, Ebling F J G, Champion R H, Burton J L eds), 4th edn, vol. 1, p. 246. Oxford: Blackwell Scientific Publications.

[3] Hanifin J M (1986) In *Clinical Reviews in Allergy* (Gershwin M E, Keslin M H eds.) **3,** p. 43. Amsterdam: Elsevier.
[4] Rajka G (1983) In *Recent Advances in Dermatology – 6* (Rook A J, Maibach H I eds), p. 105. Edinburgh: Churchill Livingstone.

Acne

Acne[1] is principally a problem of adolescence, although acneiform lesions can sometimes be seen in neonates or infants.

TREATMENT

1. Treatment is directed at removing the keratin plugs using a chemical peeling agent, such as benzoyl peroxide, available as a gel, cream or lotion in 2.5%, 5% and 10% concentrations (examples of proprietary preparations are Acetoxyl, Benoxyl, Panoxyl and Quinoderm). This is applied once daily after washing, preferably at night.
2. For moderate to severe acne, long-term low-dose antibiotic therapy is required, usually tetracycline (for 3–6 months and if necessary, longer). Tetracycline should not be given to children under 12 years of age and, if necessary, erythromycin can be substituted.

PROGNOSIS

● The prognosis is very good with resolution after the teens; only a relatively few individuals suffer with persistent acne in adult life.

FOLLOW-UP

Regular follow-up is important.

[1] Cunliffe W J, Cotterill J A. (1975) *The Acnes*. London: Saunders.

Psoriasis

Psoriasis[1] is primarily a disease of young adults but can develop for the first time at any age. In older children, it may present as guttate psoriasis: a shower of small, discrete, red, scaly lesions, predominantly on the trunk, often seen following a streptococcal sore throat.

TREATMENT

1. If a streptococcal infection is suspected (on the basis of a throat swab and antistreptolysin O titre), appropriate treatment with penicillin or erythromycin is required.
2. Treatment of chronic plaque psoriasis should be kept to a minimum with the application of 2% sulphur and salicylic acid ointment or coal tar and salicylic acid ointment.
3. For more difficult and extensive psoriasis, dithranol is the treatment of choice. It is applied accurately to the affected areas of skin in low concentrations in a cream base (Dithrocream, Psoradrate) or in salicylic acid and zinc oxide pastel (Lassar's paste). In-patient treatment may be necessary.
4. A course of ultra-violet light therapy (UVB) is often helpful.
5. Topical steroids should *not* be used for the treatment of stable plaque psoriasis.

PROGNOSIS

- Psoriasis is typically a chronic relapsing inflammatory disorder.
- There is a genetic tendency to develop psoriasis, although the mode of inheritance is unclear.
- Guttate psoriasis has a better prognosis; it usually resolves after about two months, although the typical plaques on the elbows, knees and scalp may develop at any time in the future.

FOLLOW-UP

Follow-up should be as regular as necessary.

[1] Champion R H (1986) *Br. Med. J.*, **292**, 1693.

Pityriasis Rosea

Pityriasis rosea is a common disorder of adolescence and young adults, characterised by the appearance of a single lesion called the 'herald patch', followed after 24–72 hours by numerous smaller discrete lesions on the trunk, upper arms and thighs. Typically the distribution is along the lines of the ribs, giving a 'christmas tree' appearance. It is thought to be a viral infection, although this has not been proven.

TREATMENT

Apart from the rash patients are usually asymptomatic, although there may be an associated mild flu-like illness. No treatment is usually required beyond reassurance.

PROGNOSIS

● The rash clears spontaneously in about 6 weeks.

FOLLOW-UP

Follow-up is not usually necessary.

[1] Björnberg A *et al.* (1972) *Acta Dermatovenerol.*, **42**, (suppl. 50), 1.

Granuloma Annulare

Granuloma annulare lesions[1] consist of asymptomatic skin-coloured papules occurring typically on the dorsal aspect of the hands and feet. The cause is unknown. Multiple lesions are considered to be associated with diabetes mellitus, although this is not well established.

TREATMENT

1. Record any family history of diabetes; check urinalysis and a fasting blood sugar.
2. No specific treatment is usually necessary.
3. Intralesional corticosteroids may improve disfiguring lesions, although there is the risk that this can cause permanent skin atrophy.

PROGNOSIS

● This is a harmless condition but resolution may be slow, taking years rather than months.

FOLLOW-UP

Follow-up should be as necessary.

[1] Wells R S *et al.* (1963) *Br. J. Dermatol.*, **75**, 199.

Alopecia Areata

Alopecia areata is a condition in which there are areas of well-circumscribed hair-loss on the scalp which have characteristic exclamation mark hairs. The cause is unknown, although there is an increased incidence of vitiligo and other autoimmune diseases in affected individuals and their families.

TREATMENT

1. No specific treatment for this disorder is known.
2. Many agents can induce hair regrowth to a limited extent but their effect is usually temporary; examples include intralesional and topical steroids.
3. Alopecia areata should be distinguished from habitual hair-pulling (trichotillomania) and ringworm of the scalp.

PROGNOSIS

- Alopecia areata is usually self-limiting. Most cases, with only a few small areas of hair loss, have a good prognosis and reassurance is very important.
- The earlier the onset and the more extensive the hair loss, the worse the prognosis. Occasionally the whole scalp is bald with loss of eyebrows and eyelashes (alopecia totalis) and rarely there is complete loss of all body hair (alopecia universalis).

FOLLOW-UP

Follow-up should be routine while the condition persists.

[1] Rook A J, Dawber R P R (1982) *Diseases of the Hair and Scalp*. Oxford: Blackwell Scientific Publications.

Impetigo

Impetigo[1,2] is a contagious superficial skin infection with a yellow exudate that dries and forms a honey-coloured crust. It may present as fragile blisters, particularly in neonates and infants. The condition is caused by *Staphylococcus aureus*, β-haemolytic streptococci or a mixed infection.

TREATMENT

1. Soaks, either physiological (normal) saline or potassium permanganate soaks to remove the crust, two or three times daily.
2. Topical antibiotics, such as chlortetracycline (Aureomycin), fusidic acid (Fucidin) or mupirocin (Bactroban) are useful for the treatment of early minor infections, applied three or four times daily for seven days.
3. Systemic antibiotics: most cases of impetigo require a course of an appropriate oral antibiotic, such as flucloxacillin, penicillin V or erythromycin. This is especially important for the treatment of streptococcal infections to prevent the serious complication of glomerulonephritis.
4. In patients with recurrent staphylococcal infections, screen for nasal carriers: nasal swabs should be taken not only from the patient but also from the whole family and close friends. Treatment with a nasal cream containing chlorhexidene and neomycin (Naseptin) is important to eradicate the focus of infection.

PROGNOSIS

- Patients will respond rapidly to appropriate antibiotic therapy.
- 'Impetigo' is most commonly seen as a secondary bacterial infection of a pre-existing skin condition such as atopic eczema or an infestation such as scabies or head lice. This may not become evident until after a course of antibiotics.

FOLLOW-UP

Follow-up is not usually necessary.

---

[1] Elias P M *et al.* (1977) *Arch. Dermatol.*, **113,** 207.
[2] Maibach H, Aly R (1981) *Skin Microbiology; Relevance to Clinical Infection.* New York: Springer Verlag.

Staphylococcal scalded skin syndrome

This serious complication occurs as a result of certain phage types of staphylococci (usually group II types 55 or 71) which produce an exotoxin, causing widespread toxic epidermic necrolysis.

TREATMENT

Intravenous anti-staphylococcal antibiotics, such as flucloxacillin (Floxapen) or fusidic acid (Fucidin), for 2–3 days, then orally for a further seven days.

PROGNOSIS

- Although rare, it is important that this potentially life-threatening condition is recognised early, because it responds well to appropriate systemic antibiotic therapy.

FOLLOW-UP

Follow-up should be as necessary.

Warts and Mollusca Contagiosa

Warts

Warts[1,2] are very common in schoolchildren and are caused by the human papilloma virus (HPV). It is now known that there are a number of strains of HPV (32 to date) giving rise to different clinical types of warts: the common type, plantar, plane, filiform and genital warts.

TREATMENT

1. Treatment is by daily application of a wart paint, such as 16.7% salicylic acid with 16.7% lactic acid (Salactol) or glutaraldehyde (Glutarol).
2. Cryotherapy using liquid nitrogen.
3. Plantar warts are best treated with salicylic acid plasters (40%) or formalin soaks (formaldehyde 4% in normal saline).
4. Genital warts respond to treatment with podophyllum (15, 20 or 25% in benzoin compound tincture) applied once weekly, under medical supervision, for up to six weeks.

PROGNOSIS

- A large proportion of common warts disappear spontaneously, although this can take from a few weeks to a number of years.
- Children who are immunosuppressed and those with atopic eczema are especially susceptible to warts.

FOLLOW-UP

Follow-up is necessary only if the warts are persistent, as in the immunosuppressed patient.

[1] Singer A *et al.* (1985) *Br. J. Hosp. Med.*, **34,** 104.
[2] Jablonska S *et al.* (1982) In *Recent Advances in Dermatology – 6* (Rook A, Maibach H eds), p. 1. Edinburgh: Churchill Livingstone.

Mollusca contagiosa

Mollusca contagiosa are smooth translucent papules with a characteristic central punctum, caused by a pox virus. These are common in children and tend to occur in crops. They can appear anywhere on the body and typically affect adjacent skin surfaces.

TREATMENT

1. No treatment initially is quite reasonable, especially in young children.
2. Otherwise, gentle cryotherapy using liquid nitrogen.

PROGNOSIS

- Spontaneous resolution takes place within a few weeks to several months.

FOLLOW-UP

Follow-up is usually only necessary in the immunocompromised patient.

Superficial Fungal Infections

Infection of the scalp (tinea capitis)[1] is seen as a patch of hair loss with broken hairs. Most species (in particular *Microsporum*) fluoresce green under a Wood's (long-wave UVL) lamp.

TREATMENT

1. Griseofulvin is specific for dermatophyte infections. Treatment of the scalp requires 4–6 weeks of therapy (10 mg/kg body weight daily in divided doses).
2. Topical antifungal agents are ineffective.

PROGNOSIS

- There is full recovery with total regrowth of hair, if treated promptly and correctly.

FOLLOW-UP

A routine follow-up appointment at the end of the course of treatment is usually all that is necessary.

---

[1] Roberts S O B *et al.* (1986) In *Textbook of Dermatology* (Rook A, Wilkinson D S, Ebling F J G, Champion R H, Burton J L eds) 4th edn, vol. 2, p. 885. Oxford: Blackwell Scientific Publications.

Infestations

Scabies

Scabies[1,2] is a highly contagious disorder caused by the mite, *Sarcoptes scabiei*. The typical eruption consists of intensely pruritic papules, vesicles and burrows. The distribution tends to favour the finger webs, wrists and genitalia. In infants, lesions are commonly found on the palms and soles and around the axillae.

TREATMENT

1. Gamma benzene hexachloride (Quellada) or monosulfiram lotion; two applications on consecutive nights.
2. The whole family should be treated whether or not infestation is evident.
3. Following treatment, bed linen, underwear and night clothes should be changed and all items washed.
4. Use calamine lotion for itching persisting after treatment.

PROGNOSIS

- Affected individuals will respond to treatment, although it is very important that all family members and contacts at school should be examined and treated simultaneously.
- The itching might take several weeks to settle.

FOLLOW-UP

Follow-up is not usually necessary.

Lice

Head lice[1,2] (pediculosis capitis) are common in schoolchildren. The nit is a head-louse egg which is firmly attached to a scalp hair; nits are readily recognisable as small white adherent grain-like particles. Head lice cause severe irritation of the scalp and secondary bacterial infection.

TREATMENT

1. Treatment is with malathion (Prioderm, Derbac) or carbaryl (Carylderm, Derbac) lotion applied to the entire scalp and left on for 12 hours. The hair should then be washed and the dead nits removed with a fine-tooth metal comb.

2. As with scabies, all family members should be treated simultaneously.

PROGNOSIS

- Prognosis is as for scabies.

FOLLOW-UP

Follow-up is not usually necessary.

---

[1] Hewitt M (1977) *Medicine*, **32,** 1849.
[2] Hurwitz S (1981) *Clinical Pediatric Dermatology*, p. 301. Philadelphia: Saunders.

15

Infections and Viral Diseases

J. D. M. Gould

β-Haemolytic Streptococcal Infections

Group A streptococci

Lancefield Group A streptococci are among the most common pathogenic bacteria isolated from children. More than 60 different types have been recognised. The mechanism of spread varies according to the clinical type of infection. Manifestations of disease include pharyngitis, lymphadenitis, suppurative tonsillitis, impetigo, cellulitis and puerperal sepsis. Erythrogenic (pyrogenic) toxins may lead to scarlet fever. Poorly understood immunological processes lead to the occasional development of complications such as acute rheumatic fever (p. 56) and acute glomerulonephritis (p. 122).

PREVENTION

1. Sibling contacts of cases have a 25% risk of acquisition of infection (rates as high as 50% during epidemics).
2. Approximately 50–80% culture positive contacts become ill.
3. Prophylactic antibiotic therapy of close family contacts should be considered especially with large families in crowded conditions, and where the index case has developed rheumatic fever or nephritis. Short courses of antibiotics for contacts are inappropriate.
4. Long-term prophylaxis in patients who have a well documented history of rheumatic fever (including Sydenham's chorea) is mandatory, using:

   a) Penicillin V, 125–250 mg twice daily orally (low risk).
   b) Benzathine penicillin G 750 mg i.m. every 4 weeks (high risk).
   c) Sulphadiazine 0.5–1 g once daily if the patient is penicillin intolerant.

5. Children with rheumatic valvular heart disease require additional short-term antibiotic prophylaxis at the time of dental and other surgical procedures where bacteraemia is likely:

a) Low risk surgery: erythromycin 20 mg/kg orally 1 hour before, then 10 mg/kg 6 hours later.
b) High risk surgery: amoxycillin 50 mg/kg i.m. (maximum 2 g) plus gentamicin 2 mg/kg i.m. half hour before procedure, then amoxycillin 25 mg/kg orally or i.m. 6 hours later.

TREATMENT

1. Penicillin, orally or systemically. Erythromycin if there is penicillin allergy. Oral therapy (penicillin V 125–500 mg four times daily, depending on age) must be maintained for a minimum of 10 days for pharyngitis, lymphadenitis or otitis. Any acute pharyngitis, especially if associated with tonsillar exudation (whitish yellow), cervical lymphadenopathy or systemic toxicity should be considered as being potentially of streptococcal aetiology and treated as such.
2. Surgical drainage may be indicated for peritonsillar abscess.
3. Local skin care and antiseptics should be used in addition to oral/systemic therapy for impetigo.
4. There is no clear proof that penicillin reduces the risk of development of acute nephritis[1], although it will effectively prevent rheumatic fever and suppurative complications.

PROGNOSIS

- Spontaneous recovery usually occurs from streptococcal throat infections or impetigo. There are occasional suppurative complications and non-suppurative sequelae.
- 3% develop rheumatic fever from untreated respiratory streptococcal infections under epidemic conditions by only 0.3% under endemic conditions[2].
- In those with a previous history of rheumatic fever there is a 15–50% risk of recurrence with repeat streptococcal throat infection[3]. Regular

prophylactic therapy will minimise this risk.

- 10–15% risk of acute glomerulonephritis with nephritogenic strain infection[4].
- Cellulitis can spread rapidly via lymphatics or blood stream, and needs aggressive therapy.
- Unrecognised puerperal sepsis and neonatal infections have high mortality rates.

FOLLOW-UP

No follow-up is necessary for uncomplicated streptococcal infection if adequately treated. The complications of rheumatic fever (p. 56) or glomerulonephritis (p. 122) require regular review.

[1] Weinstein L et al. (1971) J. Infect. Dis., **124,** 229.
[2] Siegel A C et al. (1961) New Eng. J. Med., **265,** 559.
[3] Wannamaker L W (1981) In Textbook of Pediatric Infectious Diseases (Feigin RD, Cherry JD eds), p. 986. Philadelphia: Saunders.
[4] Wannamaker L W (1970) New Eng. J. Med., **282,** 23, 78.

Group B streptococci

Group B streptococci are an important cause of acute bacterial infection in the perinatal period. Between 10–40% mothers are colonised around the time of birth[1]. The incidence of sepsis in the newborn is in the range of 1.5–4/1000 live births[2]. Infection in the newborn may be either early (respiratory distress, apnoea, overwhelming sepsis) or late (meningitis, osteomyelitis).

PREVENTION

1. No specific recommendation for the prevention of group B streptococcal infection in infants can be made. Any infant presenting with fever, respiratory distress, radiographic 'air bronchogram', meningitis or systemic collapse should be considered infected and treated accordingly until culture results are available.
2. Antibiotic treatment of pregnant women colonised with group B streptococci does not lead to long-term eradication, and cannot be recommended. Treatment of high risk, colonised pregnant women (e.g. those with premature or prolonged rupture of membranes, or fever), by high dose amoxycillin or ampicillin before and during labour appears to decrease the incidence of neonatal infection[3].

TREATMENT

1. Early use of antibiotics in presumed or possible neonatal sepsis is mandatory pending culture results. Combination therapy with ceftazidime/amoxycillin, ceftazidime/penicillin or penicillin/gentamicin, will provide broad spectrum cover pending confirmation of infection.
2. Specific therapy: benzylpenicillin 60 mg/kg/dose every 12 hours (preterm infant) or every 8 hours (term infant) for 10 days (sepsis) or 14 days (meningitis).

PROGNOSIS

- Early infection

  a) Factors including placentally acquired immunity, prolonged rupture of membranes and prematurity influence outcome in colonised infants. There is a 20–50% mortality with sepsis.

  b) 20–50% survivors with meningeal infection have neurological sequelae[4].

- Late onset infections 14% mortality overall. Highest mortality in those with meningitis[5].

FOLLOW-UP

Neurological or other sequelae of severe sepsis may need long-term review and reassessment.

[1] Baker C J et al. (1973) J. Pediatr., **83,** 919.
[2] Anthony B F (1981) In Textbook of Pediatric Infectious Diseases (Feigin R D, Cherry J D eds.), p. 995. Philadelphia: Saunders.
[3] Report of The Committee on Infectious Diseases (1986) Red Book 20th edn, p. 343. Illinois: American Academy of Pediatrics.
[4] Baker C J (1977) J. Infect. Dis., **136,** 137.
[5] Speck W T et al. (1979) In Care of The High-risk Neonate (Klaus M H, Fanaroff A A, eds.), p. 267. Philadelphia: Saunders.

Brucellosis

Brucellosis is primarily an infectious disease of cattle (*Brucella abortus*), goats (*B. melitensis*) and swine (*B. suis*). Occasional infections from sheep (*B. ovis*) and dogs (*B. canis*) have been described. In children most disease occurs from infected dairy products, but in adults it can commonly occur by airborne-spread in heavily contaminated areas (e.g. slaughter houses). *Brucella* species differ in degree of invasiveness and virulence, *B. melitensis* and *B. suis* producing most severe disease. In countries where compulsory pasteurisation of milk and control measures in cattle and goats are effected, the disease is rare. Following infection, there is usually an incubation period of 1–3 weeks, followed by either insidious or acute onset of fever, chills, weakness, malaise, weight loss, anorexia, arthralgia and myalgia. Lymphadenopathy is common, and hepatomegaly and splenomegaly are seen. More rarely endocarditis, pneumonia, abscesses, osteomyelitis and meningoencephalitis occur.

PREVENTION

Eradication of brucellosis in animals has proved difficult, especially in developing countries. Pasteurisation of all potentially infected dairy produce would eliminate almost all brucellosis occurring in children.

TREATMENT

1. Uncomplicated disease

   a) Tetracycline or oxytetracycline orally 25–40 mg/kg/day (maximum 2 g/day) in three or four divided doses for 3–4 weeks.
   b) If the patient is under nine years of age, to prevent staining of teeth, trimethoprim-sulfamethoxazole (10 mg/kg/day trimethoprim) for four weeks has been advised[1] but leads to a high (46%) relapse rate in adults[2].

2. Severe or complicated disease

   a) Intravenous tetracycline 15–20 mg/kg/day combined with streptomycin 20 mg/kg/day (maximum 1 g/day for two weeks) or gentamicin 6 mg/kg/day in three divided doses intravenously.
   b) Addition of rifampicin 15–20 mg/kg/day for treatment of neurological disease, endocarditis or abscess. Six weeks' combination therapy may be required for the treatment of endocarditis or abscess[3].

   c) Prednisolone 1 mg/kg/24 hours in three divided doses may prevent the Herxheimer-type reaction seen in 5–10% patients when antimicrobial therapy is commenced in severe disease, or when the diagnosis has been delayed[1].
   d) Abscesses should be drained surgically where possible and such patients should be isolated.

PROGNOSIS

- The mortality for untreated brucellosis is 2–3% overall[4].
- 84% deaths are reported associated with endocarditis[5].
- The outcome is dependent on the clinical manifestations, usually classified as:

   a) Asymptomatic brucellosis: 30–50% infection in adult vets/abbatoir workers are subclinical. No figures are available for children.
   b) Acute brucellosis: presents with acute fever, weakness and anorexia. 10–30% patients are blood culture positive. Approximately 15% have associated splenomegaly, lymphadenopathy and hepatomegaly. 1–2% develop localised disease – usually associated with complications. Untreated, symptoms commonly settle within three months, or may become chronic (especially *B. suis*), localised (especially *B. melitensis* or *B. suis*), or relaps-

ing (2–15%). With prompt therapy 96% children are afebrile within seven days[6]. Children are often thought to have mild or self-limiting disease especially if infected with *B. abortus*[7].

c) Chronic brucellosis: often associated with localised abscesses. Headaches, lassitude and depression are seen in 70% affected patients. Anxiety and emotional lability are seen in 18%[9], splenomegaly in 50%, and hepatomegaly in 25%.

d) Localised brucellosis: disease can occur in any organ including spleen, testis, liver, gallbladder and kidney but is most important in:

   i) Bones and joints (20% localised disease): commonest in spine (usually *B. melitensis*) or weight-bearing joints (especially knee). Suppurative and destructive when seen with acute disease, but aseptic reactive arthopathy may also occur in chronic disease[10,11].

   ii) Cardiovascular (20% localised disease): endocarditis, myocarditis and pericarditis can occur. Mortality in adults may be as high as 83%[5] but may not follow the same fulminant course in childhood[12].

   iii) Pulmonary (15% localised disease): bronchitis, pneumonia, pleurisy, pleural effusion, empyema and abscess can occur[13].

   iv) Neurological (10% localised disease): neurological complications may occur early or late in the disease and present as acute or subacute meningitis or encephalitis. Progress is dependent on rapid and appropriate therapy.

FOLLOW-UP

Fever should be monitored to make sure that there has been an adequate response to therapy. Most children are afebrile within seven days unless there are complications. Morbidity and mortality are low in children with prompt treatment, but relapse (2–15% with tetracycline/streptomycin therapy) can occur within three months of therapy, especially if short courses of antibiotics are given, in which case a more prolonged course of therapy including rifampicin should be considered[3]. Depression and emotional disturbances may last many weeks in adults, but are not commonly reported in children. Specific complications (e.g. cardiac, neurological or bone disease) may need prolonged monitoring and careful management (e.g. prosthetic valve replacement with endocarditis).

[1] Hall W H *et al.* (1977) In *Infectious Diseases*, 2nd edn (Hoeprich P D ed.), p. 1035. Hagerstown: Harper & Row.

[2] Ariza J *et al.* (1985) *J. Infect. Dis.*, **152**, 1358.

[3] Mandell G L *et al.* (1985) *Principles and Practice of Infectious Diseases*, 2nd edn (Mandell G L, Dougles R G, Bennett J E eds). New York: Wiley.

[4] Christie A B (1980) *Infectious Disease: Epidemiology and Clinical Practice*, 3rd edn, p. 839. Edinburgh: Churchill Livingstone.

[5] Cohen P S *et al.* (1980) *Prog. Cardiovasc. Dis.*, **22**, 205.

[6] Mandell G L *et al.* (1979) *Principles and Practice of Infectious Diseases* (Mandell G L, Dougles R G, Bennett J E eds), p. 1972. New York: Wiley.

[7] Street L Jr *et al.* (1975) *Paediatrics*, **55**, 416.

[8] Martin W J *et al.* (1961) *Arch. Int. Med.*, **107**, 75.

[9] Sacks N *et al.* (1976) *S. Afr. Med. J.*, **50**, 725.

[10] Glasgow M M S (1976) *Br. J. Surg.*, **63**, 283.

[11] Alacorn G S *et al.* (1981) *J. Rheum.*, **8**, 621.

[12] Lubani M *et al.* (1986) *Arch. Dis. Childh.*, **61**, 569.

[13] Geer A E (1956) *Dis. Chest*, **29**, 508.

Chickenpox (Varicella)

Chickenpox is a common and highly contagious infection caused by the varicella–zoster (VZ) virus, a member of the herpes group. Infection is characterised by a generalised vesicular rash usually with few systemic effects. The incubation period is 11–21 days. Infectivity lasts from one day before the rash develops until all lesions have crusted. After recovery, the virus may persist in latent form for many years, and reactivate producing a vesicular eruption localised to a sensory dermatome (zoster or shingles).

PREVENTION

1. Zoster immune globulin (ZIG) will modify or prevent illness in non-immune individuals, and should be administered to those at risk from varicella within 48 hours if possible, and preferably not more than 96 hours after exposure.
2. Candidates for ZIG provided significant exposure has occurred:

   a) Immunocompromised susceptible children.
   b) Normal susceptible children or adolescents, if hospitalised or likely to be in contact with immunocompromised children.
   c) Newborn infant of a mother who had onset of chickenpox within five days before delivery or within 48 hours after delivery.
   d) Preterm infants (> 28 weeks' gestation) whose mother lacks prior history of chickenpox.
   e) Preterm infants < 28 weeks' gestation or < 1000 g regardless of maternal history[1].

3. Dosage of ZIG

Newborn/under 1 year	100 mg
1–5 years	250 mg
6–10 years	500 mg
11–14 years	750 mg
15 years–adult	1000 mg

TREATMENT

1. Uncomplicated varicella requires no specific therapy.
2. Neonates with VZ infection should be treated with acyclovir 10 mg/kg every 8 hours i.v. for 10 days.
3. In immune suppressed children, or those with severe or atypical chickenpox, give acyclovir 250 mg/m² every 8 hours i.v. over one hour for 10 days, or in ambulant children oral acyclovir 500 mg/m² 5 times daily[2].
4. If CNS invasion suspected, give acyclovir 500 mg/m² i.v. every 8 hours. (Monitor renal function[3].) Post-exanthem encephalitis or cerebellitis is not an indication for acyclovir, and the use of dexamethasone is controversial[4,5].
5. Herpes zoster should be treated with oral or i.v. acyclovir.

PROGNOSIS

- Infection is generally mild, and sequelae are uncommon.
- Immunodeficient children and neonates can develop a fulminant viraemia, with atypical bullous or haemorrhagic lesions, hepatitis, pulmonary complications and encephalitis. Untreated, the mortality is 20–50%. The risk to neonates is greatest when delivery is within five days of onset of the maternal rash[6].
- Rare complications in apparently normal children include:

  a) Post-exanthem encephalitis, usually associated with cerebellitis. Recovery is usual, but may not be complete.
  b) Acute progressive encephalitis occurring with the exanthem, which must be differentiated from Reye's syndrome. Poor prognosis.
  c) Guillain–Barré syndrome.
  d) Idiopathic thrombocytopenic purpura.
  e) Very rarely, nephritis, myocarditis and arthritis have been reported.

FOLLOW-UP

No specific follow-up is necessary except where neurological or other complications ensue.

[1] Report of the Committee on Infectious Diseases (1986) *Red Book* 20th edn, p. 402. Illinois: American Academy of Pediatrics.
[2] Novelli V M *et al.* (1984) *J. Infect. Dis.*, **149**, 478.

[3] Bean B *et al.* (1985) *J. Infect. Dis.*, **151**, 362.
[4] Illis L S *et al.* (1984) In *Contemporary Neurology* (Harrison M J G ed.), p. 350. London: Butterworths.
[5] Boe J *et al.* (1965) *Br. Med. J.*, **i**, 1094.
[6] Meyers J D (1974) *J. Infect. Dis.*, **129**, 215.

Cytomegalovirus (CMV)

Infection with this herpes virus is commonly subclinical, but it may cause severe systemic disease (cytomegalic inclusion disease) when acquired *in utero* or perinatally, or a glandular fever-like illness in older children. Immunodeficient children may develop chronic and ultimately fatal pulmonary, hepatic or systemic disease. By adult life 20–80% possess CMV antibody[1] with a higher incidence of earlier infection in lower socio-economic groups. It is the most common virus known to be transmitted *in utero*.

PREVENTION

1. Cytomegalovirus hyperimmune globulin has been developed for prophylaxis of disease in bone marrow transplant patients, and preliminary data indicate efficacy[2].
2. Pregnant women caring for children in newborn nurseries and day care centres should be warned of the high excretion rate of CMV (1–3% in newborns, up to 70% in 1–2 year olds), and urged to practise good hygiene. The extent of risk to such workers has not been established.

TREATMENT

1. Congenital and perinatal infection
   No treatment yet evaluated is useful (acyclovir, vidarabine, transfer factor, hyperimmune globulin or interferon).
2. Acquired or reactivated infection

   a) Severe pulmonary, ocular or systemic manifestations in the immunosuppressed have shown response to some of the newer antiviral compounds, e.g. the acyclic nucleoside BW B759U[3,4] and phosphonoformate (PFA foscarnet sodium)[5], but further evaluation is required.

   b) Both prevention and treatment of infection with interferon and hyperimmune globulin require further evaluation[2,6].

PROGNOSIS

● Congenital and perinatal infection

   a) Congenital CMV infection occurs in 1–2% live births, and perinatally acquired infection is two to five times more common.

   b) Both primary and recurrent CMV infection in pregnancy can infect the fetus. The outcome is dependent upon the immune status of the mother. Clinical disease in the neonate is very unlikely with recurrent maternal infection[7].

   c) In primary maternal infection there is a 50% risk of fetal infection indicated by seropositivity, with 15% infected infants showing clinical disease[7].

   d) Less than 5% all infected infants manifest severe clinical disease (cytomegalic inclusion disease – hepatosplenomegaly, jaundice purpura, microcephaly, cerebral calcification and chorioretinitis). Mortality is 20–30%[8]. Hepatic and haematological complications usually resolve, cerebral and ocular complications persist and usually have a poor prognosis.

e) 5–15% asymptomatic congenital and perinatally acquired infections may present in the first year with pneumonitis[9] or in the pre-school years with deafness[10] or impaired cognitive function[11].

- Acquired infection

   a) Most infection is subclinical or mild. Clinical disease manifesting as a glandular fever-like illness is self-limited, but may be symptomatic for some months.

   b) Primary infection, and occasionally reactivated infection, may result in progressive fatal interstitial pneumonitis, hepatitis or gastrointestinal haemorrhage in immunosuppressed children.

FOLLOW-UP

Follow-up is usually unnecessary with CMV infection in the normal host, although recurrent low grade fever, anorexia, lethargy and depression are sometimes seen. Immunosuppressed children require careful monitoring of pulmonary function (chest x-ray, lung function studies, lung biopsy). Congenital infection requires regular monitoring of neurological function, development, and assessment of hearing in pre-school years.

[1] Krech U H et al. (1971) Cytomegalovirus Infections of Man. Basel: Karger.
[2] Blacklock H A et al. (1985) Lancet, ii, 152.
[3] Shepp D H et al. (1985) Ann. Intern. Med., 103, 368.
[4] Felsenstein D et al. (1985) Ann. Intern. Med., 103, 377.
[5] Ringden O et al. (1985) Lancet, i, 1503.
[6] Meyers J D (1985) Infection, 13 (suppl. 2), S211.
[7] Stagno S et al. (1982) New Eng. J. Med., 306, 945.
[8] Stagno S et al. (1985) New Eng. J. Med., 313, 1270.
[9] Dworsky M E et al. (1982) Pediatr. Infect. Dis., 1, 188.
[10] Melish M E et al. (1973) Am. J. Dis. Childh., 126, 190.
[11] Hanshaw J B et al. (1976) New Eng. J. Med., 295, 468.
[12] Pagano J S et al. (1975) J. Infect. Dis., 132, 114.

Dengue

Dengue fever and *dengue haemorrhagic fever* (DHF) are diseases caused by one of four antigenically distinct arthropod-borne viruses. Dengue is endemic in tropical Asia, the Pacific islands and the Caribbean. The alphavirus infections O'nyong-nyong and Chikungunya produce dengue-like disease in Africa, India and SE Asia. Non-immune children infected for the first time present with dengue fever, an acute febrile illness, characterised by biphasic fever, myalgia, arthralgia, rash, leukopenia and lymphadenopathy. The incubation period is 2–7 days. Children presenting with DHF show serological evidence of previous infection from a closely related virus, or are infants of immune mothers. Dengue haemorrhagic fever is characterised by increased capillary permeability, haemorrhagic diathesis, and in severe cases, a protein-losing shock syndrome (DSS).

PREVENTION

An attenuated vaccine for dengue type I and a killed vaccine for Chikungunya are effective, but not available for general use. The possibility exists that dengue immunisation may sensitise the recipient so that ensuing infection may result in DHF/DSS.

TREATMENT

1. Dengue fever. Treatment is supportive, with antipyretics, analgesics and fluid replacement.
2. DHF/DSS

   a) Monitor for hypovolaemia (CVP line if profound shock). Plasma expansion[1], correction of acidosis and inotropic support (e.g. dopamine) as required.
   b) Replace haemorrhagic loss with fresh blood. Consider clotting factor concentrate or fresh blood exchange transfusion to correct disseminated intravascular coagulation (DIC).
   c) Avoid salicylate therapy. Steroids are of no benefit[2].

PROGNOSIS

- Dengue fever. The primary infection is usually self-limited and benign. No significant morbidity with appropriate supportive care, but convalescence may be slow, with characteristic asthenia and depression, especially in older children.
- DHF/DSS

   a) 15–20% mortality of hospitalised cases despite intensive care[2]. Death from uncontrollable haemorrhage, DIC and irreversible shock.
   b) Long-term sequelae are uncommon, but include asthenia, depression and residual brain damage from haemorrhage or infarction.

FOLLOW-UP

Bradycardia and ventricular extrasystoles may persist for several weeks, and are not of poor prognosis. Asthenia and depression may require specific measures.

[1] Cohen S N *et al.* (1966) *J. Pediatr.*, **68,** 448.
[2] Sumarmo M D *et al.* (1982) *Paediatrics*, **69,** 45.

Diphtheria

Diphtheria is an acute infectious disease caused by *Corynebacterium diphtheriae*. Symptoms result from toxin release following infection of the upper respiratory tract. The toxin causes local tissue necrosis with resultant inflammation, oedema, exudation and mucosal membrane formation. The membrane and oedematous tissue may encroach upon the airway, resulting in respiratory obstruction. Toxin dissemination may result in widespread tissue damage, especially to heart (myocarditis), nervous system (coma, peripheral neuritis), liver (necrosis) and kidneys.

PREVENTION

Active immunisation in early childhood provides good but not complete immunity. Boosters should be given at pre-school age, and after six years of age using the adult vaccine at 10-yearly intervals or when there is contact with disease.

TREATMENT

1. Cases where there is evidence of respiratory obstruction or palatal/pharyngeal paralysis should be nursed in an intensive care unit if available.
2. Equine antitoxin should be administered as soon as possible in a single dose of 40 000–120 000 units i.v. (larger dosage for more severe disease). To avoid the risk of anaphylaxis, test for horse serum sensitivity first with 0.1 ml of 1:1000 dilution in saline intradermally (>10 mm erythema within 20 minutes indicates the need for desensitisation).
3. Penicillin or erythromycin for 7 days minimum or until three consecutive cultures negative.
4. Laryngeal obstruction may be relieved by tracheostomy if necessary.
5. Monitor for evidence of myocarditis (the risk persists for up to six weeks after onset of symptoms). The extent of the pharyngeal exudate is a significant risk factor for development of myocarditis[1].
6. Prednisolone does not influence the development of myocarditis or neuritis[1].
7. Palatal and pharyngeal paralysis will necessitate nasogastric feeding or parenteral nutrition.

PROGNOSIS

- Prognosis depends upon the virulence of the organism (the gravis strain has a poor prognosis), location and extent of diphtheritic membrane, immunisation status of host, speed of commencement of appropriate medical management, and availability of intensive care facilities for maintaining airway and monitoring for cardiac and other complications.
- 30–50% mortality overall used to occur prior to the use of antitoxin, antibiotics and intensive medical care, worse in children under four years of age. Mortality now <5%.
- 10–25% patients develop myocarditis and this is responsible for 50–60% deaths[2].
- Recovery from diphtheritic neuropathy should be complete in survivors[3].

FOLLOW-UP

Recovery from the complications of diphtheria is normally complete, and long-term follow-up is not indicated. An exception is diphtheritic myocarditis, which may lead to residual damage requiring cardiac assessment. Active immunisation should be given to all patients during convalescence, as infection does not confer lasting immunity.

[1] Thisyakorn U S A *et al.* (1984) *Pediatr. Infect. Dis.*, **3**, 126.
[2] Tahernia A C (1969) *J. Pediatr.*, **75**, 1008.
[3] Karrar Z A (1981) *J. Trop. Pediatr.*, **27**, 23.

Gonorrhoea

Gonorrhoea in childhood includes all disease caused by *Neisseria gonorrhoeae*, including ophthalmia neonatorum, disseminated sepsis and arthritis, vaginitis, proctitis and urethritis.

TREATMENT

1. Gonococcal ophthalmia.

    a) Isolate the infant. Protect staff with gloves.
    b) Benzylpenicillin 30 mg/kg 12-hourly i.v. for seven days, plus penicillin irrigation to eyes using eye drops hourly for 6 hours, then 2-hourly for 12 hours, then every 4 hours.
2. Disseminated infection and arthritis. Benzylpenicillin 60 mg/kg/24 hours divided into three or four doses i.v. Give for 10–14 days.
3. Childhood disease. Ophthalmia, arthritis or disseminated disease will require intravenous penicillin therapy for a minimum of 10 days. For local uncomplicated vulvovaginitis and urethritis give oral penicillin therapy.
4. The possibility of penicillinase-producing strains of gonococcus should be considered where response to therapy is poor. Consider use of spectinomycin[1] or systemic cephalosporin therapy[2].

PROGNOSIS

- Perinatal infection. (This includes gonococcal ophthalmia (see p. 20) and, rarely, disseminated infection with arthritis and septicaemia.)

    a) Untreated or late recognised ophthalmia may lead to perforation of the globe, panophthalmitis and permanent blindness. Early and vigorous combined topical and systemic therapy will result in complete recovery.
    b) Outcome from disseminated infection depends on early recognition and start of appropriate therapy.

- Childhood disease

    a) Infection is rare in childhood. The possibility of sexual abuse should always be considered.
    b) Uncomplicated vulvovaginitis or urethritis should respond rapidly to therapy without sequelae.
    c) Prognosis in gonococcal arthritis depends on prompt recognition and institution of therapy. Purulent arthritis of the hip may rarely lead to femoral head necrosis.

FOLLOW-UP

All patients should have follow-up cultures, and the source of infection should be identified and treated.

[1] Ward M E (1977) *J. Antimicrob. Chemother.*, **3**, 323.
[2] Collier A C *et al.* (1984) *Am. J. Med.*, **77** (suppl. symposia), 68.

Herpes Simplex

Herpes simplex virus, like other herpes viruses, is a DNA virus with a capability for reactivation following a primary infection and latent period. Many of the troublesome peri-oral, cutaneous and genital manifestations of the disease in children and adults relate to reactivation. Two types of herpes simplex virus have been identified. Type 1 is responsible for infections of the oral cavity, eye, central nervous system and skin. Type 2 is responsible for genital disease and most perinatally acquired infection.

PREVENTION

1. Patients and staff with open lesions are potentially infectious. Such lesions should be covered if possible, and any staff member with a herpetic whitlow should not have direct patient care responsibilities. Care should in particular be taken to isolate children with eczema, immunocompromised patients and neonates from known infection.
2. Neonatal infection

   a) Women found to have clinically apparent herpes simplex infections in late pregnancy or in labour should be delivered by caesarean section if possible (unless membranes have been ruptured for more than 4 hours)[1].
   b) Recently delivered mothers with active oral herpes should use a mask at times of contact with their infants but should be allowed to breast feed, so long as personal hygiene is emphasised.
   c) Treatment of active lesions in the mother with acyclovir ointment may reduce virus shedding.

TREATMENT

1. Primary gingivostomatitis and cutaneous lesions

   a) Self-limiting disease. Treatment with analgesics and fluid is usually sufficient.
   b) Acyclovir (suspension or tablets) 100–200 mg five times daily for seven days, may shorten the course of illness if given soon after the appearance of lesions, but has yet to be fully evaluated.
   c) Topical acyclovir therapy is ineffective for recurrent cold sores[2].

2. Eye infections. Acyclovir ophthalmic ointment 3% topically five times daily for seven days.
3. Genital herpes. Primary and recurrent infection: acyclovir orally 100–200 mg five times daily for seven days[3]. Early treatment may decrease recurrence risk[4].
4. CNS infection

   a) Acyclovir 500 mg/m² 8-hourly i.v. over one hour, for 10–14 days. Monitor for renal toxicity, especially if fluids are being limited.
   b) Institute standard therapy to minimise cerebral oedema – hyperventilation, mannitol, fluid limitation and possible surgical decompression.
   c) The role of dexamethasone in combination with acyclovir is yet to be evaluated, and cannot be recommended.

5. Immunodeficiency. With a risk of dissemination or eczema herpeticum use acyclovir 250 mg/m² 8-hourly i.v. over one hour or 500 mg/m² five times daily orally[5,6] for 7–10 days.
6. Perinatal infection

   a) Acyclovir 10 mg/kg 8-hourly by i.v. infusion over one hour for 10–14 days.
   b) Full supportive therapy as necessary.

PROGNOSIS

- Gingivostomatitis. A primary infection in children. 100% complete recovery after 10–14 days unless underlying immunodeficiency is present.
- Primary skin infections. Usually mild or subclinical. Spontaneous 100% recovery unless underlying immunodeficiency or eczema. Severe eczema herpeticum may become hae-

morrhagic or develop secondary bacterial infection. With supportive therapy and antiviral therapy, recovery should be complete.

- Secondary mucocutaneous infections. Recurrent vesiculation related to reactivation common, but benign. Recurrence of eczema herpeticum is seen[7].
- Eye infections. Corneal involvement results in dendritic ulceration and permanent scarring without appropriate early therapy.
- Vulvovaginitis. Usually seen in adolescent sexually active children or may be a pointer to sexual abuse except in perinatal period. Primary infection heals spontaneously, reactivation is common.
- Central nervous system. This may be a primary infection (commoner in younger children[8]) or reactivation. Except perinatally, it affects frontal and temporal lobes, and may be unilateral or bilateral.

    a) 70–80% mortality untreated in first 30 days, 90% mortality by 6 months (all age groups)[9].
    b) 30–54% mortality with antiviral therapy[10]. Morbidity often severe, with hemiparesis, cranial nerve defects, seizures, dysphasia and personality changes[10].

- Perinatal infection

    a) 80–85% mortality with disseminated infection if untreated. Major morbidity in survivors[11,12]. Antiviral chemotherapy has reduced mortality to 25%, but morbidity, especially with CNS involvement, remains high[13].
    b) Aetiology may go unrecognised, as presentation may be with disseminated viraemia, indistinguishable from overwhelming bacterial sepsis, and show no evidence of mucocutaneous lesions[14]
    c) Localised ocular or cutaneous infection is at risk of dissemination.

FOLLOW-UP

Most primary infections in normal children are self-limiting, and once healed require no specific follow-up. Disseminated infection in neonates, and CNS infection may produce profound morbidity in survivors, requiring long-term assessment and support. Recurrent or persistent infection in the immunocompromised host will require regular follow-up, with assessment of immune status, confirmation of recurrence by viral culture, and intermittent or long-term acyclovir, topically or systemically, as appropriate.

[1] Nahmias A J (1976) In *Infectious Diseases of the Fetus and Newborn Infant* (Remington J S, Klein J O eds.), p. 156. Philadelphia: Saunders.
[2] Spruance S L et al. (1982) *Am. J. Med.*, **73**, 315.
[3] Bryson Y J et al. (1983) *New Eng. J. Med.*, **308**, 916.
[4] Bryson Y J (1983) *J. Antimicrob. Chemother.*, **12**, 61.
[5] Serota F T et al. (1982) *J. Am. Med. Assoc.*, **247**, 2132.
[6] Novelli V M et al. (1984) *J. Infect. Dis.*, **149**, 478.
[7] Brain R T (1956) *Br. Med. J.*, **i**, 1061.
[8] Marshall W C (1983) In *Paediatric Neurology* (Brett F M ed.), p. 508. Edinburgh: Churchill Livingstone.
[9] Hirsch M S (1979) *New Eng. J. Med.*, **301**, 987.
[10] Ho D D et al. (1985) *Med. Clin. North Am.*, **69**, 415.
[11] Hanshaw J B et al. (1985) In *Viral Diseases in the Fetus and Newborn* (Hanshaw J B, Dudgeon J A, Marshall W C eds.), p. 139. Philadelphia: Saunders.
[12] Whitley R J et al. (1980) *Paediatrics*, **66**, 495.
[13] Corey L et al. (1986) *New Eng. J. Med.*, **314**, 749.
[14] Arvin A M et al. (1982) *J. Pediatr.*, **100**, 715.

Infectious Mononucleosis

Infectious mononucleosis results from infection by the Epstein–Barr virus (EBV) of the herpes group. It is seen most frequently in adolescents and young adults, and is characterised by fever and lymphoid hyperplasia, frequently accompanied by pharyngitis, mild hepatic dysfunction, non-specific rashes and haematological abnormalities. Infection is often mild or inapparent, but occasionally severe complications are seen.

TREATMENT

1. Short-term steroid administration (under 14 days) reduces symptoms of more severe manifestations[1], e.g. threatened airway obstruction from lymphoedema, hepatitis or severe abdominal symptoms.
2. Neurological complications (Guillain–Barré syndrome, meningoencephalitis) and haemolytic anaemia may respond to a prolonged course of steroids.
3. A number of acyclic nucleoside antiviral agents including acyclovir have been used in EBV infections in immunodeficient patients[2,3] but their clinical value has yet to be confirmed.

PROGNOSIS

- Of symptomatic patients, 85% develop pharyngitis, 95% lymphadenopathy and 50% a palpable spleen. 80% have elevated serum transaminases. If ampicillin therapy has been given, >90% will develop a macular rash.
- 10% symptomatic patients have CNS involvement, but this is often mild. Rarely convulsions, ataxia, Bell's palsy, transverse myelitis, Guillain-Barré syndrome and encephalitis are seen.

- Potentially lethal complications include:

  a) Meningoencephalitis and Guillain–Barré syndrome.
  b) Reye's syndrome.
  c) Splenic rupture (often associated with trauma).
  d) Severe pharyngitis and lymphadenopathy with respiratory obstruction.

- Severe, progressive and fatal illness is seen with some forms of immunodeficiency, including the X-linked immunoproliferative syndrome[4].
- Epstein–Barr virus appears to be a co-factor in the induction of Burkitt's lymphoma (Africa) and nasopharyngeal carcinoma (China).

FOLLOW-UP

No specific follow-up is necessary, except where neurological or other complications are seen. Some patients complain of lassitude and depression for many months in the recovery phase.

[1] Bolden K J (1972) *J. R. Coll. Gen. Practit.*, **22**, 87.
[2] Purtilo D T (1985) *Biomed. Pharmacother.*, **39**, 52.
[3] Lin J C et al. (1984) *J. Virol.*, **50**, 50.
[4] Sullivan J L (1983) *Adv. Pediatr.*, **30**, 365.

Pertussis

Pertussis is an acute infection of the respiratory tract produced by infection with *Bordetella pertussis* or *Bordetella parapertussis*. Similar symptoms are sometimes produced by adenovirus infections[1]. It is highly communicable. The incubation period of pertussis is 6–20 days. Infectivity is greatest early in the disease and lasts for about one month until all the organisms are cleared from the nasopharynx.

PREVENTION

1. Approximately 80% exposed children who have received three doses of pertussis vaccine (as DPT) will be protected. Immunisation is not routinely indicated over 6 years of age.
2. All infants and young children should be immunised against pertussis *unless*:
   a) The child has a proven or suspected neurological disorder (including seizures in the neonatal period).
   b) A first degree relative has a seizure disorder.
   c) Serious local or systemic reaction occurred to a previous immunisation with DPT.
3. Underlying cardiac or respiratory disease in the child is a strong indication *to give* pertussis immunisation.

TREATMENT

1. Infants <6 months should be hospitalised initially for nursing and observation.
2. Erythromycin 50 mg/kg/day for 10 days or co-trimoxazole is unlikely to alter the clinical course but may reduce period of infectivity[2].
3. Antispasmodics, antitussives, sedatives and physiotherapy are of no proven value[3].
4. Steroids and salbutamol need to be further evaluated[4,5].

PROGNOSIS

- The highest risk of disease, morbidity and mortality is in the young and those with pre-existing respiratory or cardiovascular disease; 90% deaths are from pneumonia. 72% deaths from pertussis in USA are in infants aged less one year[6].
- Mortality was 1:4000 cases in UK in 1977[7].
- Epistaxis and subconjuctival haemorrhage are frequent complications. Lobar or segmental collapse may occur in approximately one in six children[8].
- Previous immunisation will significantly reduce incidence and morbidity but will not provide complete protection.

FOLLOW-UP

All cases should have a chest x-ray on recovery to exclude residual lung collapse, and any residual changes treated vigorously with physiotherapy. Recurrence of a pertussis-like cough is common with subsequent respiratory infections for many months (post-pertussis syndrome). Previously non-immunised children with culture proven pertussis need not be immunised[9].

[1] Collier A M *et al.* (1966) *J. Pediatr.*, **69,** 1073.
[2] Bass J W *et al.* (1969) *J. Pediatr.*, **75,** 768.
[3] Broomhall J *et al.* (1984) *Arch. Dis. Childh.*, **59,** 185.
[4] Badr-El-Din M K *et al.* (1976) *J. Trop. Med. Hyg.*, **79,** 218.
[5] Editorial (1984) *Lancet*, **i,** 1162.
[6] Brooks G F *et al.* (1970) *J. Infect. Dis.*, **122,** 123.
[7] Pollock T M *et al.* (1984) *Arch. Dis. Childh.*, **59,** 162.
[8] Phelan P D *et al.* (1982) *Respiratory Illness in Children*, 2nd edn. (Phelan P D *et al.* eds), p. 72. Oxford: Blackwell.
[9] Report of the Committee on Infectious Diseases (1986) *Red Book* 20th edn, p. 270. Illinois: American Academy of Pediatrics.

Poliomyelitis

Poliovirus, one of the enteroviruses, is still responsible for endemic and epidemic infection in many parts of the world, although mass immunisation has made disease a rarity in western countries, and less common in most developing countries. Following infection, 4–8% children experience a 'minor illness' after 2–6 days. The 'major illness', with CNS manifestations, occurs 8–18 days after initial infection. Maximal infectivity is during the first week, but virus is excreted in the stools for several weeks. 90–95% infection remains asymptomatic. Clinical disease may manifest as: *non-paralytic poliomyelitis*, with fever, aseptic meningitis, hyperaesthesiae and paraesthesiae; *paralytic poliomyelitis*, with profound and sudden onset of paralysis affecting limbs and sometimes trunk and intercostal muscles; *bulbar poliomyelitis*, affecting cranial nerve nuclei, and sometimes associated with spinal paralysis, in which encephalitic signs are often seen.

PREVENTION

Both live attenuated oral poliovirus vaccine (OPV) and inactivated vaccine (IPV) provide excellent protection if administered as per standard immunisation schedules in developed countries. The response to OPV in children in tropical countries is often less satisfactory. OPV should not be used in immunodeficient children.

TREATMENT

1. Bed rest is always indicated. Exertion in the acute phase of the disease is correlated with more severe paralysis.
2. Muscle pain, spasm and tenderness respond to heat packs and analgesia.
3. Monitor for respiratory failure and treat appropriately with physiotherapy and ventilation if necessary.
4. Cardiovascular complications (shock, pulmonary oedema, hypertension, etc.) should be treated with standard forms of therapy.
5. Bladder paralysis may respond to bethanechol 5–10 mg orally or catheterisation may be necessary.
6. Long-term management of paralysis, muscle wasting, and skeletal deformity may require specific orthopaedic procedures and physiotherapy.

PROGNOSIS

- Recovery is complete in non-paralytic poliomyelitis, with or without muscle weakness.
- Some improvement of paralysis is expected with time (depending on the extent and localisation of the nerve cell damage), e.g. 60% of ultimate recovery by three months, 80% of ultimate recovery by six months[1].
- Mortality is 4% overall, with 10% mortality in bulbar form despite full supportive therapy. Mortality is usually from respiratory failure (both spinal and bulbar polio).
- Vasomotor centre involvement may result in cardiovascular complications (hypertension, arrhythmias, shock, pulmonary oedema).
- Bladder paralysis and urinary retention are usually temporary.

FOLLOW-UP

Some recovery of muscle function in paralytic poliomyelitis can be expected for 18 months to 2 years. Regular assessment of residual handicap or deformity by an orthopaedic surgeon and physiotherapist should be made throughout this recovery phase and during the period of subsequent skeletal growth.

---

[1] Horstmann D M (1981) In *Textbook of Pediatric Infectious Diseases* (Feigin R D, Cherry J D eds.), p. 1186. Philadelphia: Saunders.

Kala Azar

Kala azar, or visceral leishmaniasis, is caused by the protozoan haemoflagellate *Leishmania donovani* which is transmitted by various species of phlebotamine sandflies. There are three epidemiological forms: *Mediterranean type* extending from the Mediterranean littoral through Central Asia into China. This predominantly affects young children aged 1–5 years. Dogs, foxes and feral animals act as reservoirs. *Indian type*, with human reservoir, affecting children predominantly in the age range 5–15 years, and adults. *African type*, with rodents and dogs as a reservoir, affecting mainly older children and young adults.

PREVENTION

Control of sandflies by spraying, reduction of animal reservoirs (dogs) and early therapy to prevent neighbourhood transmissions.

TREATMENT

1. Sodium stibogluconate (Pentostam) 20 mg (antimony)/kg daily i.m. or i.v. (by very slow injection), maximum dose 850 mg/day (2 g sodium stibogluconate = 600 mg antimony). All forms of disease require 20–30 days therapy (depending on rapidity of response)[1]. (Note that the previous recommendation to treat Indian kala azar for 6–10 days has now been revised[2].)
2. Patients should be hospitalised. Side-effects of therapy include nausea, vomiting, urticaria, ECG changes and bradycardia.
3. In cases of apparent antimony resistance, use hydroxystilbamidine isethionate 3–4.5 mg/kg/day i.v. (three 10-day courses with intervals of seven days between them), pentamidine isethionate 2–4 mg/kg i.m. every three days for 15 doses, or amphotericin B increasing from a test dose of 0.1 mg/kg i.v. (monitor for toxic effects), gradually to 1.5 mg/kg i.v. alternate days.
4. Relapse should be treated with Pentostam (dosage as above) for 40 days[1].
5. Secondary gastrointestinal and respiratory infections are common and may require vigorous therapy.

PROGNOSIS

- Clinical illness is seen in only 3–5% those infected[3].
- Untreated established visceral leishmaniasis is fatal in 75–85% infantile and 90% adult cases[4]. Death occurs from bleeding diathesis, complications of anaemia, nephritis or secondary intestinal or respiratory infections.
- Prompt treatment results in 90–98% cure.
- Relapse after complete therapeutic course (i.e. 30 days) is rare except in the African form.

FOLLOW-UP

The criteria for cure are absence of fever, regression of hepatosplenomegaly, and a return to normal of haematological parameters and serum proteins. If the patient fails to respond satisfactorily, a second course of treatment will be necessary. It is essential that all patients are followed at a minimum of 6-monthly intervals for two years to assess cure. Fluorescent antibody (IFAT) or ELISA titres (if available) should be absent by the end of one year, and the Formol gel test negative by six months. A change to a positive leishmanin skin test (Montenegro test – intracutaneous injection of 0.5 ml suspension leptomonads in formal saline) within two months of commencing therapy signifies immunity and is also a pointer to successful treatment. Post-kala azar dermal leishmaniasis is a not uncommon sequel in India. It presents approximately one year after the initial disease. Features are erythematous or hypopigmented patches on the skin, which may ulcerate. Donovan bodies can be recovered from the skin lesions. Treatment should be reinstituted.

[1] WHO (1982) *Scientific Working Group of UNDP/World Bank/WHO, 4th annual report.* (TOR/Chem Leish/VL/82.3). Geneva: WHO.
[2] Thakur C P et al. (1984) *Br. Med. J.*, **288**, 895.
[3] Pampiglione S et al. (1975) *Trans. R. Soc. Trop. Med. Hyg.*, **69**, 60.
[4] Wittner M (1981) In *Textbook of Pediatric Infectious Diseases* (Feigin R D, Cherry J D eds.), p. 1562. Philadelphia: Saunders.

Kawasaki Disease

Kawasaki disease is an acute febrile syndrome of unknown aetiology that occurs predominantly in children under five years of age. Although the disease occurs worldwide, it appears to be most prevalent in Japan, where more than 40 000 cases have been reported since it was first described in 1967. The disease is characterised by fever, conjunctival infection, mucous membrane changes, erythema and oedema followed by desquamation of the palms and soles, rash and lymphadenopathy. Prominent cardiovascular manifestations give rise to considerable morbidity and occasional death. The disease cannot be distinguished pathologically from infantile polyarteritis nodosa[1,2].

TREATMENT

1. Initial bed rest, careful monitoring for hypertension, vasculitis and coronary artery aneurysms (serial echo cardiography and ECG). Monitor platelet count, especially in the second and third week of illness.
2. Aspirin therapy. During initial phase 100–120 mg/kg/day in three divided doses. (Beware of gastroentestinal haemorrhage. Also monitor levels because of variable absorption[3].) Thereafter 5–20 mg/kg once daily to inhibit platelet aggregation until vasculitis or coronary disease appears resolved.
3. High dose intravenous gammaglobulin 400 mg/kg daily for five days during acute phase is claimed to reduce coronary artery involvement[4].
4. Exchange transfusion should be considered for severe cardiac, cutaneous, intestinal or cerebral vascular complications[5]. Plasmapheresis might provide an alternative but has yet to be evaluated.
5. Corticosteroids may be harmful[6].

PROGNOSIS

- Frequently benign, and probably underdiagnosed.
- 20–60% diagnosed cases develop coronary arteritis and aneurysms[7-9]. 50% aneurysms regress within 18 months[10].
- 1–4% case fatality rate is mainly from coronary thrombosis or aneurysmal rupture within first 3 months of initial illness[11].
- The degree of thrombocytosis correlates with prognosis. A platelet count $> 1000 \times 10^9/l$ correlates with severe vasculitis[12].

- The greatest risk is in those under one year, and males more than females.
- Other cardiovascular complications include myocarditis, pericarditis, cardiac failure, hypertension, peripheral gangrene and cerebral thrombosis[9,13].
- Non-cardiovascular complications include sterile pyuria/meatitis (7%), hydrops of gallbladder (4%), hepatitis (3%), arthritis (3%), aseptic meningitis (2%), uveitis and small bowel obstruction.
- Clinical recovery is usually complete, but sequelae of cardiovascular damage are possible.

FOLLOW-UP

If coronary involvement is demonstrated or suspected during the acute phase, regular systematic echocardiographic analysis is needed, and consideration to selective coronary angiography given to those with persistent lesions. The optimal extent and time of analysis remains uncertain. Three-monthly blood count, platelets and ESR is necessary while on maintenance aspirin therapy.

[1] Landing B H et al. (1977) Paediatrics, **59**, 651.
[2] Larson E J (1977) In Vascular Lesions of Collagen Diseases and Related Conditions (Japan Medical Research Foundation ed.), p. 322. Tokyo: University Tokyo Press.
[3] Koren G et al. (1984) J. Pediatr., **105**, 991.
[4] Furusho K et al. (1984) Lancet, **ii**, 1055.
[5] Netter J C et al. (1984) Lancet, **i**, 452.
[6] Melish M E et al. (1979) Pediatr. Res., **13**, 451.
[7] Kato H et al. (1975) J. Pediatr., **86**, 892.
[8] Meade R H et al. (1982) J. Pediatr., **100**, 558.
[9] MMWR Report (1985) J. Am. Med. Assoc., **253**, 957.
[10] Kato H et al. (1982) Am. J. Cardiol., **49**, 1758.
[11] Tanaka N (1975) Pathol. Microbiol. (Basel), **43**, 204.
[12] Levin M et al. (1985) Br. Med. J., **290**, 1456.
[13] Novelli V M et al. (1984) Arch. Dis. Childh., **59**, 405.

Leprosy

Leprosy, a chronic infectious disease caused by *Mycobacterium leprae*, can affect children of all ages. Disease is endemic in many parts of Africa, South and SE Asia and South America. The WHO estimates that 12–15 million people are affected worldwide. Infection may commonly be subclinical[1] or may present as a variable spectrum of clinical disease from *tuberculoid leprosy* where disease is localised to a few sites in skin or peripheral nerves, producing hypopigmented or erythematous anaesthetic and anhidrotic areas, to *lepromatous leprosy*, where infection disseminates locally and by the blood stream to other organs, producing widespread diffuse nodular lesions. *Borderline leprosy* (dimorphous or intermediate leprosy) has features of both. The term *indeterminate* leprosy is used to describe the initial manifestations of clinical disease following infection where ill-defined hyperpigmented or erythematous macules with intact or only mildly altered sensation are seen. Classification of disease is important to establish both prognosis and correct therapy. The factors which determine outcome are ill understood. HLA encoded factors[2] and the level of host cell-mediated immune response (CMI) are important in determining the spectrum of disease. Cell-mediated immune response is consistently suppressed to many antigens, including *M. leprae* in lepromatous leprosy, but not in tuberculoid leprosy. The Mitsuda reaction (read 3–4 weeks after injection of intradermal lepromin) can be used as an aid to classification of the clinical form of leprosy[3,4] but is *not* an aid to diagnosis. Serological tests for leprosy are now available, but seropositivity appears to indicate exposure rather than clinical disease[5].

PREVENTION

Vaccination against leprosy is not yet of proven value, but is on trial[6]. Chemoprophylaxis with dapsone of close contacts may have limited value, but is not recommended for endemic areas because of development of dapsone resistance.

TREATMENT

1. Therapy must be commenced in all cases, using combination therapy[7]. There is no uniform opinion on duration of therapy, but development of drug resistance, combined with poor patient compliance to therapy, has led to the WHO recommending short therapeutic courses. Where practical, response to therapy should be assessed regularly both clinically and by histopathological evaluation.
2. Tuberculoid/borderline tuberculoid

    a) Minimum 6 months therapy with:
       i) Dapsone 1–2 mg/kg/day.
       ii) Rifampicin 10–20 mg/kg/once weekly.
    b) For treatment in endemic areas use dapsone daily (unsupervised) with rifampicin monthly (supervised) if weekly therapy is impractical.

3. Lepromatous/borderline-lepromatous

    a) Minimum two years' therapy with above *plus* clofazimine 50–100 mg daily for first six months of therapy.
    b) If dapsone resistance is suspected, give clofazimine 50–100 mg/day combined with rifampicin 10 mg/kg/day.
    c) Therapy with dapsone should not be discontinued with erythema nodosum leprosum (ENL)[8].
    d) Toxic reactions to therapy are common, especially to dapsone, causing haemolytic anaemia, in patients with G6PD deficiency; rifampicin causing hepatotoxicity, and clofazimine causing skin pigmentation and enteritis.
    e) Drug resistance or patient intolerance may necessitate other drug combinations. Ethionamide, prothionamide and isoprodian in combination with either rifampicin or dapsone are being evaluated.

4. Lepra reactions

    a) Maintain chemotherapy and include clofazimine.

b) Adequate analgesia.

c) Prednisolone 1–2 mg/kg/day, tapering to minimum effective dose in severe cases.

5. ENL

a) Treat as with lepra reactions.

b) The addition of thalidomide (adult dose 100–400 mg/day, paediatric dose not established) may be of value in relief of pain.

6. The eye

a) Effective systemic chemotherapy as above.

b) General ophthalmic measures to reduce inflammation (topical steroids, antibiotics if indicated).

c) Protection of globe if facial weakness exists.

7. Surgical treatment and general measures

a) Protection from secondary deformity related to anaesthesia.

b) Correction of deformity by special surgical or orthopaedic techniques[9].

c) Prevention and treatment of skin ulceration with immobilisation, appliances, dressings, etc.

PROGNOSIS

- Indeterminate leprosy. 75% spontaneous healing, without development of significant clinical disease[10]. The remainder progress to other clinical forms.
- Tuberculoid leprosy

a) Macular form: the prognosis after treatment is excellent. Severe hypopigmentation and/or areas of anaesthesia may remain.

b) Infiltrated form: swelling of nerve trunks and areas of anaesthesia and/or paresis may be permanent in advanced cases. There is a subsequent risk of mutilation.

- Lepromatous leprosy

a) Advanced disease is rare in children. Prognosis is guarded and depends on disease involvement at the start of therapy, response to therapy and compliance to therapy. Severe debility and deformity are related to diffuse skin infiltration or persistence of anaesthesia or paresis.

b) Relapse is commonest in lepromatous leprosy (watch for drug resistant strains, poor therapy compliance).

c) 50% cases on therapy develop ENL[11] after commencing chemotherapy (tender subcutaneous nodules, fever, sinovitis, iridocyclitis, skin ulceration, occasional glomerulonephritis). Erythema nodosum leprosum may also be precipitated by nutritional factors or intercurrent infection[12].

d) Ocular involvement may be severe, and associated with direct invasion of the globe or an acute inflammatory reaction related to ENL or a 'lepra reaction' (see below)[13].

- Borderline leprosy

a) The prognosis is variable and guarded. Serious deformities and relapse are common. Alterations in immunological balance may lead to a lepra reaction:

i) Downgrading reaction: unfavourable prognosis, associated with clinical change towards lepromatous leprosy.

ii) Reversal or upgrading reaction: favourable prognosis, associated with improved host immunity, and often accompanies therapy.

b) Clinical features of downgrading and reversal reactions are similar – fever, erythema and swelling of skin, new skin lesions, swelling and tenderness of nerves.

FOLLOW-UP

Response to therapy must be assessed both clinically and (where indicated) by histopathological evaluation of skin biopsies, smears or nerve biopsies. Nasal scrapings may also be of value in assessing infectivity and compliance with therapy. The frequency and duration of review depends on the type and severity of the disease. Relapse is common, and frequently associated with poor compliance with therapy, or insufficient therapy.

[1] Abe M et al. (1980) Int. J. Lepr., **48**, 109.
[2] Van Eden W et al. (1984) Leprosy Review, **55**, 89.
[3] Mitsuda K (1919) (in Japanese) Jap. J. Dermatol Urol., **19**, 697 (in English) (1953) Int. J. Leprosy., **21**, 347.
[4] Melsome R et al. (1983) Int J. Lepr., **51**, 235.
[5] Editorial (1986) Lancet, **i**, 533.
[6] Anon (1985) Nature, **317**, 665.
[7] World Health Organisation (1982) Leprosy (WHO Tech. Rep. Series no. 675). Geneva: WHO.
[8] World Health Organisation (1977) Leprosy (WHO Tech. Rep. Series no. 607). Geneva: WHO.
[9] McDowell F et al. (1974) Surgical Rehabilitation in Leprosy and in Other Peripheral Nerve Disorders. Baltimore: Williams and Wilkins.
[10] Dhamendra (1975) quoted by Karat A B A (1978) in Disease of Children in Subtropics and Tropics, 3rd edn (Jelliffe D B, Stanfield J P eds.) p. 813. London: Edward Arnold.
[11] Meyers W M (1981) In Textbook of Pediatric Infectious Diseases (Feigin R D, Cherry J D eds.), p. 880. Philadelphia: Saunders.
[12] Jolliffe D S (1977) Br. J. Dermatol., **97**, 345.
[13] ffytche T J et al. (1985) J. Roy. Soc. Med., **78**, 397.

Lyme Disease

Lyme disease is an illness with a seasonal incidence transmitted by ixodid ticks and caused by the spirochaete *Borrelia burgdorferi* in the USA or antigenically similar spirochaetes in Europe[1-3]. The first stage of the clinical illness, usually lasting several weeks, starts with a spreading erythematous rash centred on the tick bite, followed by multiple secondary lesions (erythema chronica migrans), accompanied by headache, stiff neck, myalgia, arthralgia, malaise, fatigue and lymphadenopathy[4]. Weeks or months later, the second stage of the illness may develop, with neurological or cardiac symptoms, and weeks to years later, many patients develop arthritis (third stage).

TREATMENT

1. Treatment with antibiotics in the first stage of the illness usually stops progression of the disease[5].
2. For children over 10 years of age, tetracycline 250 mg q.d.s. is recommended. Penicillin V 50 mg/kg orally daily in four divided doses for 10 days for younger children.
3. Children presenting with second stage meningoencephalitis should be treated with penicillin G 200 mg/kg/day i.v. in four divided doses for 10 days.
4. Peripheral or cranial neuritis, including Bell's palsy, should be treated with oral penicillin if no previous treatment is given. Prednisolone should be considered for Bell's palsy but will not alter the duration of other neurological manifestations[6].

PROGNOSIS

- Symptoms and signs of second and third stage disease may develop weeks to years after the tick bite unless adequate treatment is given in the first stage.
- 15% patients develop neurological problems, usually meningoencephalitis, with 40% developing cranial neuritis (usually Bell's palsy) or peripheral neuritis[6].
- 8% patients develop heart problems, most commonly atrioventricular block. Cardiomegaly and cardiac muscle damage have also been described.
- Arthritis develops in about 60% untreated patients usually months or even years after the tick bite.

FOLLOW-UP

Early treatment is likely to prevent major second or third stage manifestations, but all patients should be reviewed periodically for evidence of cardiac, neurological and joint signs. Although clinically normal, 50% complain of persistent symptoms including headache, fatigue, muscle and joint pains for several weeks despite early therapy, and 5% have persisting symptoms for 1–2 years. Those presenting with second or third stage disease are both more refractory to treatment and more likely to have prolonged symptoms or signs requiring review.

[1] Steere A C et al. (1979) Ann. Intern. Med., **91,** 730.
[2] Stanek G et al. (1985) Lancet, **i,** 401.
[3] Johnson R C et al. (1984) Int. J. Systemic Bacteriol., **34,** 496.
[4] Steere A C et al. (1983) Ann. Intern. Med., **99,** 76.
[5] Steere A C et al. (1983) Ann. Intern. Med., **99,** 22.
[6] Pachner A R et al. (1985) Neurology, **35,** 47.
[7] Parke A (1987) Br. Med. J., **294,** 525.

Malaria

Malaria is a febrile disease caused by the asexual reproduction of protozoan parasites in erythrocytes. One billion people are at risk, 96 million cases occur annually in Africa, with 1 million deaths. Most deaths occur in children aged 1–5 years[1]. Malaria is re-emerging in some countries in which it previously had been under control. Multiple drug resistance has recently made both acute therapy and prophylaxis more difficult. Four species of malaria parasite belonging to the genus *Plasmodium* are responsible for disease: *P. falciparum* is common in all malarial areas (chloroquine resistance SE Asia, S. America, E. Africa and central America); *P. vivax* is common in all malarial areas; *P. malariae* is found in SE Asia and E. Africa; and *P. ovale* occurs mainly in W. Africa.

PREVENTION

1. Reduction of contact with mosquitoes through the use of insect repellents, protective clothes and screens, elimination of the insect vector through the use of insecticides, etc., are vital. Chemoprophylaxis in malaria emdemic areas is also necessary.

2. Chemoprophylaxis: dosage given is based on a 60 kg adult (reduction table below)[2]:
   a) Areas with no chloroquine resistance: chloroquine or amodiaquine 300 mg (base) weekly.
   b) Areas of low chloroquine resistance: chloroquine or amodiaquine weekly *plus* proguanil 200 mg (base) daily.
   c) Areas of high degree chloroquine resistance: chloroquine or amodiaquine weekly *plus* either proguanil 200 mg (base) daily or dapsone/pyrimethamine (Maloprim) one tablet weekly.
   d) Dosage reduction for age[7]:

Age	Child's dose	
	Chloroquine, proguanil	Maloprim
<5 weeks	1/8 adult dose	Not recommended
6 weeks– 5 months	1/4 adult dose	1/8 adult dose
6 months– 1 year	1/4 adult dose	1/4 adult dose
1–5 years (5–20 kg)	1/2 adult dose	1/2 adult dose
6–12 years (20–40 kg)	3/4 adult dose	3/4 adult dose
>12 years (40 kg)	Adult dose	Adult dose

TREATMENT

1. *P. falciparum*

a) Chloroquine phosphate or chloroquine sulphate. Dosage related to chloroquine *base*, i.e. 100 mg chloroquine base = 161 mg chloroquine phosphate = 136 mg chloroquine sulphate. Dosage: 25 mg/kg chloroquine *base* in four divided doses:

   DAY 1 10 mg/kg stat.
             5 mg/kg at 6 hours.
   DAY 2 5 mg/kg
   DAY 3 5 mg/kg

   Note: cardiac arrhythmia may occur if above dosage is exceeded.

b) If chloroquine resistance is suspected, give quinine. Dosage: 20 mg/kg quinine sulphate daily for 10–14 days, orally in three divided daily doses, or intravenously for five days if not tolerated orally (see below) or if there is a high parasite count. In addition give pyrimethamine and sulphonamide, e.g. Fansidar: dosage 1.0 mg/kg pyrimethamine/day for the last three days of quinine therapy.

c) For severely ill patients with cerebral malaria or blackwater fever give:

   i) Quinine dihydrochloride by intravenous infusion 10 mg/kg in 10 ml fluid/kg over four hours at intervals of 12 hours for 4–12 doses, as indicated. This must *not* be given by rapid injection, and is *not* effective by i.m. injection. Monitor carefully for hypotension, hypoglycaemia, cardiac arrhythmias, neurotoxicity and respiratory depression.

   ii) If there are signs of hepatic or renal failure, reduce above infusion frequency to one every 24 hours.

   iii) A dosage increase of 50% is necessary if quinine resistance is suspected (seen especially in SE Asia), but beware of drug toxicity[3,4].

   iv) Fluid limitation to 40 ml/kg/24 hours unless there is clinical hypovolaemia.

   v) Supportive therapy with ventilation for pulmonary oedema may be required.

   vi) Anticonvulsants when clinically indicated.

   vii) Steroids are contraindicated in cerebral malaria[5].

2. *P. vivax, P. ovale and P. malariae.*

Combine oral chloroquine therapy as outlined in 1(a) above, with primaquine phosphate, to eliminate exoerythrocytic parasites and effect a radical cure. (30 mg primaquine base = 50 mg primaquine phosphate.) Dosage 0.3 mg primaquine base/kg/day orally for 14 days. Beware of acute haemolysis in patients with G6PD deficiency – check level first if there is a high risk.

PROGNOSIS

● *P. falciparum*

a) Always life threatening in non-immune patients, with potential for massive parasitaemia, delirium, coma, hyperpyrexia or convulsions (cerebral malaria); haemoglobinuria and acute renal failure (blackwater fever); hepatic failure (bilious remittent fever); extensive vascular involvement of the gastrointestinal tract, accompanied by nausea, vomiting, diarrhoea and prostration (algid malaria); or acute pulmonary oedema.

b) Mortality from the above pernicious forms untreated is 50%. If treated 0.5%[6].

c) 2% patients with *P. falciparum* malaria develop cerebral symptoms. The death rate in cerebral malaria is still around 20%[5].

d) There is no recurrence of *P. falciparum* if treated appropriately, as no persistence of exoerythrocytic stage in the liver.

● *P. vivax and P. ovale*

a) Untreated disease is self limiting. Parasitaemia may last several days to three months.

b) Recurrences (short term relapse) may occur from persistent parasitaemia.

c) Recurrences (long-term relapse) occur from persisting parasites in liver parenchyma.

● *P. malariae*

a) Untreated, it is a relatively mild disease.

b) Chronic membranoproliferative glomerulonephritis and/or nephrotic syndrome is often seen with long-term disease.

Blood film examination for malaria parasites should be performed at the end of therapy. If chloroquine resistant falciparum suspected, repeat the blood film 10 and 20 days later, or if clinically indicated. Complications of cerebral malaria or blackwater fever may need long-term monitoring and support.

[1] WHO (1976) *WHO Chron.*, **30**, 3.
[2] WHO (1986) *Vaccination Certificate Requirements for International Travel*, p. 45. Geneva: WHO.
[3] Hall A (1985) *Lancet*, **i**, 1453.
[4] Warrell D A et al. (1985) *Lancet*, **i**, 1453.
[5] Warrell D A et al. (1982) *New Eng. J. Med.*, **306**, 313.
[6] Walzer P D et al. (1974) *Am. J. Trop. Med. Hyg.*, **23**, 328.
[7] Pulse (1986) *Travel Guide: Immunisation Recommendations*. London: Morgan Grampian.

Measles

Measles is a contagious viral disease characterised by fever, coryza, conjunctivitis, cough, Koplik's spots, and a distinctive maculopapular rash. The incubation period is 10–14 days and infection is greatest just before the rash appears. The disease occurs endemically and epidemically throughout the world, although where widespread active immunisation has been implemented the incidence has been reduced dramatically.

PREVENTION

1. Non-immune children with immunodeficiency should be protected by human immune globulin (see *dosage* below) immediately on contact with measles. Consideration should be given to active immunisation in some of these children and to normal non-immune children if within three days of measles exposure. Children should normally be immunised at 12–18 months, but earlier in developing countries (9–12 months). Serious complications associated with measles vaccine are very rare.

2. Dosage of normal immunoglobulin to protect against measles:

<1 year	250 mg
1–2 years	500 mg
3 years +	750 mg

TREATMENT

1. There is no specific treatment for measles infection. Bed rest, antipyretics and adequate fluid intake are indicated. Isolate from non-immune children until five days after the rash has appeared.

2. Pulmonary complications often relate to secondary bacterial infection and should be treated vigorously with antibiotics and physiotherapy.

3. Secondary complications, as seen in developing countries, may require intensive medical support with enteral or parenteral feeding, vitamin supplements, systemic antibiotics and careful monitoring for cardiac involvement.

4. Inosiplex (isoprinosine) has been used in the long-term treatment of subacute sclerosing panencephalitis (SSPE) and is claimed to improve survival[1], but further evaluation is required.

PROGNOSIS

- In the western world, unusual manifestations and complications of measles are rare. In developing countries, a number of factors, of which relative protein malnutrition is probably the most important, lead to widespread morbidity and mortality, especially in children between the ages of 8 months and 3 years.

- Prognosis and likelihood of both unusual manifestations and complication of disease is dependent upon:

  a) Age: if less than three years the disease is more severe.

b) Immune response: both humoral (passive transplacental antibody or antibody from previous vaccination) and T-cell immunity (affected by immunosuppressives or protein malnutrition) are important. Deficiency of either or both will lead to more severe measles.
c) Underlying disease, especially pre-existing cardiac or pulmonary disease.
d) Availability of supportive medical care.

• Around 10% hospitalised cases die in developing countries[2]. Death is usually from either fulminant toxic illness or secondary pulmonary and intestinal complications, but rarely from myocarditis or acute encephalitis.
• In the western world serious morbidity and mortality are rare (1.5/10 000 notifications died in UK 1970–83[3]) but is seen with:

a) Immunodeficiency: measles is severe and protracted, giant cell pneumonia or encephalitis is usually fatal[4-6].
b) Acute neurological complications in around 0.1% cases. Mortality is 10–20%[7]. 20–40% who recover will have residual damage[8].
c) Subacute sclerosing panencephalitis is seen in around 1/100 000 natural infections, 1/1 000 000 following measles immunisation. It is most commonly seen following measles contracted under 2 years of age. It has a variable time of onset after initial infection (mean 7 years) with variably progressive neurological deterioration sometimes accompanied by partial remission but inevitable death.

FOLLOW-UP

Uncomplicated measles does not require follow-up. Secondary complications such as seen in developing countries may require specific review, and the nutritional state of the child in the recovery phase should be monitored.

[1] Jones C E et al. (1982) Lancet, i, 1034.
[2] O'Donovan C (1971) East Afr. Med. J., 48, 526.
[3] Miller C L (1985) Br. Med. J., 290, 443.
[4] Mitus A et al. (1959) New Eng. J. Med., 261, 882.
[5] Siegel M M et al. (1977) Paediatrics, 60, 38.
[6] Murphy J V et al. (1976) J. Pediatr., 88, 937.
[7] Miller H G et al. (1956) Q. J. Med., 25, 427.
[8] Cherry J D (1981) In Textbook of Pediatric Infectious Diseases (Feigin R D, Cherry J D eds.), p. 1210. Philadelphia: Saunders.

Mumps

Mumps is a common contagious infection caused by a myxovirus, and spread by the respiratory route. It is characterised by painful, tender swelling of the parotid or other salivary glands. The testes, ovaries, pancreas and CNS may also be affected. The incubation period is 14–24 days with infectivity for six days before, and up to nine days after the appearance of salivary gland swelling. In countries where childhood vaccination is not carried out, mumps is common, with 50% of children being infected before school age.

PREVENTION

A live, attenuated mumps virus vaccine is now used in many countries, usually in combination with measles and rubella. The preparation is virtually without side-effects, and has a protective efficacy of about 97% against natural infection.

TREATMENT

1. No specific therapy is available. Treatment is symptomatic including local support for orchitis.
2. Steroids are not of proven benefit in any of the complications of mumps.
3. Passive immunisation with immunoglobulin is ineffective[1].
4. Although of relatively low infectivity, children with clinical disease should be isolated when possible.

PROGNOSIS

- 20–40% infection is subclinical.
- Severe systemic manifestations are uncommon.
- Involvement of the CNS is common, but usually mild. In 50% hospitalised cases CSF pleocytosis occurs, with clinical meningitis in around 10%, often with some encephalitic features (delirium, convulsions)[2]. Prognosis is good.

- Deafness occurs in around 4% cases acutely, due to eighth nerve neuritis but recovery is usual[3].
- Orchitis occurs in 30% post-pubertal males, less common in young children. 15–40% orchitis may be bilateral and may lead to impaired fertility, estimated at 13%, but absolute infertility is rare. Oophoritis has been recorded in 7% post-pubertal females[1].
- Mastitis, thyroiditis, pancreatitis and arthritis are occasional complications.
- There is no clear relationship of mumps to the pathogenesis of insulin dependent diabetes mellitus[4].

FOLLOW-UP

No follow-up is indicated in uncomplicated mumps, and most complications are self-limiting and temporary. A check for residual high tone deafness in children suspected of hearing loss in the acute phase of the disease should be made.

[1] Reed D et al. (1967) J. Am. Med. Assoc., **199,** 967.
[2] Azimi P H et al. (1969) J. Am. Med. Assoc., **207,** 505.
[3] Vuori M et al. (1962) Acta Oto-Laryngol., **55,** 231.
[4] Ratzmann K P et al. (1984) Diabetes Care, **7,** 170.

Rabies

Rabies is a viral infection of the CNS transmitted from animals by bite, scratch or aerosol inhalation. Domestic animals, especially dogs and cats, comprise the largest source of human exposure in most parts of the world. Other animal vectors include rats (N. Africa), foxes (Europe and USA), skunk (USA) and bats (N. and S. America, Denmark). Vaccination, domestic pet control measures and quarantine laws have limited human rabies in Europe and the USA, but 15 000 deaths due to rabies are estimated to occur yearly in India and Pakistan. Infection with rabies virus is followed by an incubation period ranging from nine days up to more than one year (two months average in adults, less in children), followed by an acute febrile illness with central nervous system manifestations, inducing anxiety, dysphagia, convulsions and death.

PREVENTION

Pre-exposure immunisation is recommended for adults and children living in areas where rabies is a constant threat. Three injections of human diploid cell vaccine (HDCV) should be given i.m. on days 0, 7, and 28. Booster doses of 1 ml i.m. every two years have been recommended, but give rise to a 6–10% risk of allergic reaction[1]. A variety of public control measures including oral vaccination of wild animals are used or are being studied.

TREATMENT

1. All patients known to be exposed to saliva from an infected animal, or one likely to be infected (either by bite, scratch or contamination of mucous membrane) should receive local wound care and immunoprophylaxis. When a child is bitten by an animal suspected of having rabies, the animal should if possible be captured and confined for a 10-day period by a veterinary surgeon if a domestic animal, and killed and examined if signs of rabies develop. A suspect wild animal should be killed at once, and the brain examined for evidence of rabies. In cases of doubt, the decision to immunise an exposed child should normally be made in consultation with the local health department who can provide information on the risk of rabies in a particular area for each species of animal.
2. Local wound care. The immediate objective is to prevent virus from entering neural tissue. All wounds should be flushed and cleaned with soap and water. Tetanus prophylaxis should be administered if indicated and measures taken to control bacterial infection. The wound should not be sutured if possible.
3. Immunoprophylaxis. Combined active immunisation with HDVC and passive immunisation with human rabies immune globulin (HRIG) should be given.

   a) HDCV 1 ml i.m. on day 1. Repeat doses on days 3, 7, 14 and 28. A sixth dose is often advised. Approximately 25% recipients develop local pain erythema and swelling. 20% develop mild systemic reactions – muscle aches, abdominal pains, headache and nausea.

   b) HRIG 20 i.u./kg in one dose, given at same time as HDCV but in a different site. If not available immediately, can be given up to 8 days after HDCV. Give half volume as infiltrate around wound, the remainder intramuscularly.

PROGNOSIS

- Progressive encephalitis leading to death despite intensive supportive care, is almost certain in any patient presenting with symptoms. Reported survivors have in almost all cases received either post-exposure or pre-exposure prophylaxis before the onset of clinical illness[2,3]. The severity of the brainstem encephalitis is thought to determine outcome.

[1] Marwick C (1985) *J. Am. Med. Assoc.*, **254**, 13.
[2] Mandell G L *et al.* (1985) In *Principles and Practice of Infectious Disease* 2nd edn (Mandell G L, Douglas R G, Bennett J E eds), p. 897. New York: Wiley.
[3] Hattwick M A W *et al.* (1972) *Ann. Intern. Med.*, **76**, 931.

Rubella

Rubella (German measles) is a common communicable disease of childhood usually characterised by mild constitutional symptoms, macular rash (often faint) and enlargement of postoccipital, retroauricular and posterior cervical lymph nodes. Aggressive immunisation programmes in early childhood in the USA and some other countries has resulted in a marked decline in incidence. Rubella in early pregnancy may cause abortion or severe congenital anomalies in the newborn infant.

PREVENTION

Active immunisation with live attenuated rubella vaccine provides protection to 95% those immunised.

TREATMENT

1. Postnatal infection

   a) No specific treatment is indicated or possible in uncomplicated rubella.
   b) Arthritis usually responds to aspirin therapy.
   c) Steroid therapy is of no proven benefit for complications such as arthritis, encephalitis or thrombocytopenia.

2. Congenital infection

   a) Immune serum globulin (20 ml) may be effective in preventing disease if administered to a non-immune pregnant woman within 72 hours of exposure to rubella[1].
   b) Termination of pregnancy should be considered for serologically proven rubella in early pregnancy.
   c) Most babies with congenital rubella are contagious, and should be isolated if hospitalised. Some may excrete virus for more than one year.

PROGNOSIS

- Postnatally acquired infection

   a) Transient arthritis or arthralgia can occur. Incidence varies and may be as high as 18%[2].
   b) Encephalitis may occur with the rash or post-exanthem and is very rare (around 1/ 6000 cases[3]). Clinical recovery is usually complete.
   c) Other rare neurological complications include progressive panencephalitis, which may at times resemble SSPE[4], optic neuritis, peripheral neuritis and Guillain–Barré syndrome.
   d) Thrombocytopenia, which is usually transient, occurs in 1/3000 cases[5].

- Congenital infection. Congenital rubella syndrome is the result of fetal infection in the first 12 weeks of pregnancy. The prognosis is dependent on the degree of multisystem involvement. The most common manifestations are[1]:

   a) 50–85% growth retardation < 2500 g at birth.
   b) 35% congenital cataracts; 5% congenital glaucoma.
   c) 90% sensorineural hearing loss.
   d) 10–20% active meningoencephalitis.
   e) 30% cardiac defects.

- Many other features can be seen in congenital rubella syndrome, including pneumonitis, hepatitis, nephritis, bone changes, purpura, and immunodeficiency. The overall mortality of those severely affected is 10–20% in first year[1].

FOLLOW-UP

Uncomplicated rubella does not require follow-up. Complications are usually transient and mild. The widespread effects of congenital infection will require regular monitoring and specific assessment and intervention by ophthalmologist, cardiologist and developmental paediatrician.

[1] Cherry J D (1981) In *Textbook of Paediatric Infectious Diseases* (Feigin R D, Cherry J D eds.), p. 1370. Philadelphia: Saunders.

[2] Judelsohn R G et al. (1973) *J. Am. Med. Assoc.*, **223**, 401.
[3] Margolis F J et al. (1943) *J. Pediatr.*, **23**, 158.
[4] Wolinsky J S et al. (1976) *Arch. Neurol.*, **33**, 722.
[5] Bayer W L et al. (1965) *New Eng. J. Med.*, **273**, 1362

Syphilis

Syphilis is caused by infection with the spirochaete *Treponema pallidum*. Infection occurs through sexual contact, or transplacentally producing congenital syphilis. Presentation in the pre-pubertal or early pubertal child may be a pointer to sexual abuse. Fortunately congenital syphilis remains rare in developed countries where maternal serological screening is routinely carried out, although the incidence is increasing in the USA in minority groups receiving poor antenatal care[1]. It may present in the neonatal period with multiple signs and symptoms, including fever, anaemia, jaundice, purpura, rhinitis, lymphadenopathy, mucosal lesions, periostitis and meningoencephalitis. Many children with the disease have no abnormal findings at birth and can present later with neurosyphilis which may masquerade as a behavioural disorder, paresis or mental retardation.

TREATMENT

1. Congenital syphilis

   a) All infants born to mothers who receive inadequate or no therapy, whose therapy is unknown or receive drugs other than penicillin should be treated.
   b) Those with symptoms of CNS involvement, or who are asymptomatic but with abnormal CSF (positive VDRL, increased protein or pleocytosis) should receive benzylpenicillin 30 mg/kg/day for 14–21 days.
   c) Asymptomatic or symptomatic patients with normal CSF should receive benzathine penicillin G 30 mg/kg in a single dose.

2. Syphilis in childhood

   a) Early (<1 year duration): procaine penicillin G 360 mg daily for 8 days.
   b) Late (>1 year duration): Procaine penicillin G 360 mg daily for 15 days.
   c) Neurosyphilis in older children: benzylpenicillin 25 mg/kg/6-hourly for 10 days or procaine penicillin G 360 mg daily for 15 days.

PROGNOSIS

● Congenital syphilis

   a) 25% untreated cases abort or are stillbirths.
   b) 25–30% untreated die in perinatal period[2].
   c) Prognosis in those presenting with clinical disease at birth depends upon:
      i) Severity of disease.
      ii) Involvement of the CNS.
      iii) Rapidity of introduction of therapy.
   d) 40% untreated infants develop late manifestations of infection[3].
   e) Up to 20% untreated infants develop neurosyphilis at later date[4].

● Primary syphilis in childhood

   a) No sequelae with early diagnosis and prompt treatment.
   b) Untreated may develop secondary disease 2–10 weeks after primary disease.
   c) 40% untreated will develop tertiary disease after latent period of 3–10 years, which may include gummas, cardiovascular syphilis or neurosyphilis.

291

Children with early syphilis and congenital syphilis should have repeat clinical evaluation and serology at 3, 6, 9 and 12 months of age, with repeat CSF examination (if previously abnormal) at 6 months. Patients with neurosyphilis should have repeat serology and CSF examination at 6-monthly intervals for at least 3 years[5].

[1] Mascola L et al. (1984) J. Am. Med. Assoc., **252,** 1719.
[2] Nabarro J N D (1954) Congenital Syphilis. Baltimore: Williams and Wilkins.
[3] Thomas F W (1949) Syphilis; Its Course and Management. New York: Macmillan.
[4] Dodge P R (1981) In Textbook of Pediatric Infectious Diseases (Feigin R D, Cherry J D eds.), p. 308. Philadelphia: Saunders.
[5] Report of the Committee of Infectious Diseases (1986) Red book 20th edn, p. 351. Illinois: American Academy of Paediatrics.

Tetanus

Tetanus is caused by the anaerobic, spore-forming bacillus *Clostridium tetani*, an organism present in soil and human and animal faeces. Clinical symptoms are produced by a toxin which acts primarily on the spinal cord, but also on brain, motor end plates and autonomic nerves. Features of the disease include trismus, toxic spasms of skeletal muscles, spasm of glottis and larynx and hydrophobia. The disease remains an important and theoretically preventable cause of morbidity and mortality in developing countries. It has been estimated that three-quarters of a million newborn infants die of tetanus every year[1].

PREVENTION

Tetanus is preventable by full active immunisation as per the standard vaccination schedules. Boosters should be given every 10 years, or in those exposed to the risk of tetanus if more than 5 years have elapsed since last immunisation reduced to one year if severe injury with high risk and combined with human hyperimmune globulin (HTIG). Neonatal tetanus can be prevented by two injections of toxoid one month apart to non-immune pregnant women.

TREATMENT

1. As the disease may progress very rapidly, all patients should be admitted to intensive care facilities in regional centres if available.
2. Neutralisation of toxin by administration of HTIG 30–300 units/kg i.m., as soon as disease suspected or confirmed.
3. The wound must be identified and widely excised, then packed with gauze soaked in hydrogen peroxide or antibacterial agent. Delayed closure at a later date.
4. Benzylpenicillin 30 mg/kg 6-hourly i.v. or i.m.

for one week, or alternative anaerobic antibiotic.

5. Full symptomatic and supportive treatment according to severity of case:

a) Mild cases (no dysphagia or respiratory difficulty): sedate with phenobarbitone 10.0 mg/kg loading dose then 7.5 mg/kg/day in two divided doses as maintenance, or diazepam 2–10 mg/kg/day by nasogastric route or i.v. by continuous infusion.

b) Intermediate cases (some dysphagia or respiratory difficulty): above measures plus establish airway, either by nasotracheal (NT) intubation or consider tracheostomy in older child. The average duration of symptoms is 3–4 weeks[2]. Relaxation for intubation may require suxamethonium chloride 1 mg/kg.

c) Severe cases: NT intubation or tracheostomy followed by intermittent positive pressure ventilation (IPPV) and muscle paralysis (vecuronium may produce the fewest cardiovascular effects[3]) until symptoms abate.

6. Very severe tetanus is characterised by cardio-vascular instability and autonomic disturbance. Under these circumstances give deep sedation and consider use of labetalol[4] or magnesium sulphate by continuous infusion[5].
7. Intrathecal administration of HTIG combined with parenteral corticosteroids has been suggested in severe cases[6] but is not of proven benefit.

PROGNOSIS

- With full intensive care facilities applied early, theoretical recovery should be 100%.
- Without facilities for intensive care, the fatality rate is 45–55%, higher in neonates[7].
- Localised tetanus has a good prognosis.
- Pointers to severe disease include a short time interval between injury and development of symptoms (2–10 days) and cephalic disease. Determination of the 'severity index' of each case may prove useful[8].

FOLLOW-UP

Children making a complete recovery from tetanus do not require specific follow-up. They should be actively immunised.

[1] Cook R et al. (1985) Arch. Dis. Childh., 60, 401.
[2] Edmondson R S et al. (1979) Br. Med. J., i, 1401.
[3] Powles A B et al. (1985) Anaesthesia, 40, 879.
[4] Dundee J W et al. (1979) Br. Med. J., i, 1121.
[5] James M F M et al. (1985) Intensive Care Med., II, 5.
[6] Shann F (1983) Med. J. Aust., 2, 604.
[7] Weinstein L (1981) In Textbook of Pediatric Infectious Diseases (Feigin R D, Cherry J D eds.), p. 843. Philadelphia: Saunders.
[8] Phillips L A (1967) Lancet i, 1216.

Toxoplasmosis

Infection with the protozoon *Toxoplasma gondii* is widespread in animals and man: by adult life 20–40% people have antibody in the UK and USA[1]. Infection is usually acquired from eating uncooked meat or handling faeces from infected cats. Human toxoplasma infections may be acquired, congenital, or recrudescent.

PREVENTION

Cat litter should be disposed of daily. Pregnant women with negative or unknown immunity should avoid contact with cats and undercooked meat.

TREATMENT

1. Clinically active, generalised or localised toxoplasmosis are all indications for treatment. Congenital toxoplasmosis should be treated including asymptomatic infections.
2. Give sulphadiazine or sulfamethoxazole 25 mg/kg four times daily *plus* pyrimethamine (Daraprim) 1 mg/kg/day, or sulphadoxine and pyrimethamine (Fansidar)[2]. Give for 6–8 months in asymptomatic congenital infection, 12–15 months in symptomatic congenital infection. In acquired infection, give for twice the time taken to abate symptoms or until a good immune response can be demonstrated.
3. Monitor for bone marrow suppression and/or give folinic acid 3 mg twice weekly *or* fresh brewer's yeast 100 mg/day.
4. The use of corticosteroids (in conjunction with antimicrobials) in the management of ocular complications is controversial, and is reserved for acute, progressive chorioretinal lesions in the region of the macula.
5. Treatment of acquired *Toxoplasma* infection in pregnancy is controversial, but usually advised. Give sulphadiazine and pyrimethamine or spiramycin[3,4].

PROGNOSIS

● Acquired

a) Almost all cases are asymptomatic. Rarely symptomatic, usually with self-limiting glandular fever-like illness.
b) 1% symptomatic cases develop retinochoroiditis, usually unilateral. Vision is preserved if macula is unaffected.
c) Extremely rare myocardial involvement can cause death.

● Congenital

a) Congenital infection occurs only at the time of acute maternal infection. Risk of seroconversion in pregnancy is 0.2–0.7%[5,6].
b) Therapeutic abortion should be considered for serologically proven acute toxoplasmosis in early pregnancy[4,6].
c) 60% congenitally infected babies are asymptomatic at birth[7], but may develop recurrent posterior uveitis and neurological sequelae later[8].
d) With symptomatic congenital infection, prognosis relates to severity of symptoms, and especially neurological manifestations.

Mortality is around 12%, mental retardation 86%, convulsions 81%, cerebral palsy 20%, severely impaired vision 63%[3].

FOLLOW-UP

Symptomatic congenital infection will need long-term follow-up and regular assessment of vision and developmental progress. Retinochoroiditis will need close review, at least monthly, until quiescent. Long-term sequelae of the disease are uncommon, but recurrent episodes of posterior uveitis can occur, especially during adolescence.

[1] Editorial (1984) *Lancet*, **i**, 605.
[2] Maisonneuve H *et al.* (1984) *Presse Med.*, **13**, 859.
[3] Remington J S *et al.* (1983) *Infectious Diseases of the Fetus and Newborn* (Remington J S, Klein J O eds.), p. 143. Philadelphia: Saunders.
[4] Frenkel J K (1985) *Ped. Clin. North Am.*, **32**, 917.
[5] Williams K A B *et al.* (1981) *J. Infect.*, **3**, 219.
[6] Foulon W *et al.* (1984) *Br. J. Obstet. Gynaecol.*, **91**, 419.
[7] Eichenwald H F (1960) In *Human Toxoplasmosis* (Siim J C ed.), p. 41. Copenhagen: Munksgaard.
[8] Feldman H A (1981) *Textbook of Pediatric Infectious Diseases* (Feigin R D, Cherry J D eds.), p. 722. Philadelphia: Saunders.

Tuberculosis

Infection with *Mycobacterium tuberculosis* produces chronic disease characterised by an extremely variable clinical course. Most primary infection is asymptomatic. Clinical disease, which takes many forms, can result from complications of primary disease, failure to contain primary infection with lymphohaematogenous spread, progressive primary disease or reactivation of primary disease. Pulmonary, meningitic, renal and skeletal tuberculosis (TB) are the most commonly seen and important forms of disease. Although there was a rapid decline in incidence and mortality from *M. tuberculosis* until the early 1970s in Europe and the USA, changing population immunity and immigration from India and the Middle East, where the disease remains endemic, has resulted in continuing notification of new cases.

PREVENTION

1. Isoniazid (INAH) preventive therapy should be given for 2–3 months to all children exposed to active disease. Therapy discontinued at that time only if tuberculin sensitivity has not developed.
2. Bacille Calmette–Guérin (BCG) vaccine should be considered as a control measure in countries of low incidence of tuberculosis for:

   a) Children, particularly infants, where there is possible household exposure to tuberculosis.
   b) Groups in which an excessive rate of new infection can be demonstrated, and where usual surveillance and treatment programmes have failed or are not feasible.

3. BCG can be given to newborn infants, but after two months of age should only be given where purified protein derivative (PPD) testing is negative. Testing should be repeated 2–3 months after immunisation, and immunisation repeated if PPD remains negative. BCG should not be given to children with burns, skin infections, immunodeficiency or children receiving immunosuppressives including steroids. Data on whether or not INAH inhibits effectiveness of standard BCG are conflicting, and efficacy of INAH resistant BCG is in some doubt. If possible, BCG should be given after the course of prophylactic INAH has been completed. INAH, which has well documented efficacy should not be pre-empted by BCG, which does not.

TREATMENT

1. Therapy should be commenced not only in all cases of overt clinical disease, but also:

   a) All children and adolescents with a positive tuberculin test > 10 mm induration (PPD 5TU).
   b) Children exposed to active disease (therapy for 2–3 months until clear that tuberculin sensitivity has not developed).
   c) 'Prophylactic' treatment to neonates and young children for 8 weeks in combination with INAH resistant BCG where there is a high risk of direct TB contact, see above.
   d) Treatment of asymptomatic, radiologically normal children with positive tuberculin test and possible recent TB contact.

2. Standard therapy is isoniazid 10 mg/kg/day *plus* rifampicin 15–20 mg/kg/day. Therapy lasts for one year. If a third drug is used in combination initially, total duration may be shortened to nine months. Pyridoxine 10 mg/day should be given to prevent peripheral neuritis. Hepatic enzymes should be monitored.
3. With serious disease, tuberculous meningitis, or where there is possible drug resistance, combine above with a third drug:

   a) Streptomycin 20 mg/kg/day by i.m. injection for up to 3 months.
   b) Pyrazinamide 20 mg/kg/day in four divided doses for up to 6 months.

c) Ethambutol 15–20 mg/day in children over 13 years age only (beware of possible optic neuritis).

4. Use ethionamide 15–20 mg/kg/day orally as a *substitute* for INAH if INAH resistance is suspected.

5. Corticosteroids may be useful in suppressing inflammatory response, and should be considered for:

a) Tuberculous meningitis with complications[1,2].
b) Acute pericardial effusion[3].
c) Pleural effusion where mediastinal shift is producing respiratory embarrassment[1].
d) Miliary tuberculosis associated with severe alveolocapillary block and cyanosis.
e) Major symptoms related to mediastinal lymph node enlargement.

6. Isolation of children with tuberculosis once therapy established is only necessary if there is:

a) Productive cough.
b) Demonstrable cavitation on x-ray.
c) A draining sinus.
d) Renal tuberculosis.

PROGNOSIS

- Pulmonary tuberculosis

a) 80–90% primary pulmonary infections in children older than 1 year are asymptomatic. 40–50% primary pulmonary infections in children under 1 year of age are asymptomatic.
b) All children with primary pulmonary TB are at risk of developing complications of the primary complex, or of developing secondary disease.
c) Bronchial obstruction from a primary focus can lead to obstructive hyperinflation, sudden death by asphyxia (rare), segmental pulmonary lesions, (decreasing risk with age)[4].
d) 60% segmental lesions result in permanent anatomical sequelae[2].

e) 75–80% primary pulmonary infection calcifies[4].
f) Pleural effusion occurs when a primary complex involves the pleura. This can be localised, generalised, unilateral or bilateral.
g) Rare pulmonary complications include left phrenic nerve paresis and progressive cavitating tuberculosis (rare with good nutrition, fatal if not treated).

- Non-pulmonary tuberculosis

a) Myocardial and pericardial tuberculosis occur in 0.4–4% cases[5].
b) Miliary tuberculosis is commonest in infants <1 year (up to 16% risk in primary infection[4]), but no age is exempt. Untreated it leads to death in 4–8 weeks.
c) Tuberculous meningitis occurs in 0.3% primary infections. It accompanies miliary TB in 50% cases. Rare below 4 months of age, but usually occurs before the age of six years. Poor prognosis <18 months or if coma or convulsions develop. Long-term sequelae are numerous including blindness, deafness, mental retardation, paresis and hypothalamic/pituitary disturbance.
d) Tuberculomas, tuberculous brain abscess and spinal tuberculous leptomeningitis may rarely occur.
e) Bone and joint tuberculosis is seen in 1–6% untreated cases. Commonly affects vertebrae, knee or hip. In infants, tuberculous dactylitis is the commonest form of skeletal TB.
f) Renal tuberculosis usually occurs in adolescence[6]. May be unilateral or bilateral. Often asymptomatic until late in course of disease.
g) Congenital and neonatal tuberculosis have been reported. Prognosis is dependent on early recognition. Stillbirth may occur.

FOLLOW-UP

Follow-up should be monthly initially, to encourage and ensure therapy compliance. Hepatic enzymes should be monitored (slight rise above normal values acceptable initially). Optic neuritis should be checked for regularly if treatment includes ethambutol. A chest x-ray is required at one month and at completion of therapy in pulmonary tuberculosis. Follow-up beyond termination of therapy is not necessary except with sequelae of disease, e.g. meningitis.

[1] Smith M H D (1958) *Paediatrics*, **22,** 774.

[2] Smith M H D *et al.* (1981) *Textbook of Pediatric Infectious Diseases* (Feigin R D, Cherry J D eds.), p. 1016. Philadelphia: Saunders.

[3] Rooney J J *et al.* (1970) *Ann. Intern. Med.*, **72,** 73.

[4] Payne M (1959) MD Thesis. Quoted by Smith *et al.* (1981)[2].

[5] Boyd G L (1953) *Am. J. Dis. Childh.*, **86,** 293.

[6] Ehrlich R M *et al.* (1971) *J. Urol.*, **105,** 461.

16

Disorders of the Blood

J. Graham-Pole

Iron Deficiency Anaemia

Iron deficiency anaemia is the commonest childhood nutritional deficiency, particularly affecting infants between the ages of six months and three years, with a second smaller peak during adolescence. The causes are inadequate iron in the diet, increasing requirements with accelerating growth, limited intestinal absorption, and blood loss, particularly from the bowel and through menstruation.

TREATMENT

1. Prophylaxis

   a) A recommended iron intake for children ranges from 7 mg/day at 6 months to 15 mg/day at 18 years of age, or about 0.5 mg/100 kcal of diet.
   b) Artificially fed infants should receive 10–15 mg elemental iron per reconstituted quart during the first year of life[1].
   c) Use of iron-fortified cereals should be encouraged during infancy.
   d) Children's diets should contain iron-rich foods, including red meat, green leaf vegetables, fruit, eggs, and fortified cereals.
   e) Some authorities recommend withholding iron supplementation during the first two to three months in severely preterm infants, because of the risk of haemolysis from vitamin E deficiency.
   f) Maternal iron supplementation during pregnancy is important for the mother-to-be, because the fetus stores iron at the expense of the mother. It is rare for a baby to be born iron-deficient, even in the face of severe maternal iron deficiency.

2. Oral iron

   a) Any form of ferrous salt is effective in treating simple iron deficiency, but ferric iron is poorly absorbed. The recommended oral dose is 6 mg/kg/day of elemental iron; larger doses increase the severity of gastrointestinal side-effects. It should be continued for 8 weeks after the haemoglobin level returns to normal.
   b) The reticulocyte count peaks at 5–10 days after starting therapy, depending on the severity of the anaemia, and the haematocrit rises initially by 1% daily, slowing to 0.5% daily.
   c) Failure to respond indicates:
      i) Non-administration.
      ii) Persistent blood loss.
      iii) Incorrect diagnosis.

3. Parenteral iron

   a) Intramuscular iron-dextran complex (Imferon: 50 mg iron/ml) as a source of elemental iron, should be used for:
      i) Inflammatory bowel disease or malabsorption;
      ii) Severe intolerance of oral iron;
      iii) Non-compliant families.
   b) It is given by deep intramuscular injection in the thigh, and may rarely cause generalised reactions including arthralgia and angioneurotic oedema.

4. Blood transfusion

   a) This is indicated when the haemoglobin level is less than 0.93 mmol/l (6 g/dl) (haematocrit < 20%), with the attendant risk of cardiac failure.
   b) If cardiac failure is present, exchange transfusion is safer in small children.

PROGNOSIS

- 30–60% children in industrial and underdeveloped communities are chronically iron-deficient.
- Prognosis depends on public education about nutrition, general provision of iron supplementation in milks and infant foods, and recognition and treatment of non-dietary causes, such as blood loss and malabsorption.

- Failure to respond to iron therapy may indicate other coexistent disease.

FOLLOW-UP

Follow-up haemoglobin (Hb) and reticulocyte counts should be measured one week after initiating treatment. Subsequent monthly checks of Hb and red cell indices should continue for 6 months, as well as monitoring growth and development, and excluding continuing gastrointestinal blood loss where appropriate.

[1] Report of 62nd Ross Conference on Pediatric Research (1970) Columbus, Ohio: Ross Laboratories.

Megaloblastic Anaemia

In children, megaloblastic anaemia is usually due to deficiency of folic acid, less commonly of cyanocobalamin (vitamin B_{12}). Both function as essential coenzymes in normal metabolic processes. Deficiency is most apparent in the erythropoietic pathway, but also produces abnormalities in other marrow functions. The commonest causes are dietary deficiency with increased requirements (e.g. accelerated growth, chronic haemolysis), malabsorption affecting the small bowel, and less commonly metabolic disorders[1].

TREATMENT

1. Prophylaxis: in conditions where there is a risk of developing megaloblastic anaemia, e.g. following gastric or small bowel resection, preterm birth[2], or chronic haemolysis, folic acid and sometimes B_{12} should be prescribed.
2. Treatment depends upon correcting the deficiency; relieving any underlying disorder; improving the diet.
3. Most patients respond to folic acid 100–200 μg daily, but the usual treatment dose is 5 mg, reducing to 1 mg daily after seven days, and this should be continued for at least 3 months.
4. Hydroxocobalamin (B_{12}) should be injected in a dose of 25–100 μg daily, depending on age, for several doses and maintained with monthly doses of 100–1000 μg. Patients with metabolic defects may require more frequent doses.

PROGNOSIS

- Prognosis depends on correct and early diagnosis and recognition of underlying diseases.
- Persistent deficiency may lead to chronically slow growth in early childhood.
- B_{12} deficiency can also lead to serious CNS derangements. Folic acid therapy may accelerate this if there is concurrent B_{12} deficiency.

FOLLOW-UP

A reasonable follow-up is to obtain FBC and reticulocytes weekly for one month, monthly for 6 months, then every 3 months for 2 years. Growth and development should also be followed. Although early post-treatment folate or B_{12} levels should be obtained, they are unnecessary once there has been a satisfactory response to treatment. Follow-up evaluation of B_{12} deficiency is particularly important to prevent or detect relapse.

[1] Willoughby M L N (1977) Paediatric Haematology, p. 21. Edinburgh: Churchill Livingstone.
[2] Shojania A M et al. (1964) J. Pediatr., 63, 323.

Bone Marrow Failure

Bone marrow failure is a condition in which the normal haematopoietic cells are reduced in number, most often resulting in pancytopenia due to reduction in megakaryocytes, erythroblasts and myeloblasts. It may be constitutional and associated with other congenital defects, or acquired, either secondary to infections or toxins (e.g. radiation, chloramphenicol, benzene), but most often it is idiopathic[1].

TREATMENT

1. Initial transfusion of blood products is indicated for haemoglobin levels less than 1.24 mmol/l (8 mg/dl) and platelet counts less than 30×10^9/l if symptoms are present, and these transfusions may have to be repeated.

2. A useful formula for transfusion of packed red blood cells (which have a haematocrit of about 70%) is[2]:

$$\text{Volume (ml) required} = \frac{\text{Desired–Actual Hb(g)}}{0.23(g)}$$

3. One unit of platelets contains about 5×10^{11} platelets, and should raise the recipient count by about 20×10^9/l/m^2 body surface area[2].

4. Regular screens should be performed to detect developing antibodies to red cells and platelets. Use of washed or frozen cells and minimising transfusions may lessen such sensitisation.

5. Isolation in a protected environment and prompt use of systemic antibiotics for suspected sepsis, pending the results of blood and other cultures, helps to counter the high risk of fatal infections.

6. Traditional treatment with androgenic and corticosteroids has produced disappointing results in both European and American studies[3,4] but long-term androgen treatment may help in a minority of cases. The usual doses are: prednisolone 1 mg/kg/day and oxymethalone 5 mg/kg/day.

7. Antithymocyte globulin has been tested in recent clinical trials with some beneficial results, based on the autoimmune nature of some cases of bone marrow failure[5].

8. Bone marrow transplantation from a histocompatible sibling is the treatment of choice for the severe disease[6], producing long-term survival in 50–80% in reported series. Graft rejection is a significant problem in frequently transfused cases, the remaining failures being due to fatal opportunistic infections and/or graft-versus-host disease.

PROGNOSIS

- Most deaths occur in the first 3 months after diagnosis, in patients with generally severe aplastic anaemia (neutrophil count $< 1000 \times 10^6$/l, platelet count $< 20 \times 10^9$/l, reticulocytes $< 1\%$).
- Initial severity is generally greater in children than adults, and greater in acquired than in genetic forms[7].
- Long-term improvement may occur in less severe cases, either spontaneously or following treatment.

FOLLOW-UP

Frequent follow-up after discharge from hospital is essential (e.g. once or twice weekly initially) to exclude infections, complications and check blood counts. Monthly follow-up for FBC and 3–6 monthly marrow examinations should continue for a minimum of two years.

[1] Ather B P et al. (1978) Clin. Hematol., 7, 431.
[2] Luban N L C (1984) In Blood Diseases of Infancy and Childhood (Miller D, Baehner R, McMillan C eds.), ch. 3. St Louis: Mosby.
[3] Li F P et al. (1972) Blood, 40, 153.
[4] Davis S et al. (1972) Lancet, i, 871.
[5] Champlin R et al. (1983) New Eng. J. Med., 308, 113.
[6] Gale R P (1981) Ann. Int. Med., 95, 477.
[7] Najean Y et al. (1982) Am. J. Pediatr. Hematol. Oncol., 4, 273.

Haemolytic Anaemia

Haemolytic anaemia is characterised by a shortened red blood cell life-span with a compensatory increase in bone marrow activity, changes in red cell morphology (spherocytes, schistocytes, polychromasia), and increased bilirubin metabolism[1]. The cause may be constitutional (e.g. spherocytosis, red cell enzyme deficiencies, haemoglobinopathies) or acquired (e.g. autoimmune, hypersplenism), and will be considered under the following headings: membrane defects, metabolic defects, haemoglobin abnormalities, immune defects.

Membrane defects

The primary function of the red blood cell membrane is to separate the finely tuned internal environment from the more random exterior. This it achieves by energy-requiring processes brought about by interaction between the internal cellular metabolism and the complex structure of the red cell membrane. Intrinsic structural membrane defects include hereditary spherocytosis, elliptocytosis, stomatocytosis and pyropoikilocytosis. Membrane failure occurs because these cells do not have the characteristic biconcave disc form and are more fragile and inefficient.

TREATMENT

1. Transfusions are necessary in early life if the haemolysis is not well compensated, and particularly for aplastic crises.
2. Splenectomy is the treatment of choice for chronic haemolysis, since it prolongs red cell survival to 80% of normal[2]. It should be postponed if possible until at least 5 years of age to reduce the risk of fatal infections.
3. Post-splenectomy penicillin 125–250 mg b.d. (erythromycin or a cephalosporin in the case of penicillin hypersensitivity) should be taken throughout childhood.
4. Folic acid should be given in a dose of 1 mg daily until splenectomy is performed.
5. Polyvalent pneumococcal vaccine should be given just before splenectomy.

PROGNOSIS

- Patients vary greatly in the severity of their haemolytic tendency and, particularly with hereditary elliptocytosis and stomatocytosis, may be asymptomatic.
- Most patients will have a normal life-span if recognised early and appropriately treated.
- Crises, either haemolytic or aplastic, may occur, particularly in spherocytosis. These are usually precipitated by infections, and may be life-threatening.
- As in all chronic haemolytic conditions, pigmentary gallstones occur, with a frequency correlating with the severity of haemolysis.
- If splenectomy is necessary to control haemolysis, overwhelming post-splenectomy infections with encapsulated organisms are a recognised hazard, particularly in young children.

FOLLOW-UP

Monthly Hb and reticulocytes are usually adequate, but parents should be alerted to the need for physician supervision of any infections, particularly in pre-school children.

---

[1] Pearson H A et al. (1984) In Blood Diseases of Infancy and Childhood, 5th edn. (Miller D, Baehner R, McMillan C eds.), ch. 8. St Louis: Mosby.
[2] Chapman R G (1968) J. Clin. Invest., **47,** 2263.

Metabolic defects

Inborn enzyme deficiencies affect both major metabolic routes of glycolytic metabolism, i.e. the anaerobic (Embden-Meyerhof) and aerobic (hexose-monophosphate shunt) pathways. Since glycolysis is essential for the production of energy, to maintain the red cell's shape and deformability, to deliver oxygen from lungs to tissues, to reduce haemoglobin, and synthesise prime nucleotides, any enzyme deficiency produces major metabolic derangements and shortened red cell survival. Although a large number of enzyme deficiencies is now described[1], the commonest are glucose-6-phosphate dehydrogenase (G6PD) deficiency, affecting aerobic metabolism, and pyruvate kinase (PK) deficiency, affecting anaerobic metabolism.

TREATMENT

1. Exchange transfusion may be necessary for neonatal hyperbilirubinaemia.
2. Intermittent transfusions are indicated for chronic haemolysis or haemolytic/aplastic crises.
3. Splenectomy may lessen transfusion frequency, but it is not as effective as for spherocytosis.
4. Post-splenectomy penicillin (or equivalent) prophylaxis should be given throughout childhood.
5. Avoidance of all potentially toxic oxidative drugs (antimalarials, antipyretics, sulphonamides) is essential for G6PD-deficient subjects.
6. Folic acid administration is indicated for patients experiencing chronic haemolysis.

PROGNOSIS

- G6PD deficiency is heterogeneous in its clinical severity, depending on the ethnic group and biochemical variant. The most severe forms are seen in Mediterranean and northern European races, who experience chronic lifelong haemolysis.
- Avoidance of oxidative drugs and prompt treatment of infections will avert haemolytic and aplastic crises.
- Patients suffering chronic haemolysis and/or repeated crises may be growth-retarded.

FOLLOW-UP

Monthly Hb and reticulocytes are usually adequate, but parents should be alerted to the need for physician supervision of any infections, particularly in pre-school children.

---

[1] Miller D R (1984) In *Blood Diseases of Infancy and Childhood* 5th edn. (Miller D, Baehner R, McMillan C, eds.), ch. 11. St Louis: Mosby.

Haemoglobin abnormalities

There are two major inherited abnormalities affecting synthesis of the globin chains of human haemoglobin: (a) the haemoglobinopathies, most notably the sickling syndromes, in which there is an abnormal amino acid substitution in the chain; and (b) an absence or deficiency of one or more globin chain, which characterises the thalassaemia syndromes.

Sickle cell anaemia

The sickle cell gene is present in 8–40% of black people, depending on geographic region. The homozygous (SS) state is associated with a wide spectrum of clinical features, including chronic haemolytic anaemia, frequent painful vasocclusive crises, and haemolytic, aplastic and sequestration crises, usually triggered by infections, to which sickle cell patients are highly susceptible.

TREATMENT

1. In spite of extensive research[1], there is currently no specific treatment for sickle cell disease.
2. Sickling may be lessened by avoiding dehydration, acidosis, hypoxia, and infections as far as possible.
3. Whole blood (usually exchange) transfusions are indicated for all severe crises, to improve oxygenation and suppress further sickle cell production by the marrow.
4. Analgesics should be given freely for vasocclusive pain crises.
5. Systemic antibiotics must be given immediately in any case of suspected sepsis.
6. Prophylactic penicillin (or equivalent) treatment should be given throughout childhood.
7. Folic acid supplements are also indicated as in any chronic haemolytic state.
8. Immunisation with pneumococcal polyvalent vaccine should be given at two years of age.

PROGNOSIS

- Survival beyond 40 years has been unusual until recently, since when there has been greater attention and supervision of this population.
- Death in early life is not uncommon due to overwhelming sepsis and sequestration crises.
- Damage to major organs, including heart, liver, kidneys and nervous system, often results from

repeated vasocclusive episodes and/or transfusion haemosiderosis.

- Normal growth, development and pubertal changes are often markedly delayed.

FOLLOW-UP

Sickle cell patients must be followed frequently (e.g. monthly) preferably in a specialised clinic for monitoring growth, development of complications and FBC.

---

[1] Dean J et al. (1978) New Eng. J. Med., **299**, 752.

Thalassaemia

The thalassaemia syndromes affect predominantly Mediterranean, middle eastern and oriental races. Either β-globin or α-globin chains may be deficient, and homozygous subjects suffer from lifelong hypochromic microcytic anaemia with severely shortened red cell life-span.

TREATMENT

1. The mainstay of treatment is transfusion of packed red blood cells[1] aimed at maintaining the haemoglobin level above 1.55 mmol/l (10 g/dl), usually requiring monthly or more frequent transfusions.
2. The use of 'neocytes' (specially prepared units of blood containing only the youngest red blood cells) increases the survival of transfused cells, although this is an expensive technology.
3. Chelation treatment with desferrioxamine or similar chelators is essential to remove excess iron. Desferrioxamine 1–2 g can result in excretion of as much as 100 mg urinary iron daily, when given via a 8–10 hour overnight subcutaneous infusion pump[2].
4. Splenectomy is sometimes indicated if transfusion requirements seem to be increasing and there is evidence of hypersplenism. This should, if possible, be postponed until school age, and post-splenectomy antibiotic prophylaxis is indicated.
5. Gallstones may occasionally require cholecystectomy in older patients.
6. Ascorbic acid has been shown to increase iron excretion and daily doses up to 500 mg may be a useful and safe adjunctive treatment[3].
7. Bone marrow transplantation has been increasingly tested in Italy and the USA, as a curative approach. The indications and justifications are the subject of continuing research.

PROGNOSIS

- Life-span is usually markedly shortened, due to the life-long severe anaemia and transfusion-induced haemosiderosis.
- Growth, development and pubertal changes are usually retarded.
- The recent use of more intensive 'hypertransfusion' programmes has greatly improved this prognosis[1], without worsening the problems of iron overload.
- It is too early to know if modern treatment approaches will result in patients achieving a normal life-span.

FOLLOW-UP

Patients with thalassaemia should be seen at least monthly, preferably at a specialised clinic for medical assessment and for checking of Hb and iron stores. Education of parents and children in the use of long-term chelation therapy is essential.

---

[1] Kattarius C et al. (1970) Arch. Dis. Childh., **45**, 502.
[2] Hussain M A M et al. (1977) Lancet, **i**, 977.
[3] Neinhuis A W (1983) New Eng. J. Med., **304**, 170.

Immune defects

Immune haemolysis is due to the deposition of specific IgG or IgM antibody on the red cell surface. This may be caused by blood group incompatibility (ABO, Rhesus), drugs, infections, or autoimmune disease. It may be of warm or cold antibody type, and haemolysis may be intravascular or extravascular.

TREATMENT

1. Transfusion of red cells is necessary for adequate cardiovascular function and tissue oxygenation. The 'least incompatible' red cells must be used in cases where completely compatible blood cannot be found.

2. Corticosteroids (e.g. prednisolone 1–2 mg/kg/day) are effective particularly in IgG-mediated haemolysis.
3. Other immunosuppressive drugs, such as azathioprine[1] and cyclophosphamide, may be effective in steroid-dependent patients.
4. Splenectomy may be indicated for either acute or chronic haemolysis uncontrolled by other measures.
5. Plasma exchange may be effective in patients with large quantities of circulating IgM antibody producing intravascular haemolysis.

PROGNOSIS

- Post-infective cases in young children are usually acute and short-lived, rarely recurrent, and the prognosis is excellent.
- Intravascular haemolysis may be associated with severe haemoglobinuria and renal failure.
- The course is often more chronic in older children, and may be life-threatening if associated with aplastic crises.

FOLLOW-UP

Patients must be followed closely after hospital discharge for evidence of persistent or recurrent haemolysis, with weekly then monthly Hb, reticulocyte count and Coombs' tests.

[1] Hitzig W H *et al.* (1966) *Blood*, **28,** 840.

Purpuras

Purpuras are characterised by multiple spontaneous haemorrhages in the skin and mucous membranes, ranging from pinpoint petechiae to extensive bruises (ecchymoses). The lesions are non-raised and non-blanching, and are due to either capillary or platelet deficiency. The causes may be classified according to whether the platelet count is normal (vascular or platelet dysfunction) or low (thrombocytopenia).

Anaphylactoid (Henoch-Schönlein) purpura

Anaphylactoid purpura is the commonest vascular purpura in paediatrics. The rash is initially urticarial, then purpuric, and is almost confined to the lower limbs and buttocks, often associated with periarticular arthropathy, oedema, and abdominal pain, indicating intestinal involvement. Intussusception is a not uncommon complication. Rarely, there may be testicular torsion or central nervous system involvement. It is probably caused by a hypersensitivity reaction resulting in a vasculitis that is immunologically mediated, but there are no consistent haematological abnormalities.

TREATMENT

1. Treatment is symptomatic. No specific therapy has been described which is consistently beneficial.

2. Bed rest during the acute phase may shorten the course and lessen the risk of renal complications.
3. Corticosteroids are sometimes used for gut and renal involvement, but are not consistently helpful[1].

PROGNOSIS

- Prognosis depends largely on the presence or absence of renal involvement. Chronic renal involvement is seen in 25–30% of patients, although only about 50% progress to chronic glomerulonephritis and renal failure[1].
- About 60% of patients suffer a single self-limited episode.

FOLLOW-UP

Follow-up is weekly for the first month, then monthly for FBC, ESR, and renal function studies for patients with renal involvement. Continuing follow-up is not needed for patients without complications.

[1] Allen D M *et al.* (1960) *Am. J. Dis. Childh.*, **99**, 833.

Purpura fulminans

Purpura fulminans may complicate severe systemic infections, including meningococcaemia, typhoid, smallpox, measles and diphtheria, and is primarily vascular but may be complicated by the haematological abnormalities of disseminated intravascular coagulation (DIC, see p. 308).

TREATMENT

Treatment iş as for *DIC* (see p. 308).

PROGNOSIS

● With improved supportive care and the use of heparin, the previous 50% mortality rate has been greatly lowered.

FOLLOW-UP

Close follow-up is necessary in the immediate post-hospital period (e.g. weekly FBC and renal function studies). Fully recovered cases do not require prolonged follow-up.

Platelet dysfunction

This may be congenital (von Willebrand's disease, thrombasthenia) or acquired (salicylate ingestion, renal or hepatic insufficiency), and is associated with a prolonged bleeding time due to faulty platelet plug formation.

TREATMENT

These patients should be transfused with fresh normal platelets either prophylactically (before surgery), or in the event of severe bleeding.

PROGNOSIS

● Prognosis is generally good in the congenital forms, which are rarely life-threatening.

● Prognosis is dependent on the underlying condition in the acquired forms.

FOLLOW-UP

Three monthly check-ups with occasional bleeding times are usually sufficient. Patients should be more fully evaluated before any elective surgery.

Idiopathic thrombocytopenia purpura

Idiopathic thrombocytopenia purpura (ITP) is an immunologically based disorder associated with destruction of platelets by an antiplatelet IgG antibody in the plasma. It develops acutely in children usually between the age of 2 and 8 years following a recent viral infection, with bleeding into the skin and mucosal surfaces[1]. The more chronic 'adult' form sometimes affects older children. The platelet count is often less than $20 \times 10^9/l$ and bone marrow examination reveals increased young megakaryocytes.

TREATMENT

1. Protection: young children with severe manifestations should be protected from injury and should probably be admitted to hospital for a short initial stay.
2. Corticosteroids: this remains a controversial issue. Some experts still favour conservative management of the acute disease without steroids. A recent American controlled trial[2] concluded that steroids produced no significant benefit over placebo, while a recent European study reported a significantly shorter duration of thrombocytopenia and capillary fragility in treated patients, without serious side-effects[3]. The usual dose of prednisone prescribed is 2 mg/kg/day for 14–21 days, which may be repeated for recurrences.
3. Intravenous gammaglobulin in a special high dose formulation has recently been reported to produce responses in refractory cases, through an uncertain mechanism[4]. The recommended dose is 400 mg/kg/day for five days.
4. Splenectomy is indicated in severe cases not responsive to the above measures, and this is usually rapidly successful in slowing down

platelet destruction. Long-term penicillin is indicated postoperatively, because of the risk of overwhelming sepsis.

5. Other immunosuppresive drugs (e.g. vincristine, azathioprine) may be effective in refractory cases[5].

PROGNOSIS

- This is a self-limited condition in 80% cases, with complete recovery within 6 months.
- In the minority (most often older children) the disease becomes chronic.
- Mortality is 1% or less, usually from CNS bleeding at the time of initial onset of the disease.

FOLLOW-UP

Follow-up should be monthly for platelet counts for the first 12 months. Prolonged follow-up is not needed in the uncomplicated case.

[1] Lusher J M et al. (1966) J. Pediatr., **68,** 971.
[2] Buchanan G R et al. (1984) Am. J. Pediatr. Hematol. Oncol., **6,** 355.
[3] Sartorius J A (1984) Am. J. Pediatr. Hematol. Oncol., **6,** 165.
[4] Imbach P (1981) Lancet, **i,** 1228.
[5] Ahn Y S (1974) New Eng. J. Med., **291,** 376.

Disseminated intravascular coagulation

There are several conditions in which platelets and other coagulation factors, including fibrinogen and factors V and VIII, may be consumed acutely in the circulation due to widespread endothelial deposition and subsequent fibrinolysis. They include purpura fulminans, Gram-negative sepsis, incompatible blood transfusions, haemolytic uraemic syndrome, and giant haemangiomas. There may be widespread purpura and bleeding from venepuncture sites, and there is a high risk of major internal bleeding. The condition is identified by the development of thrombocytopenia, a prolonged prothrombin time, elevated plasma fibrin degradation products, and deficiency of individual clotting factors.

TREATMENT

1. Replacement therapy: fresh frozen plasma is the main source of replacement of consumed coagulation factors. The usual dose is 10 ml/kg i.v. infusion, which may need to be repeated every 12–24 hours. The volume of plasma required may be a problem particularly in infants, and individual factors such as fibrinogen can be given as concentrates. Cryoprecipitate is a useful alternative but probably has no particular advantage over fresh frozen plasma.
2. Fresh platelet transfusions should be given to try to maintain the platelet count above $30 \times 10^9/l$, and they may be required daily or more often in severe cases.
3. Heparin therapy: replacement of missing coagulation factors has little effect on the underlying pathogenesis of DIC and there is some evidence that it may exacerbate it[1]. Continuous intravenous infusion of heparin in a dose of 25 units/kg may arrest the triggering mechanism responsible for its onset and prevent further deposition of clotting factors in the vasculature. This is a controversial topic, but when used with caution and with close monitoring of the clotting indices, heparin may be effective in arresting purpura fulminans.
4. Corticosteroids: these are usually given to severely ill and shocked patients, in a dose of 1–2 mg/kg/day prednisolone or equivalent, but there is no clear evidence of their effectiveness in arresting DIC.

PROGNOSIS

- This is a severe condition, with a high (>50%) mortality in cases of acute onset.
- The prognosis depends largely on the outcome of the underlying disease.

FOLLOW-UP

Follow-up is dictated by the underlying disease. Patients must be followed frequently after hospital discharge if there is evidence of continuing haematological or renal abnormalities. Haemoglobin, platelet count, prothrombin time, partial thromboplastin time and renal function studies should be checked frequently.

[1] Hathaway W E (1973) J. Pediatr., **82,** 900.

Haemophilia A and B (Factor VIII and IX Deficiency)

Haemophilia A and B are X-linked recessive conditions and occur almost exclusively in males. Von Willebrand's disease has an autosomal dominant pattern of inheritance and is seen equally in boys and girls. Clinical manifestations are most commonly subcutaneous and intramuscular haematomas and haemarthroses and less commonly bleeding from mucosal surfaces. These findings result from failure of the plasma phase of haemostasis.

TREATMENT

1. Prophylaxis

   a) These children and their families should be educated early in the avoidance of unnecessary trauma including contact sports.
   b) Rest and subsequent graded exercises should be prescribed for affected musculoskeletal sites of bleeding.
   c) Education should be directed toward occupations not requiring great physical activity.
   d) Intramuscular injections and aspirin-containing drugs must be avoided.
   e) Regular prophylactic dental care is needed to minimise the need for extractions.
   f) These patients should be registered with a clinic specialising in their care and with the local haemophilia organisation.
   g) Home treatment with self-administration of factor concentrates can be taught to school-age children and their parents[1].

2. Replacement therapy: therapeutic sources of factors VIII and IX are fresh frozen plasma, cryoprecipitate and factor concentrates. A factor level from 25% to 50% will arrest spontaneous haemorrhage, but for surgery and for severe bleeding deep to mucosal surfaces the level should be kept between 50% and 100%. Factor VIII 1 unit/kg and factor IX 2 units/kg raise the respective factor levels by approximately 2%. Cryoprecipitate is commonly used for factor VIII deficiency but fresh frozen plasma must be used for factor IX deficiency, and these often need to be infused at 8–24 hour intervals (because of their short plasma half-life), according to the severity of the bleeding problem and its response. Commercial concentrates have the advantage of convenience but may carry an increased risk of blood-borne viral infections (e.g. hepatitis, HIV).

3. Haemarthroses may require temporary splinting and even joint aspiration under cover of adequate factor replacement. Vigorous physical therapy is indicated subsequently.

4. Antifibrinolytic therapy: these agents (e.g. ε-amino caproic acid) may be useful in short courses for the prevention and treatment of superficial (e.g. dental) bleeding, by inhibiting plasminogen activity. A recommended dose is 100 mg/kg 6 hourly for 7 days[2]. These drugs are not advocated for treating haemarthroses, since clots may form that are not possible to dissolve and so contribute to contractures.

5. Surgery: synovectomy and even prosthetic joint replacement have been increasingly advocated for severely damaged joints, since the ready availability of replacement factors can now maintain adequate plasma levels over prolonged periods. Factor levels must be maintained at 60–80% for at least 4 days postoperatively, and at 20–30% for 2–3 weeks thereafter during rehabilitation.

PROGNOSIS

- Prognosis is closely related to the basal level of the deficient plasma factor, patients with less than 1% having much more severe haemorrhagic problems than those with 5% or greater.
- In general, patients with 'classical' haemophilia have a more severe clinical course than patients with von Willebrand's disease.
- The prognosis is less favourable for patients who develop circulating inhibitors particularly

of factor VIII, since treatment is much more difficult.

- There may be permanent disability from joint contractures, renal and hepatic impairment.
- Recent reports of positive post-transfusion serological tests for the acquired human immunodeficiency virus (HIV) in some haemophiliacs is of major concern.

FOLLOW-UP

Long-term 1–3 monthly visits to a specialised clinic are essential to monitor growth and development, dental, hepatic, renal and musculoskeletal function. Evidence of increased bleeding severity or frequency is an indication to screen for circulating inhibitors (found in 10–20% patients with factor VIII deficiency).

[1] Levine P H (1974) *New Eng. J. Med.*, **291,** 1381.
[2] Walsh P N *et al.* (1971) *Br. J. Haematol.*, **20,** 463.

Haemorrhagic Disease of the Newborn

Factors II, VII, IX and X make up the prothrombin complex, synthesised in the liver and dependent on vitamin K. Deficiency of this vitamin in the newborn results in haemorrhagic manifestations between the second and fourth day of life. Hepatic immaturity, hypoxia and infection may worsen the condition, which is more common in breast-fed infants.

TREATMENT

1. Prophylaxis: vitamin K 1 mg i.m. or i.v. is now routinely given to all newborns, with the result that today this condition rarely manifests itself.
2. Treatment

   a) For the established condition, vitamin K 1–2 mg i.v. (avoiding i.m. injections) usually corrects the coagulation disorder rapidly.
   b) For severe cases, particularly those with hepatic insufficiency, an infusion of fresh frozen plasma 10–15 ml/kg is indicated.
   c) Early feeding, avoiding breast milk initially, is also important.

PROGNOSIS

- Although serious and even fatal bleeding may complicate this condition, with prompt recognition and treatment it resolves rapidly and permanently.

FOLLOW-UP

Return visits should be arranged during the early post-hospital period, but long-term follow-up is not necessary.

Neutropenia

Neutropenia is defined as a circulating absolute neutrophil count less than $1500 \times 10^6/l$. Severe infections become progressively more common as the neutrophil count drops below $500 \times 10^6/l$. It may be an isolated condition, which is either congenital or acquired, and caused either by marrow non-production or increased destruction. Or it may be part of a pancytopenic picture associated with marrow suppression or replacement, or with hypersplenism.

TREATMENT

1. Withdrawal of offending cause (e.g. drug).
2. Isolation from sources of infection in the acute phase.
3. Prompt cultures and use of systemic antibiotics for suspected sepsis.
4. Neutrophil transfusions (daily for 5–7 days, or until recovery) for documented sepsis not responsive to systemic antibiotics.
5. Prednisolone (1–2 mg/kg/day) or other immunosuppressive therapy (e.g. antithymocyte globulin) may be effective in immunologically mediated cases.
6. In autoimmune cases, high doses of intravenous immunoglobulin (300–500 mg/kg) have recently been reported to be beneficial[1].

PROGNOSIS

- Severe neutropenias are associated with a high mortality and death rate from systemic sepsis if not treated quickly.
- Other forms of neutropenia, including cyclic neutropenia, often have a more indolent course and may even be self-limited.

FOLLOW-UP

Follow-up should be weekly for clinical check-ups and FBC during the acute phase, then long-term monthly follow-ups for the chronic but uncomplicated case.

---

[1] Pollack S et al. (1982) New Eng. J. Med., **307,** 253.

Lymphocytosis

A relative lymphocytosis is the norm in the infant and young child, a gradual fall in the lymphocyte count and rise in the neutrophil count occurring over the first decade of life. This is of no pathological significance. An absolute lymphocytosis is commonly seen in children with non-bacterial infections, and this may rise as high as $50\,000 \times 10^6/l$ in acute pertussis. Most viral infections induce a lesser rise in the lymphocytes, which are often atypical, notably infectious mononucleosis. These conditions must be distinguished from acute leukaemia.

TREATMENT AND PROGNOSIS

Treatment and prognosis depend upon the underlying condition, but these disorders are usually self-limited and the outlook is good.

FOLLOW-UP

Follow-up is generally not indicated.

Lymphopenia

Lymphopenia is usually a sign of immunodeficiency, and may be congenital or acquired. The congenital forms may be part of a more generalised syndrome, in which the absolute lymphocyte count may be persistently less than $500 \times 10^6/l$. The acquired form usually arises secondarily to drug treatment, notably with corticosteroids and cytotoxic drugs.

TREATMENT

1. For congenital immunodeficiencies associated with lymphopenia, some form of immune reconstitution with fetal thymic implants or bone marrow transplantation has had some success in recent years[1].
2. Acquired lymphopenia usually reverses when the offending agent is withdrawn.
3. Vigorous treatment of complicating viral or fungal infections is indicated, using specific agents (e.g. amphotericin, acyclovir) if available.

PROGNOSIS

- Lymphopenia is a serious disorder, as it is associated with life-threatening viral and fungal infections, and the prognosis is very guarded unless there is treatment available for the underlying disorder.

FOLLOW-UP

Frequent follow-up visits are essential for physical examination, FBC and immunological testing. This should be at a specialised clinic, weekly initially, then monthly as the condition allows.

---

[1] Soothill J F (1984) In *Textbook of Paediatrics* (Forfar J O, Arneil G C eds.) p. 1333. Edinburgh: Churchill Livingstone.

Acute Leukaemia

Acute leukaemia is the commonest malignant condition of children, the leukaemias combined accounting for about 30% childhood cancer. There are few established facts about its aetiology, but genetic predisposition, slow-growing viruses, and radiation have all been implicated. About 70% childhood leukaemias are of the acute lymphoblastic type (ALL), about 20% the acute myeloblastic type (AML) or its variants. ALL is in turn divided by immunological subtyping into 'common' (CALLA-antigen-positive), T-cell, B-cell and pre-B-cell ALL. These subgroupings affect both prognosis and treatment planning. The greatest incidence of leukaemia is in pre-school children. The symptoms and signs are largely the result of replacement of the normal bone marrow by neoplastic cells.

TREATMENT

1. General supportive measures: these are particularly important at the time of initial diagnosis when the marrow is completely replaced by leukaemic cells, but apply throughout the course of treatment, particularly at times of drug-induced marrow suppression.

   a) Isolation: children with severe neutropenia should be isolated, particularly when in hospital, to protect them from exogenous infection.
   b) Antibiotics should be administered systemically and in combination immediately on development of clinical signs of infection, and after appropriate cultures have been collected. They should include an antistaphylococcal agent, an aminoglycoside, and a penicillin having good coverage against *Pseudomonas*.
   c) Blood component transfusion: red cells, platelets, and occasionally white cells, may all be needed repeatedly, particularly in the early phases of the disease.
   d) Correction of metabolic abnormalities: establishment of adequate hydration and renal blood flow, correction of hyperuricaemia, metabolic acidosis, hyperkalaemia, hyperphosphataemia and hypocalcaemia, may all be important early on. These problems are often exacerbated by rapid breakdown of leukaemic cells with chemotherapy. Fluids should be given at a rate of 3000 ml/m^2/day, the urine should be alkalinised with sodium bicarbonate 50 mmol/l, and allopurinol should be given in a dose of 300 mg/m^2/day. Occasionally metabolic disturbances may be so severe as to require renal dialysis.
   e) Psychological and social support: the diagnosis of cancer in childhood puts a very stressful burden on the affected family, and adequate support in this regard from the paediatric team is essential.

3. Specific treatment: ALL

   a) Remission of the disease can be induced in 90% or more cases with the combination of prednisone (1 mg/kg/day for 28 days) plus vincristine (1.5 mg/m^2/week for four doses). L-Asparaginase as a third induction agent has been shown in several studies to improve both the remission rate and overall duration of remission; a commonly used regimen is 6000 units/m^2/day for 14 days. Other drugs are used to induce remissions in refractory and relapsed cases. These include antimetabolites (cytosine arabinoside), anthracyclines (daunomycin), plant alkaloids (VM26), and alkylating agents (cyclophosphamide).
   b) Prophylaxis against the development of CNS leukaemic infiltration is routinely given after remission induction, and has reduced the incidence of CNS leukaemia from over 50% to less than 10%. Intrathecal injections with the triple combination of methotrexate, hydrocortisone and cytosine arabinoside is preferable to the previously used cranial irradiation and intrathecal methotrexate, since the latter is more likely to produce learning difficulties in young children[1]. Intrathecal drugs should

probably be repeated every 2–3 months during maintenance treatment.

c) Maintenance treatment: this remains the most controversial part of treatment, but there is general consensus that it should continue for three years, and should include the antimetabolites, 6-mercaptopurine (50–75 mg/m²/day orally) plus methotrexate (20 mg/m²/week orally), together with pulses of additional therapy every 1–3 months, usually including prednisolone and vincristine. Many current clinical trials are testing the role of a consolidation phase of treatment using several of the drugs mentioned above. The intensity of treatment is generally dictated by the spectrum of prognostic features already listed.

d) Treatment of other 'sanctuary' sites of disease: boys should have testicular biopsies performed, probably towards the end of the maintenance phase of treatment, because the incidence of testicular leukaemic infiltration is close to 20%[2]. If this is found the testes should be irradiated, usually to about 1500 cGy, and maintenance therapy continued, probably for another 2–3 years. Although this inevitably produces sterility, no other long-term effects (e.g. testicular cancer) have been reported.

3. Specific treatment: AML

a) Induction: this group of leukaemias is more resistant and must generally be treated more intensively than ALL. The most effective induction regimen is with doxorubicin (adriamycin) or rubidomycin, thioguanine and cytosine arabinoside in combination, repeated at 2–4 week intervals until marrow examination documents remission. CNS prophylaxis is usually used in a similar way as for ALL, but the incidence seems to be lower in AML.

b) Maintenance treatment: the optimal treatment for maintaining a remission in AML remains to be defined, but generally it combines or alternates the above combinations of induction agents with corticosteroids, plant alkaloids and other antimetabolites[3].

4. Bone marrow transplantation: for children with more refractory forms of leukaemia, including AML, B-cell ALL, and other forms of leukaemia that have proved refractory to conventional treatment, bone marrow transplantation from a histocompatible sibling is the treatment of choice. This has achieved prolonged disease-free remissions in 30–50% such patients, who would otherwise have been expected to suffer inevitable further relapses[4].

PROGNOSIS

- The outlook for children with leukaemia has steadily improved over the last 30 years, with the increasing understanding and use of chemotherapy, such that about 60% of those diagnosed today can be expected to be alive and disease-free six years from now. From this improved outcome several prognostic factors have emerged, which are recognisable at the time of diagnosis[5].
- Cytological type: ALL has a better prognosis than AML and its variants.
- Age: patients under one year and greater than eight years do less well than children between these ages.
- Sex: boys fare less well than girls.
- Race: black children seem to have a less favourable outcome than white children.
- Immunological type: common ALL is the most favourable type, followed by T-cell and pre-B-cell types, then by B-cell ALL.
- Blast cell count: the prognosis is inversely correlated with the height of the initial circulating white cell count.
- Chromosomal abnormalities: leukaemic cells with marked chromosomal abnormalities, notably hypodiploidy, are associated with less favourable prognosis.
- CNS involvement. The presence of CNS leukaemic infiltrates at diagnosis is an unfavourable feature.

FOLLOW-UP

Close long-term follow-up for assessment and treatment are essential, initially weekly, then 2–4 weekly during maintenance treatment. Physical examination, FBC, bone marrow aspirations, renal and hepatic function must all be checked regularly. Follow-up should be at a specialised clinic.

[1] Rowland J H et al. (1984) *J. Clin. Oncol.*, **2,** 1327.
[2] Tiedmann K et al. (1982) *Br. Med. J.*, **285,** 1614.
[3] Weinstein H J et al. (1983) *Blood*, **62,** 315.
[4] Gale R P et al. (1983) *Lancet*, **ii,** 633.
[5] Simone J V (1975) *Cancer*, **36,** 2099.

17
Diseases of the Lymphatic System

G. du Mont

Hodgkin's Disease

Hodgkin's disease is rare in children, accounting for 10% all lymphoma cases. It is three times more common in boys, occurring from middle childhood onwards. Multifocal malignant proliferation of reticulum cells of the lymphoreticular system occurs. The diagnosis is based on the presence of binucleated giant cells characterised histologically as Sternberg-Reed cells. The histological classification is determined by the relative proportions of infiltrated lymphocytes, eosinophils and macrophages, and by the presence of collagen. In increasing order of malignancy the categories are lymphocyte predominance, nodular sclerosis, mixed cellularity and lymphocyte depletion.

TREATMENT

1. Treatment depends on the clinical staging, histology and disease volume.
2. Radiotherapy

   a) Alone: local radiotherapy, to a dose of 30 Gy is used in children with clinical stage IA disease with cervical or inguinal nodes affected only (excluding lymphocyte depletion category).
   b) With combination chemotherapy for bulky mediastinal disease.

3. Combination chemotherapy

   a) In the majority of cases combination chemotherapy is first line treatment. It is also effective in reclaiming relapses.
   b) Chlorambucil, vinblastine, procarbazine and prednisolone (ChlVPP) is the combination of choice, using between three and six courses. ChlVPP is well tolerated.
   c) Alternative combinations can be used in poor responders. MOPP consisting of mustine, vincristine (Oncovin), procarbazine and prednisolone is a toxic combination causing severe nausea and vomiting, and infertility in males[1]. Less toxic regimens substitute cyclophosphamide for mustine (C-MOPP), or vinblastine for vincristine (MVPP).

4. Modification of treatment

   a) Since extensive radiotherapy with chemotherapy is associated with an increased risk of a secondary primary malignancy[2], reduced irradiation fields and doses are now used.
   b) Extended field radiation which includes bony epiphyses affects growth and can result in musculoskeletal deformity[3].
   c) Splenectomy, for staging, is not recommended in children because of the high risk of fulminant septicaemia in up to 10%[4].

PROGNOSIS

- 80–90% patients have the prospect of long-term survival[3].
- The staging of the disease and the histological category affect the prognosis.

- Histological category (Rye)

Histological category (Rye)	Incidence (%)	Prognosis
Lymphocyte predominance	16	Very Good
Nodular sclerosis	60	Good
Mixed cellularity	23	Good
Lymphocyte depletion	1	Poor

- Staging (Arbor)

Staging (Arbor)	Cases(%)	5-year relapse-free survival rate (%)[5]
Stage I	20	100
Stage II	39	85
Stage III	25	77
Stage IV	16	67

A: without constitutional symptoms
B: with fever, nightsweats or weight loss.

- Poorer prognosis is associated with constitutional symptoms and increased disease volume. 'Bulk' disease is defined as a node mass with diameter greater than 5 cm or mediastinal mass greater than one-third thoracic transverse diameter.

FOLLOW-UP

Monthly to 3-monthly follow-up is necessary depending on the regimen being followed, with regular checks on FBC and platelets.

[1] Whitehead E et al. (1982) Arch. Dis. Childh., 57, 287.
[2] Donaldson S S et al. (1982) Cancer Treat. Rep., 66, 977.
[3] Mauch P M et al. (1983) Cancer, 51, 925.
[4] Chilcote R R et al. (1976) New Eng. J. Med., 295, 798.
[5] Robinson B et al. (1984) Arch. Dis. Childh., 59, 1162.

Non-Hodgkin's Lymphoma

Non-Hodgkin's lymphoma (NHL) is rare in children accounting for approximately 5% all malignant disease in childhood. It is more common in boys than girls, affecting school age children mainly. The characteristic feature is multicentric malignant proliferation of lymphocytes or reticulum cells of the lymphoreticularendothelial system. It may involve multiple nodal sites or extranodal sites, e.g. bone marrow, gut and CNS. The disease is frequently widely disseminated with eventual bone marrow involvement.

TREATMENT

1. With bone marrow involvement treatment is usually the same as for poor prognosis acute lymphoblastic leukaemia, i.e. anti-leukaemic drugs, intrathecal chemotherapy and cranial irradiation.
2. Patients with localised disease are treated with combined chemotherapy and radiotherapy.
3. Accurate histological classification is essential for assessing the efficacy of new treatment regimens.
4. Metabolic disturbances produced by the tumour and its treatment commonly occur. These include hyperuricaemia, xanthinuria, hypercalcaemia, hyperphosphataemia, hyperkalaemia and lactic acidosis.

PROGNOSIS

- In childhood NHL is of a poor prognostic type in two-thirds of patients at diagnosis.
- Poor prognostic types are non-localised and present with diffuse abdominal or mediastinal disease, frequently with bone marrow and/or CNS involvement.
- Prognosis depends on morphology, immunotype and clinical staging.

- Morphological type   Immunotype

Lymphoblastic	T or null
True histiocytic	Phagocytic
Burkitt	B
Non-Burkitt	B or null
Immunoblastic	B or null or T

- Staging (Arbor)   2-year disease-free survival (%)[1]

| Stages I and II | 90 |
| Stages III and IV | 39 |

- Prognosis for children with NHL was poor until the introduction of improved diagnostic and staging procedures combined with the use of intensive chemotherapy with additional radiation for bulk disease and CNS prophylaxis.

FOLLOW-UP

Follow-up is monthly to 3-monthly depending on the severity of the disease and the regimen being followed. Regular checks on FBC and platelets are required during chemotherapy.

---

[1] Murphy S B et al. (1980) Cancer, **45,** 630.

18
Immunodeficiency Diseases
G. du Mont

Severe Combined Immunodeficiency

Severe combined immunodeficiency (SCID) is characterised by a severe defect in cellular and humoral immunity leading to potentially fatal bacterial, fungal, protozoal or viral infections. Failure to thrive and diarrhoea frequently occur. The condition is familial with both X-linked and autosomal recessive forms described. A deficiency in one of two enzymes concerned with purine metabolism, either adenosine deaminase (ADA) or purinonucleoside phosphorylase (PNP), is recognised in some patients.

TREATMENT

1. Specific therapy

   a) Bone marrow transplant is the treatment of choice with a good success rate if there is a histocompatible sibling donor[1,2].
   b) Red cell transfusions may be useful for some patients with ADA or PNP deficiency.
   c) Thymus grafts have benefited some patients[3,4].
   d) Thymic hormone injections have benefited some patients[5,6].

2. Non-specific therapy

   a) Infections: early treatment with antibiotics, antiviral agents and antifungal agents as appropriate, higher doses and longer courses may be needed than in immuno-competent patients.
   b) Blood transfusions may result in graft-versus-host disease as these patients are unable to kill infused lymphocytes, which remain viable for at least 14 days in acid citrate dextrose blood. Blood for transfusion should be irradiated to avoid these reactions.

PROGNOSIS

- Invariably fatal in the first few years of life if no specific therapy given.
- Following bone marrow transplant (BMT) probability of survival is 59%[1].

a)

Type of transplant	Disease-free survival (%)	Number of cases
HLA-matched	68.1	41
HLA-mismatched T-cell depleted	57.1	46
HLA-mismatched no T-cell depletion	18.2	11

b) In HLA-identical BMT:
   i) Genotypically identical marrow associated with higher disease-free survival than phenotypically identical marrow (77% versus 50%).
   ii) Age below 6 months associated with higher disease-free survival than age over 6 months (78.2% versus 42.4%).
   iii) Type of SCID does not affect disease-free survival.
   iv) Acute and chronic graft-versus-host disease (GVHD) is rare.
   v) Immunological reconstitution complete and stable within 6 months.

c) In HLA-mismatched T-cell depleted transplants:
   i) Outcome influenced by diagnosis – patients with ADA deficiency have a worse prognosis than the other SCIDs.
   ii) Age above 6 months results in a poorer prognosis.
   iii) Acute GVHD occurs in 25% but is usually not severe. Chronic GVHD occurs in approximately 20% of cases.
   iv) Immunological reconstitution takes longer than in matched transplants (6–18 months).

d) Infection is the main complication of BMT with a significant mortality. The majority of infections are due to pathogens acquired early in life and present at the time of transplantation.

- Thymus grafts, thymic hormone injections and fetal liver grafts have been used successfully, but none of these procedures is as satisfactory in producing lymphoid chimerism as BMT.

FOLLOW-UP

Due to recurrent infections the child requires frequent assessment and treatment. Following BMT, when recovery of immune function is complete, 3-monthly follow-up initially then 6–12 monthly is required.

[1] Fischer A et al. (1986) Lancet, ii, 1080.
[2] Good R A et al. (1980) In Immunology IV (Fougerau M, Dausset J eds.) p. 906. New York: Academic Press.
[3] Daga S R et al. (1984) Postgrad. Med. J., 60, 537.
[4] Businco L et al. (1975) Clin. Exp. Immunol., 21, 32.
[5] Auiti F. (1983) Lancet, i, 551.
[6] Davies E G et al. (1982) Paediatr. Res., 16, 573.

Purine Nucleoside Phosphorylase Deficiency

Purine nucleoside phosphorylase (PNP) deficiency is an uncommon autosomal recessive condition, with symptoms occurring in infancy or early childhood. Absence of PNP leads to an accumulation of deoxyguanosine which inhibits proliferation of T lymphocytes. Overwhelming varicella and cytomegalovirus infections may occur. Associated conditions include CNS disease, megaloblastic anaemia and a predisposition to develop autoimmune blood dyscrasias.

TREATMENT

1. Enzyme replacement therapy, given in the form of normal red cell infusions, improves the immunological defect by metabolising the excess deoxyguanosine, with clinical benefit in some patients. However, in the majority of patients, this treatment does not produce a satisfactory clinical improvement.
2. Bone marrow transplant (BMT) is the treatment of choice if a histocompatible sibling is available.

PROGNOSIS

- Without treatment the outcome is usually fatal.

- Survival following BMT has still to be evaluated[1].

FOLLOW-UP

Due to recurrent infections the child requires frequent assessment and treatment. Following BMT when recovery of immune function is complete, 3-monthly follow-up initially then 6–12 monthly is required.

[1] Fischer A et al. (1986) Lancet, ii, 1080.

Antibody Deficiency

X-linked hypogammaglobulinaemia

This has a prevalence of about 2:1 000 000 males. It is characterised by low levels of all the serum immunoglobulins and absent circulating 'mature' B cells. Patients present with recurrent upper and lower respiratory tract infections in infancy. Septic arthritis or meningitis due to *Haemophilus influenzae* or pneumococcus commonly occurs. Other prominent clinical features are arthritis (non-infected) and diarrhoea. Patients do not show evidence of impaired T-cell function.

TREATMENT

1. Specific therapy

   a) Intramuscular immunoglobulin (which contains only IgG) 25–50 mg/kg weekly.
   b) Newer intravenous immunoglobulin preparations now being used, with the advantage that higher doses can be given less often.
   c) Fresh frozen plasma should be given when diagnosed and at 2–3 weekly intervals if recurrent infection occurs.

2. Non-specific therapy

   a) Infections: early treatment with appropriate antibiotics, higher doses and longer courses may be required than in immunocompetent patients.
   b) Regular physiotherapy for patients who develop chest infections.

PROGNOSIS

- Overwhelming infection may prove fatal in young children prior to diagnosis.
- Patients are at particular risk from developing vaccine-associated poliomyelitis and an unusual form of persistent, potentially fatal enterovirus encephalitis (usually echovirus).
- With replacement therapy of gammaglobulin and plasma, survival to adulthood occurs.

FOLLOW-UP

Follow-up should be 2–3 monthly while on maintenance therapy. More frequent review is required during and following infective episodes.

Primary or late onset hypogammaglobulinaemia

This is a heterogeneous group of conditions and is included in the 'varied category' by WHO. In most cases, there is no evidence of inheritance, although occasionally more than one member of a family is affected in a non-X-linked pattern. Age of onset varies from 1 to 70 years. Clinical features are the same as for X-linked hypogammaglobulinaemia.

TREATMENT AND PROGNOSIS

Treatment and prognosis are the same as for X-linked hypogammaglobulinaemia.

Transient hypogammaglobulinaemia

This occurs in infancy following the decline of passively transferred maternal IgG antibodies and before the child's own immunoglobulin production has reached normal levels. Recurrent bacterial infections occur in the first few years of life with spontaneous recovery by the age of five years.

TREATMENT

Antibiotics for specific infections.

PROGNOSIS

- All patients recover spontaneously.

FOLLOW-UP

Follow-up should be 2–3 monthly until spontaneous resolution occurs. More frequent review is required during infective episodes.

Selective Immunoglobulin Deficiencies

IgA deficiency

IgA, the principal immunoglobulin of mucous secretions, is below 0.01 g/litre (lower limit of normal 0.4–0.5 g IgA/litre) in 1:700 of the general population. Recurrent lower respiratory tract infections may occur, although most patients are asymptomatic.

TREATMENT

1. Give antibiotics for specific infections.
2. Occasionally, patients who also fail to produce IgM and IgG antibody benefit from immunoglobulin replacement therapy.

PROGNOSIS

- Patients usually have a normal life span.

FOLLOW-UP

Follow-up is 3-monthly if maintenance therapy is required; more frequently during infective episodes.

T-cell defects: thymic aplasia (DiGeorge syndrome)

Developmental defects in structures arising from the third and fourth pharyngeal pouches and branchial arches can cause complete or partial thymic aplasia, absent parathyroid glands and hypocalcaemia. T-cell function is lacking, resulting in recurrent fungal and bacterial infections. Other associated anomalies include mid-line defects, micrognathia, cleft palate, and congenital heart disease involving the aortic arch.

TREATMENT

1. Hypocalcaemia

   a) Oral calcium supplements and dihydrotachysterol.
   b) 1 α-hydroxycholecalciferol.

2. Infections

   a) Prevent viral infections (e.g. measles, varicella) by giving monthly immunoglobulin.
   b) Give antibiotics for specific bacterial infections.
   c) Thymus grafts reverse the immunological defect in some patients[1].
   d) Thymic hormone injections benefit some patients.

PROGNOSIS

- Those with a complete deficiency die within a few weeks of birth.
- In those with partial deficiency the immunological defect and hypocalcaemia usually improve spontaneously and resolve by 6–9 months of age.

FOLLOW-UP

Frequent follow-up is required initially due to recurrent infective episodes. When immunological defect and hypocalcaemia have resolved, as required for associated congenital defects.

---

[1] Good R A et al. (1980) In Immunology IV (Fougerau M, Dausset J eds.) p. 906. New York: Academic Press.

Partial T-Cell Defects

Ataxia telangiectasia

This presents with progressive neurological defect with ataxia, tremor, choreoathetosis and mental deterioration associated with conjunctival telangiectasia and recurrent infections. The condition is familial with an autosomal recessive inheritance. The immunological status is variable, 50% have selective IgA and IgG$_2$ subclass deficiency and a few have panhypogammaglobulinaemia. T-cell function is also defective. There is defective DNA repair which makes cells particularly susceptible to ionising radiation and an increased incidence of lymphoid tumours.

TREATMENT

1. Immunoglobulin replacement therapy if hypogammaglobulinaemia exists.
2. Give antibiotics for specific infections.
3. Ionising radiation, particularly x-rays should be avoided.
4. Give combination chemotherapy for malignant disease.

PROGNOSIS

- Ataxia and choreoathetosis are progressive and the child is frequently chairbound by adolescence.
- The condition is usually fatal, with tumours of the lymphoreticular system the most common cause of death.

FOLLOW-UP

Three-monthly follow-up is necessary while on maintenance therapy. More frequent review is indicated during acute infections.

Wiskott-Aldrich syndrome

This is an X-linked recessive disorder affecting boys, presenting with a combination of eczema, bloody diarrhoea, thrombocytopenia and increased susceptibility to infection. Immunoglobulins are usually present in normal concentrations, but there is an inability to make IgM antibodies to polysaccharide antigens. IgE levels are high, with an increased incidence of food allergies, especially milk. B-cell lymphomas frequently occur.

TREATMENT

1. Bone marrow transplant is the treatment of choice if a histocompatible sibling donor is available.
2. Splenectomy improves the thrombocytopenia.
3. Antigen avoidance diets, e.g. cow's milk-free, may improve eczema.
4. Give antibiotics for specific infections.

PROGNOSIS

- Without specific treatment death usually occurs in childhood or young adulthood as a result of infection, haemorrhage, or a lymphoreticular malignant lesion.
- Following bone marrow transplant probability of survival is 46% (62% for HLA matched transplant and 20% for HLA mismatched transplant)[1].

FOLLOW-UP

Frequent follow-up is required depending on the severity of the condition.

---

[1] Fischer A *et al.* (1986) *Lancet*, **ii**, 1080.

Neutrophil Defects

Primary chronic neutropenia

This is a heterogeneous group of conditions of varying severity, some of which have a familial inheritance. Some patients develop severe recurrent infections, while others have few problems. A neutrophil count below 0.5×10^9/litre is associated with recurrent infections.

TREATMENT

Give antibiotics for specific infections.

PROGNOSIS

- Severe infection may be fatal.
- Most patients respond well to antibiotic treatment.

FOLLOW-UP

Close supervision is necessary during episodes of infection.

Cyclical neutropenia

Familial, autosomal dominant, and non-familial types are recognised. Low neutrophil counts occur at approximately 3-week intervals associated with fever, mouth ulcers and staphylococcal infections.

TREATMENT

1. Prophylactic antibiotics are recommended.
2. Prednisolone, 20–30 mg alternate days, may be useful in severe cases.

PROGNOSIS

- Most patients do well and may become asymptomatic for long periods when the neutropenic 'trough' becomes less severe.

FOLLOW-UP

Follow-up should be 2–3 monthly while on maintenance therapy. More frequent review is necessary during episodes of infection.

Chronic granulomatous disease

Chronic granulomatous disease (CGD) is an X-linked recessive disorder characterised by failure of neutrophils to kill catalase-positive organisms, such as *Staphylococcus aureus*. Affected males present in childhood with recurrent staphylococcal abscesses, resulting in skin and lung lesions, and discharging sinuses from lymph nodes, liver and bones. Malabsorption due to granulomatous gut involvement and salmonella infection also occurs.

TREATMENT

1. Prophylactic antibiotics.
2. High dose antibiotics for prolonged periods should be used for specific infections.
3. Early surgical intervention and prolonged drainage of abscess sites is recommended.
4. Irradiated leucocyte transfusions are a useful adjunct to therapy when life threatening infections occur[1].
5. Bone marrow transplant should be considered in severely affected patients.

PROGNOSIS

- Severe infections may be fatal in infancy if inadequately treated.
- The majority of patients respond well to treatment and survive to adult life.

FOLLOW-UP

Follow-up should be 2–3 monthly while on maintenance therapy. More frequent review is necessary during infective episodes.

---

[1] Gallin J T *et al.* (1983) *Ann. Intern. Med.*, **99**, 657.

Secondary Immunodeficiency

Loss of immunocompetence may result from a number of conditions including infection (e.g. acquired immunodeficiency syndrome), protein-losing states, drugs (e.g. steroids and cytotoxic drugs), malignancy (lymphoreticular tumours) and splenectomy.

Acquired immunodeficiency syndrome

Acquired immunodeficiency syndrome (AIDS) is due to infection with the human immunodeficiency virus (HIV). Affected infants are usually born to mothers in high risk groups, i.e. intravenous drug abusers, recipients of blood or blood products, Haitians and the heterosexual partners of individuals in these groups or of bisexuals. Other children have acquired the disease from blood transfusions. Two-thirds of pregnancies in HIV infected mothers result in infection in the infant. Of these, 50% develop AIDS. Affected infants suffer from interstitial pneumonitis, recurrent bacterial infections, mucocutaneous candidiasis, develop hepatosplenomegaly and fail to thrive.

TREATMENT

1. Interstitial pneumonia

   a) *Pneumocystis carinii*: trimethoprim (20 mg/kg/day) and sulphamethoxazole (100 mg/kg/day).
   b) Cytomegalovirus: treatment is mostly ineffective, acyclovir is either not effective or has only limited benefit. *In vitro* tests of arildone appear promising.

2. Give antibiotics for specific bacterial infections.
3. Give ketoconazole or amphotericin B for fungal infections.
4. Monthly parenteral immunoglobulin may be of benefit[1].
5. Blood products should be irradiated prior to transfusion.

PROGNOSIS

- There is a very high mortality.
- The long-term prognosis for infected survivors is not yet known.

FOLLOW-UP

Frequent follow-up is required as the course of the illness is not yet well documented.

[1] Rubinstein A (1984) *Clin. Immunol. Today*, **7**, 1.

Protein-losing states

Loss of protein in children with nephrotic syndrome, protein-losing enteropathies and following burns results in increased susceptibility to infection.

TREATMENT

1. Give prophylactic antibiotics, e.g. in nephrotic syndrome with ascites.
2. Give antibiotics for specific infections.

PROGNOSIS

- Prognosis relates to the primary condition.
- Severe infections may be fatal.

FOLLOW-UP

Follow-up is as required for the primary disease state.

Malignancy

Invasion of malignant cells into immunological tissues results in immunosuppression. Treatment with cytotoxic drugs and irradiation has additional effects on suppressing normal bone marrow function.

TREATMENT

1. Give antibiotics for specific infections.

2. Prophylactic antibiotics may be beneficial e.g. co-trimoxazole as prophylaxis against *P. carinii* infection.

PROGNOSIS

- Infection is a common cause of death in disseminated malignancy.

FOLLOW-UP

Follow-up is as required for the primary disease state.

Splenectomy

Splenectomy results in removal of a significant amount of lymphoid tissue predisposing to septicaemia, particularly pneumococcal.

TREATMENT

1. Pneumococcal vaccine may be beneficial, although evidence is not conclusive.
2. Prophylactic antibiotics (penicillin or amoxycillin) should be given.

PROGNOSIS

- Severe infection may be fatal.

FOLLOW-UP

Follow-up should be 3–6 monthly.

19
Nutritional Disorders

K. Simmer

Anorexia Nervosa

Anorexia nervosa is a serious psychological disorder characterised by voluntary starvation and severe weight loss. Food restriction may give way to 'bingeing', vomiting and laxative abuse. It usually occurs in adolescent girls and is accompanied by amenorrhoea and a relatively high level of physical activity. There are at least 10 000 severely affected patients in the UK at any one time[1].

TREATMENT

1. Psychotherapy aimed at evoking awareness of impulses, feelings and needs, and leading to a meaningful change in the personality, to stop abusing the eating function, is essential. Effective psychotherapy must be accompanied by a restoration of normal body weight but enforcing weight gain without attention to the underlying problems is useless[2].
2. Psychiatric hospitalisation is indicated when outpatient psychotherapy has failed. The parents should also be involved in treatment to improve the psychological interaction of the family[2].
3. Small doses of phenothiazines or benzodiazepines may be helpful. However, the use of psychoactive drugs may be counter-productive in the long term, by reinforcing the psychopathological state, and feelings of lack of control[3].

PROGNOSIS

- The prognosis is poor. 50% remain chronically ill and the average length of illness even in those who eventually recover is four years[3].
- 5% with severe anorexia nervosa will die from suicide, emaciation, acute infection or serious disturbances in electrolyte balance.
- Factors associated with a poor prognosis include chronicity at presentation, premorbid obesity with a vomiting pattern, low social class (although rare), inability to secure peer relationships during childhood and evidence of neurosis in the parents[3].
- A significant proportion will develop chronic schizophrenia.

FOLLOW-UP

Long-term follow-up for at least 3–5 years is essential as up to half the patients relapse. Eating habits and psychological and sexual adjustment should be reviewed.

[1] Crisp A M et al. (1976) Br. J. Psychiatr., **128,** 549.
[2] Bruch M (1974) Eating Disorders. London: Routledge and Kegan Paul.
[3] Crisp A M (1983) Br. Med. J., **287,** 855.

Obesity

Obesity is the most prevalent nutritional disorder in the developed world. The diagnosis is usually made visually and confirmed by a triceps skinfold measurement of above the 85th centile, and a weight for height greater than 120% the mean controlled for age and sex. The causes are mainly environmental. The normal mechanisms of hunger and satiety will never develop in a child who is fed for reasons other than the need for food; he will grow to regard food for emotional reasons rather than for hunger[1]. Organic disease accounts for less than 1% childhood obesity.

TREATMENT

1. Calorie restriction and exercise are essential. Fat restriction is usually sufficient, however, more aggressive diets are occasionally needed[2]. In children who are more than 50–60% above the expected weight, an initial period of hospitalisation is often necessary to achieve satisfactory weight reduction.
2. Appetite suppressants are of limited value in the management of childhood obesity.
3. The adolescent should be counselled about the cosmetic, social and medical risks of obesity.
4. A positive family-orientated approach is important for compliance.
5. Sleep apnoea and hypertension should be excluded. If the child is short and the bone age delayed, further investigations, including thyroid function tests, urea and electrolytes, and an x-ray of the pituitary fossa, are indicated.

PROGNOSIS

- There is a strong tendency for obesity to recur after initial weight reduction, and then persist into adult life. Approximately 80% obese adolescents become obese adults[3]; however, only 21% obese adults have been obese children[4].
- Ultimate height is significantly below standard, even though height is above the standard before the onset of puberty[3].
- Obesity is more common in lower socio-economic classes and where there is a family history of obesity. The outlook is better for boys than for girls. The later the onset, and the greater the severity of the obesity, the worse the prognosis.

FOLLOW-UP

Dietary and exercise advice, psychological support and family counselling are required until late adolescence. The dietician may act as the primary therapist.

[1] Bruch M (1974) *Eating Disorders*. London: Routledge and Kegan Paul.
[2] Dietz W M (1983) *J. Pediatr.*, **103,** 676.
[3] Lloyd J K et al. (1961) *Br. Med. J.*, **2,** 145.
[4] Braddon F E M et al. (1986) *Br. Med. J.*, **293,** 299.

Protein Energy Malnutrition

The diagnosis of protein energy malnutrition is made when the weight for age is less than 50%, the weight for height is less than 60% of the Boston median, or when there is nutritional oedema. It is often divided into marasmus or kwashiorkor, although most malnourished children have features of both. Marasmus is characterised by generalised wasting and is especially common in infancy. Kwashiorkor is characterised by anorexia, lethargy, dermatitis, sparse hair, hepatomegaly and oedema, and is due to a relative protein deficiency and often occurs in the second or third year of life. Pneumonia, gastroenteritis, tuberculosis and vitamin A deficiency are major associated problems.

TREATMENT

1. Correction of dehydration, hypothermia, hypoglycaemia and anaemia. These complications may be secondary to aggressive early feeding.
2. The children are fed a diet of dried skimmed milk and locally available food (e.g. in Bangladesh, rice is used as the major staple, and dal as a source of protein, with pumpkin and leafy greens). Oil is added as an additional source of calories[1].
3. Supplementation with multivitamins, potassium, iodine and magnesium.
4. Psychological stimulation.

PROGNOSIS

- Following adequate nutritional rehabilitation and treatment of the underlying infections:

  a) 5–10 g/kg/day weight gain is possible.

  b) 85% maintain a weight/height over 80% of the Boston median.

  c) There is still a 5% mortality (Save the Children Fund, Bangladesh).

- Chronic malnutrition may reduce brain growth but the developmental delay seen in many malnourished children mainly reflects associated social deprivation.

FOLLOW-UP

Follow-up for several years is required to ensure continued gain in weight and height. Nutritional rehabilitation of the whole family is necessary; the mothers must be taught how to cook locally available foods and to teach and stimulate their children.

---

[1] Khanum S (1978) *Bangladesh Paediatr.*, **4**, 3.

Vitamin D Deficiency: Rickets

Vitamin D is obtained from animal fat or ultraviolet radiation, which converts 7-dihydrocholesterol into cholecalciferol (D) in the skin, which is then mobilised in the liver to 25(OH)D and finally, in the kidney, to $1-25(OH_2)D$. Vitamin D increases the intestinal absorption of calcium and phosphorus, decreases the urinary excretion of phosphorus, decreases the faecal excretion of calcium and, therefore, facilitates the development of bone. Maternal vitamin D deficiency has been implicated in the development of neonatal rickets. However, rickets is far more often due to nutritional deficiencies in preterm infants, in whom the incidence may be as high as 32%[1]. Substrate (phosphorus) deficiency is an important factor[2]. During childhood, rickets occurs rarely in Caucasian toddlers, but is alarmingly frequent (12.5%) in Asian schoolchildren in the UK[3]. The Asian diet includes chappatis, which are unleavened and have a high content of phytate: both factors reduce calcium absorption. Their diet also includes ghee and vitamin D is destroyed when butter is made into ghee. Vitamin D-dependent rickets is an autosomal recessive condition which presents as nutritional rickets in the first year of life. Clinical signs include thickened epiphyses, delayed closure of fontanelles, costochondral beading, delayed walking, coxa vara, genu valgus and kyphoscoliosis. X-ray changes include widening, cupping and fraying of epiphyses and costochondral junctions, delayed appearance of centres of ossification, and decalcification of bone. Plasma levels of alkaline phosphatase are high, while those of calcium, inorganic phosphorus, parathormone and 25(OH)D are low.

TREATMENT

1. Prevention: breastfed babies should receive additional vitamin D (400 IU/day if term and 1000 IU/day if preterm). Very low birth-weight babies being fed on breast-milk often need additional phosphate (1 mmol/kg/day).
2. Children: vitamin D 3000 IU/day orally for 4–6 weeks, then 400 IU/day until radiological healing has occurred or an adequate dietary intake is assured. Alternatively give 600 000 IU i.m. as a single dose. For vitamin D dependent rickets treatment is with vitamin D 10 000–40 000 IU/day for life.
3. Neonates: vitamin D 2000 IU/day for 4–6 weeks, with adequate dietary calcium and phosphate.
4. Vitamin D toxicity is characterised by anorexia, nausea, vomiting, constipation and failure to thrive. Plasma urea, creatinine, calcium and phosphorus are raised and there are deposits of dense bone on x-ray. Treatment consists of a short course of steroids, a low calcium diet for a few weeks, and withdrawal of vitamin D.

PROGNOSIS

- Radiological evidence of healing occurs after 2–3 weeks of treatment.
- Bony deformities in infants and toddlers heal spontaneously. Surgical correction may be needed in adolescents.

FOLLOW-UP

Healing of rickets can be confirmed by x-ray and a falling alkaline phosphatase level. Serum calcium and phosphate levels should be monitored while children are receiving vitamin D. Follow-up should be for two years and an adequate diet assured.

[1] Callenbach J C et al. (1981) J. Pediatr., **98**, 800.
[2] McIntosh N et al. (1982) Arch. Dis. Childh., **57**, 848.
[3] Goel K M et al. (1976) Lancet, **i**, 1141.

Vitamin A Deficiency

Vitamin A occurs in such foods as milk, butter, egg yolk and cod liver oil. Its precursors are found in yellow and green plants. Vitamin A is important for the function of rod cells in the retina and for the integrity of epithelial tissues and mucous membranes. Signs of deficiency include Bitot's spots, xerophthalmia and keratomalacia.

TREATMENT

1. Prevention includes vitamin A supplementation during pregnancy.
2. Treatment is by 200 000 IU vitamin A i.m. followed by 400 IU/day orally with nutritional rehabilitation. (The dose is halved in infancy.)

PROGNOSIS

- Vitamin A deficiency is the commonest cause of childhood blindness in the world. The children are usually malnourished and the disease advanced. Mortality is high and increases in a linear fashion with the severity of the xerophthalmia[1].

- Early conjunctival signs respond to supplementation within 2 weeks, whereas advanced disease is irreversible.

FOLLOW-UP

Children should be examined every two months for at least 6–12 months. Impaired dark adaptation is a sensitive measure of continued deficiency. Supplementation with cod liver oil may be required if the diet remains inadequate.

[1] Sommer A *et al.* (1983) *Lancet*, **ii,** 585.

Vitamin B Deficiency

Infantile beri-beri (thiamine deficiency) occurs mainly in breast-fed infants of thiamine deficient mothers, e.g. those who eat a polished rice diet. It usually presents as acute cardiac failure in a young infant, but can present later as encephalopathy, or severe muscle wasting and paralysis. Riboflavin deficiency causes angular stomatitis, cheilosis and a painful magenta-coloured tongue. Niacin deficiency results in pellagra. Signs include a desquamating dermatitis affecting exposed skin and, rarely, a sore mouth, diarrhoea and mental disorders.

TREATMENT

1. Thiamine deficiency is treated by thiamine 25 mg i.m. daily for three days, then 10 mg orally twice daily.
2. Riboflavin deficiency is treated by riboflavin 5–15 mg orally daily.
3. Niacin deficiency is treated by nicotinamide 50 mg orally three times daily.

PROGNOSIS

- Prognosis depends on the adequacy of treatment of the associated malnutrition.

FOLLOW-UP

An adequate diet should be assured. Thiamine: children should be examined at least monthly for two years for muscle weakness or cardiac failure. Riboflavin: children should be reviewed monthly for at least three months. Niacin: weight gain should be checked and the neurological system examined every few months for at least two years.

Vitamin C Deficiency: Scurvy

Vitamin C is obtained from citrus fruits, berries and green vegetables. Deficiency results in impaired collagen synthesis. Signs include painful swelling and pseudoparalysis of limbs caused by subperiosteal bleeding, petechial haemorrhages, pallor, irritability and impaired growth. Capillary haemorrhages, in relation to erupted teeth, may occur and the teeth may become loosened. The peak incidence is at 8–9 months of age. X-ray changes include ground glass appearance of bones with thin cortex, pencil line 'ringing' of epiphyses and periosteal elevation from subperiosteal bleeds which later form callus.

TREATMENT

1. Prevention: vitamin C supplements (25 mg/day) should be given during the first years of life.
2. Vitamin C 300 mg daily.

PROGNOSIS

- There is rapid clinical recovery within 24 hours once supplements have begun.

- Subperiosteal bleeds may take months to resolve.

FOLLOW-UP

A diet adequate in fresh fruit and vegetables should be assured and the dietitian involved in follow-up. Weight gain and activity should be reviewed every few months; x-rays may take a year to improve.

Fluorosis

Fluorine is a normal body constituent which enhances the resistance of teeth to caries. Since 1945, artificial fluoridation of water supplies has been used successfully in many countries to prevent dental caries. Acute overdosage results from accidental or deliberate ingestion, or from professionally applied fluoride preparations. Accidental mass poisoning has also occurred[1].

TREATMENT (of acute toxicity)

1. Give milk and induce vomiting.
2. If severe, give 10 ml 10% calcium gluconate i.v. stat.

PROGNOSIS

- Chronic exposure results in the adult teeth becoming mottled and stained.

- Acute intoxication leads to abdominal pain, diarrhoea and vomiting, convulsions and cardiorespiratory failure[2].
- Artificial fluoridation of water supplies does not increase the risk of cancer[3].

[1] Waldbott G L (1981) *Clin. Toxicol.*, **18,** 531.
[2] Duxbury A J *et al.* (1981) *Br. Dent. J.*, **153,** 64.
[3] Clemmese J (1983) *Bull. WHO*, **61,** 871.

Total Parenteral Nutrition

Total parenteral nutrition (TPN) is used to provide sufficient energy, protein and other essential nutrients for maintenance and growth in very low birthweight (VLBW) babies who cannot tolerate oral feeds, and in infants with severe gut disorders or critical illness.

TREATMENT

1. Total parenteral nutrition is infused through a silastic catheter, which is introduced through a butterfly needle into a peripheral vein and positioned in the inferior or superior vena cava or right atrium. A bacterial filter is commonly used.
2. Requirements are 150 ml/kg/day and 100 kcal/kg/day.
3. Glucose is the preferred carbohydrate (12–20 g/kg/day).
4. Nitrogen is provided as crystalline amino acid solution (2–3 g/kg/day).
5. The composition of the amino acid infusate is controversial; the most commonly used reference standard is that of whole egg (Vamin).
6. Cysteine, tyrosine, histidine and arginine are necessary in addition to the recognised essential amino acids for preterm infants to achieve optimal growth.
7. Fat (1–3 g/kg/day) is necessary to provide extra calories and to prevent vitamin D and essential fatty acid deficiencies, but is contraindicated if there is severe septicaemia, hyperbilirubinaemia (200 µmol/l) or thrombocytopenia.
8. Water and fat soluble vitamins are added.
9. Calcium and phosphate requirements may need to be given on alternate days because of precipitation problems.
10. Plasma levels of sodium, chloride, potassium, glucose, phosphate, magnesium, ammonia and amino acids are monitored.
11. Serum triglycerides should not exceed 2.28 mmol/l.
12. Enteral feeds are introduced as soon as possible, as luminal nutrition is important for the normal development of the gut[1,2]. Breast-milk is used initially, as it is better digested. If 'bank' breast-milk is used, the baby is changed to an artificial feed after 1–2 weeks. A special low birthweight formula – containing increased amounts of protein, calcium, phosphate and sodium – should be considered in babies weighing less than 1.5 kg, to increase the rate of weight gain[3]. Breast-milk alone is probably insufficient to maintain adequate growth in preterm babies and so the mother's own milk may be fortified with sodium, phosphate, potassium and calories (glucose polymer or medium chain triglycerides). Oral feeds of preterm babies should be supplemented with multivitamins (including 800 IU/day vitamin D), folic acid 0.2 mg/day, and iron 2.5–5.0 mg/day.

PROGNOSIS

- Total parenteral nutrition increases the daily weight gain of VLBW babies[4].
- Complications include infection, thrombosis, fat overload, cholestasis and deficiency states, e.g. hypophosphataemia.

[1] Weaver L T et al. (1984) Arch. Dis. Childh., 59, 236.
[2] Lucas A et al. (1981) Clin. Sci., 60, 349.
[3] Lucas A et al. (1984) Arch. Dis. Childh., 59, 722.
[4] Yu V Y M et al. (1979) Arch. Dis. Childh., 54, 653.

20
Psychological Disorders

S. N. Wolkind

Mental Retardation

Severe retardation (IQ below 50) is found in 4 children per 1000. In most cases there is a recognisable biological cause. Mild retardation (IQ between 50 and 70) occurs in 2% of the population. It is caused both by socio-economic factors and biological influences.

TREATMENT[1,2]

1. There is no cure for mental retardation, but a great deal can be done to help the child reach its full potential and to support its family.
2. The family require the support of a district handicap team who will have available the range of resources needed for any individual child[3].
3. For each child a profile of the handicap is drawn up and remedial help is offered in all areas needing attention. This can include physiotherapy, speech therapy, paediatric or psychiatric treatment.
4. Medical advice must be given to the Education Authority (Education Act 1981) to ensure that appropriate schooling is found for the child.
5. Behaviour modification has an important role to play in both teaching new skills (e.g. toileting) or removing damaging symptoms (e.g. self-injury).
6. Severe agitation and overactivity can be decreased with phenothiazines. The drug of choice is pericyazine. Start with 0.5 mg per year of child, adjusting continuously according to the response, to a maximum of 1 mg per year of child in divided dose.

PROGNOSIS

- With only rare exceptions, children with severe retardation will need care and support throughout their lives.
- Most mildly retarded children will eventually live independently.
- Severe retardation is often accompanied by additional physical problems. The life expectancy is lower than that of the remainder of the population.
- The mentally retarded child is liable to develop behavioural or emotional problems, 50% in the case of the severely retarded, 30% for those mildly affected.

FOLLOW-UP

Review every six months to ensure that the total educational and medical programme is meeting the child's needs. If on a phenothiazine review blood pressure, skin (for light sensitivity) and movements every three weeks. If long-term treatment is necessary, arrange for several week breaks from medication every six months and ensure additional care is available during this period.

[1] Kirman B (1975) *Mental Handicap: A Brief Guide.* St. Albans: Crosby Lockwood Staple.
[2] James F E *et al.* (1979) *Psychiatric Illness and Mental Handicap.* London: Gaskell Press.
[3] Macfarlane J A (1980) *Child Health Pocket Consultant.* London: Grant Macintyre.

Autism

Autism is a gross deviation of normal development characterised by abnormal social relationships, serious impairment of language and stereotyped patterns of play. Most autistic children are intellectually retarded, although autistic-like disorders without retardation and language disorders are seen (Asperger's syndrome). Autism is found in 2 children in every 10 000, with boys outnumbering girls 3:1.

TREATMENT[1-3]

1. There is no cure for autism and treatment is directed at encouraging the child's potential and reducing socially obtrusive symptoms.
2. Language can be fostered by behavioural programmes.
3. The teaching of self-care should be done through the mastery of a series of small steps.
4. Social interaction should be encouraged by forcing the child to interact in order to engage in preferred activities.
5. The associated behavioural difficulties will respond to simple techniques of behaviour modification.
6. Phenothiazines may reduce tension and overactivity, but they may impair the capacity to learn. One good possibility is thioridazine 1.5–3 mg/kg in divided dose.

PROGNOSIS

- Two-thirds of those with autism will remain permanently handicapped requiring institutional care.
- Approximately 50% will gain some form of useful language.
- 30% will develop epilepsy during adolescence.
- An initial non-verbal IQ below 50 or severe language impairment beyond the age of five indicates a particularly poor prognosis.
- Most children with Asperger's syndrome or other milder variants of autism will develop into adults with major difficulties with social relationships.

FOLLOW-UP

Review every six months to ensure that the total educational and medical programme is meeting the child's needs. If the child is on thioridazine review blood pressure, check sight, skin (for light sensitivity) and movements every three weeks. If long-term treatment is necessary, arrange for several week breaks from medication every six months and ensure additional medical care is available during this period.

[1] Rutter M (1985) *J. Child Psychol. Psychiatr.*, **26,** 193.
[2] Howlin P (1981) *J. Autism Dev. Disord.*, **11,** 89.
[3] Murphy G (1982) *J. Autism Dev. Disord.*, **12,** 265.
[4] Lotter V (1974) *J. Autism Child Schiz.*, **4,** 263.

Specific Reading Retardation

Specific reading retardation is present when a child's reading ability is significantly (two standard errors of measurement) below what would be expected from his IQ. It occurs in 3–10% of the population, being more common in those from deprived areas. Boys outnumber girls 3:1. The term dyslexia which is often used tends to imply a specific neurological deficit. As the aetiology is multifactorial this can be misleading.

TREATMENT

1. Remedial help will produce short-term gains in most children, but long-term improvement is rare.
2. Attempts to increase motivation may produce improvement[1].

PROGNOSIS[2]

- The outcome is poor. Less than 10% of the children will develop reading abilities above the mean. Few will achieve skilled employment.
- The outcome is best in children with a high IQ from advantaged backgrounds.

- 25% children with reading retardation will also have conduct disorders.

FOLLOW-UP

Obtain a school progress report every year to ensure that progress is being made. If not ask for a full review by the Educational Authority.

---

[1] Levere R (1977) *Bull. Brit. Assoc. Behav. Psychother.*, **5**, 66.
[2] Maughan B *et al.* (1985) *J. Child Psychol. Psychiatr.*, **26**, 741.

Emotional Disorders

Emotional disorders occur in 2.5–6% pre-adolescent children. Symptoms include shyness, anxiety, long-standing sadness and sometimes obsessions or phobias. The sex ratio is equal in younger children, but far more girls are affected in adolescence.

TREATMENT[1]

1. Although it is difficult to give precise figures most trials of treatment indicate a good response to either goal-orientated psychotherapy or behaviour modification.
2. Behavioural techniques of desensitisation or modelling will successfully deal with the majority of phobic symptoms. They may have some success with obsessions.

PROGNOSIS[2]

- Approximately 50% pre-adolescent children with emotional disorders will continue to have marked difficulties during adolescence.

- Most will make a satisfactory adjustment in adult life.
- If obsessional symptoms are present they will continue to adulthood in 70%.
- Phobic symptoms will be almost as persistent.

FOLLOW-UP

Ensure the child is reviewed every six months to check that no worsening of the condition is occurring.

[1] Rutter M (1982) *Psychol. Med.*, **12,** 723.
[2] Berg I *et al.* (1974) *Psychol. Med.*, **4,** 428.

Enuresis

Nocturnal enuresis is the involuntary passage of urine during sleep, in the absence of physical disorder, in children aged four years or more. Rates vary greatly between different communities, but it is more common in children in disadvantaged circumstances. Boys are affected twice as often as girls.

TREATMENT

1. Although in most cases enuresis will eventually resolve spontaneously treatment will produce a faster recovery.
2. Night lifting and fluid restriction will produce a temporary improvement in most, but the majority will relapse.
3. Tricylic antidepressant drugs will rapidly reduce the frequency of wetting in 85% and totally suppress it in 30%. There is a high relapse rate on stopping medication. This is a useful procedure for a child going away on an organised holiday[1]. A good choice is imipramine from 25 mg for a six year old to 75 mg for an adolescent. Give nocte for no longer than three months.
4. Behavioural techniques[2]:

   a) The use of a star chart will often be effective not only in providing a baseline record, but also as a method of stopping the wetting.
   b) Between 50 and 100% of children will achieve dryness within two months of starting treatment with a pad and buzzer.

PROGNOSIS

- At age 7 approximately 17% children wet the

bed at least once a week, by age 10, 7% children and by age 14 only 2%. Less than 1% will continue into adulthood.

- The condition is more likely to resolve spontaneously in girls and in those who are not wet every night.
- Those who have never been dry (primary enuresis) respond better to treatment than do those who have relapsed after a period of being dry (secondary).
- Of those who remain wet 25% will develop other signs of psychological disturbance.

FOLLOW-UP

If any particular treatment is not producing improvement within three months re-evaluate and attempt a new approach.

[1] Rapoport J et al. (1980) Arch. Gen. Psychiatr., **37**, 1146.
[2] Dische S et al. (1983) Dev. Med. Child Neurol., **25**, 67.
[3] Forsythe W et al. (1974) Arch. Dis. Childh., **48**, 259.

Stammer

Stammering is a disorder involving repetitions of sound and tense blockages of speech, often with visible tremors of the tongue or jaw. Mild stammer develops in 4% children between ages 2 and 6 years.

TREATMENT[1]

1. Programmed learning such as speaking with a rhythm or controlling respiration can help 75% sufferers to cope in public.
2. Haloperidol will reduce stammer in 80%, but as relapse after stopping the medication is the norm and extrapyramidal side-effects may be severe, it should not normally be used.

PROGNOSIS

- 75% will lose their stammer by puberty. In the remaining 25% it will continue and become more severe.

FOLLOW-UP

Review every six months. If the child remains handicapped, ensure appropriate speech therapy is available.

[1] Andrews G et al. (1980) J. Speech Hear. Disor., **45**, 287.

Tics

Tics are sudden, rapid, involuntary purposeless movements of circumscribed muscle groups. They vary from transient disorders to severe multiple tics with vocalisations (Tourette's syndrome). Facial muscles are most often involved.

TREATMENT

1. Psychotherapy does not produce improvement.
2. Behaviour therapy using massed practice of the tic in which the child is taught consciously to carry out and then stop the abnormal movement, or relaxation produces definite improvement in 30%[1].
3. Haloperidol is justified if tics are severe and handicapping. It will produce substantial improvement in 70%. Start with the lowest dose which is effective. This may be approximately 0.05–0.1 mg/kg/day. Anti-parkinsonian drugs (e.g. benztropine mesylate 0.5–2 mg/day) are needed[2].

PROGNOSIS

- Tics are seen in 20% children. The vast majority are transient and disappear rapidly.
- In 1% the tics will spread. Of these 50% will eventually improve at adolescence, with 30% recovering completely.
- If tics persist, the earlier the onset the poorer the prognosis.

FOLLOW-UP

Monitor the child's general progress; if on haloperidol, examine for extrapyramidal effects every three months.

[1] Turpin G (1983) *Adv. Behav. Res. Ther.*, **5**, 203.
[2] Shapiro A *et al.* (1981) *Comp. Psychiatr.*, **22**, 193.

Conduct Disorders

Conduct disorders occur in 5–10% pre-adolescent children. Boys outnumber girls 3:1. Symptoms include aggression, stealing and poor relationships. The condition is associated with family disruption and dysharmony.

TREATMENT

1. Due to the associated family and social problems all treatments have a high failure rate.
2. There is evidence that both brief psychotherapy and behavioural treatment can be effective if gross family disturbance is absent[1].

PROGNOSIS[2]

- Two-thirds of 10–11-year-old children with conduct disorders will continue to have difficulties during adolescence.
- One-third will have major problems of adjustment during adult life.
- Severely aggressive behaviour is associated with a particularly poor outcome.

FOLLOW-UP

Monitor the child's general social functioning every six months. If condition is worsening and the family cannot meet the child's needs, social services and other welfare agencies may need to be involved to protect the child and arrange for a change of environment, such as foster care or boarding school.

[1] McAuley R (1982) *J. Child Psychol. Psychiatr.*, **23**, 335.
[2] Robins L N (1978) *Psychol. Med.*, **8**, 611.

Overactivity and Attention Deficit Disorder

Many children with conduct disorders show overactivity and poor concentration and impulse control. In a small number these symptoms are the main problem. As a pure syndrome, overactivity is overdiagnosed in the USA and underdiagnosed in the UK.

TREATMENT[1,2]

1. Stimulant drugs (pemoline 0.5–2 mg/kg) will lower impulsiveness and improve concentration. Symptoms will usually recur when they are stopped. They should only be used as part of an overall treatment plan.
2. Feedback programmes can help the child gain control over its impulsiveness.
3. A small number of children have shown an improvement on an additive-free diet. It is not possible to predict which children will respond.

PROGNOSIS

- Most affected children will have difficulties throughout their childhood and adolescence.
- The majority will remain accident prone and impulsive in adult life, but only a minority will have severe psychiatric illness.
- The presence of aggression or low IQ predicts a particularly poor outcome.

FOLLOW-UP

If on medication, review every month. Review general progress with family and school every six months.

[1] Taylor E (1979) *Neuropharmacol.*, **18**, 951.
[2] Weiss G (1979) *Arch. Gen. Psychiatr.*, **36**, 675.

21
Poisoning

T. J. Meredith and J. A. Vale

Paediatric Poisoning[1-4]

In the UK, USA and Australia, most children who are poisoned ingest therapeutic agents. 20% ingest analgesics; a further 60% ingest other pharmaceutical preparations, notably benzodiazepines, iron, anti-epileptic drugs, tricyclic antidepressants, Lomotil and the contraceptive pill. The remainder are poisoned by a variety of household products, particularly bleach, various hydrocarbons, garden plants and seeds. Approximately 1000 children under 15 years of age are admitted to hospital in England and Wales each year suffering from acute ethanol intoxication which may be associated with duress and sexual abuse. In non-developed countries, the ingestion of kerosene (paraffin) is far more common than in Europe and the USA and may account for up to 40% of total ingestions. In all cases of intoxication, advice should be given to the parents on prevention of further episodes such as locking medicines and substances away, and using child-resistant containers. In the older child who has taken a substance deliberately psychiatric referral is important.

[1] Blumer J L et al. (1986) Pediatr. Clin. North Am., **33,** 245, 665.
[2] Tenenbein M (1986) Curr. Prob. Pediatr., **16,** 186.
[3] Vale J A, Meredith T J (1985) A Concise Guide to the Management of Acute Poisoning 3rd edn. Edinburgh: Churchill Livingstone.
[4] Vale J A et al. (1987) Poisoning. In Oxford Textbook of Medicine, 2nd edn (Weatherall D J, Ledingham J G G, Warrell D A eds.). Oxford: OUP.

Paracetamol Poisoning

Paracetamol-induced liver and renal damage in children appears to be uncommon both because of early presentation at hospital and ingestion of only small quantities of the drug.

TREATMENT

1. Prevention of absorption

   a) No method is very effective more than 1–2 hours after overdose.

   b) Activated charcoal 25–50 g is more efficient than syrup of ipecacuanha 10–30 ml in preventing absorption. However, charcoal is difficult to administer to young children.

   c) The value of gastric lavage in paracetamol poisoning has not been formally assessed but is probably as useful as activated charcoal.

2. Use of protective agents

   a) Specific therapy is required if the plasma paracetamol concentration falls above the 'treatment line'[1].

   b) Administer either: methionine 1–2.5 g (36 mg/kg body weight) orally, 4-hourly for four doses (i.e. 4–10 g over 12 hours) or N-acetylcysteine 150 mg/kg i.v. over 15 minutes, followed by an infusion of 50 mg/kg in 500 ml of 5% dextrose in 4 hours and 100 mg/kg in a litre of 5% dextrose over the next 16 hours (total dose 500 mg/kg in 20 hours).

   c) If the child is vomiting or unconscious, i.v. N-acetylcysteine is the treatment of choice.

   d) Both agents are of little value if administered more than 15 hours after overdose.

   e) Around 8% those treated with i.v. N-acetylcysteine develop a rash, angioedema, hypotension and bronchospasm.

3. Treatment of hepatorenal failure

   a) Infuse dextrose (10%) i.v. to prevent hypoglycaemia.

   b) Give fresh frozen plasma to maintain prothrombin time (PT) < 60 seconds.

   c) Give i.v. mannitol 1 g/kg body weight to decrease intracranial pressure if hepatic encephalopathy supervenes.

   d) Correct acidosis and maintain electrolyte balance.

   e) Dialysis may be necessary.

PROGNOSIS

- The outcome depends on:
  a) The dose of paracetamol ingested or, more accurately, the dose absorbed.
  b) Whether a protective agent (oral methionine or intravenous *N*-acetylcysteine) has been administered early enough after overdose to prevent liver and/or renal damage.

- The severity of poisoning may be asssessed by measurement of the plasma paracetamol concentration more than 4 hours after overdose and interpreting the result by reference to the figure:

- Children less than 6 years old usually swallow only very small amounts of paracetamol.
- Without treatment, nearly two-thirds of children with a plasma paracetamol concentration above the 'treatment line' will develop severe liver and/or renal damage and about 5% will die.
- If treatment with protective agents is instituted less than 15 hours after overdose the prognosis is excellent.
- If a child presents more than 15 hours after overdose and the plasma paracetamol concentration is > 10 mg/l, measure PT, hepatorenal function and acid–base status (venous sample is satisfactory). Similar investigations should also be undertaken if the history suggests that > 150 mg/kg paracetamol has been ingested. A PT > 20 s at 24 hours or > 37 s at 48 hours suggests that severe liver damage is likely.

FOLLOW-UP

Follow-up is not required once hepatic and renal function have returned to normal.

---

[1] Vale J A, Meredith T J (1985) *A Concise Guide to the Management of Poisoning* 3rd edn. Edinburgh: Churchill Livingstone.

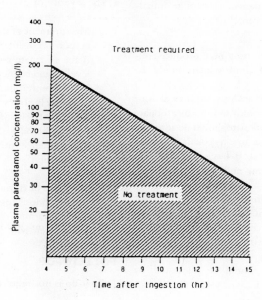

Salicylate Poisoning

Although the ingestion of aspirin is the most frequent cause of salicylate poisoning, percutaneous absorption of salicylic acid and methyl salicylate may result in toxicity. Methyl salicylate is particularly toxic because it is rapidly absorbed and one teaspoonful contains the equivalent of 6.9 g salicylate. In neonates, infants and children, salicylate intoxication may occur inadvertently through placental transfer, breast milk or by the application of teething gels to the gums.

TREATMENT

1. Prevention of absorption

   a) Gastric lavage is effective in preventing absorption of salicylate possibly up to 12 hours after overdose.
   b) Activated charcoal 10–50 g (dependent on the magnitude of the overdose) will significantly decrease absorption if administered within 1–2 hours of overdose, although its administration in young children may be difficult.
   c) Syrup of ipecacuanha is inappropriate because it induces vomiting which may be persistent and thus prevent the use of repeat dose activated charcoal therapy (see below).

2. Correction of fluid deficit, electrolyte imbalance and acid–base disturbance

   a) Vomiting and sweating may produce considerable loss of fluid which should be replaced.
   b) Severe metabolic acidosis requires at least partial correction with sodium bicarbonate i.v. Sodium bicarbonate should be administered with care because hypokalaemia may be aggravated and, if large quantities are given, the sodium and water load may precipitate or exacerbate pulmonary oedema if it is already present.
   c) Hypokalaemia is invariably present in moderately or severely intoxicated children and should be corrected with potassium supplementation.
   d) Hypoglycaemia should be alleviated by 5–10% dextrose i.v.

3. Methods to increase salicylate excretion

   a) Alkaline diuresis is of proven efficacy but it is metabolically invasive.
   b) Repeat doses of oral activated charcoal 10–50 g 4-hourly will significantly increase salicylate elimination; charcoal is best administered by nasogastric tube.
   c) Haemodialysis is more efficient than peritoneal dialysis in increasing salicylate excretion and may be required in the presence of severe intoxication and/or renal failure.

PROGNOSIS

- Salicylate poisoning in children less than 4 years old is often more serious than in older children because of the early development of metabolic acidosis. However, such young children are only occasionally severely intoxicated.
- The severity of overdose may be assessed by:

   a) Measurement of the salicylate concentration as soon as possible, repeated two hours later. If the salicylate concentration has risen the level should be measured again. If the salicylate concentration is > 500 mg/l the child is moderately to severely poisoned.
   b) Determination of the acid–base balance (venous blood is satisfactory).
   c) The presence of the clinical features of intoxication.

- The presence of coma (due to salicylate), severe metabolic acidosis together with plasma salicylate concentration > 900 mg/l indicates a poor prognosis even with energetic treatment.

FOLLOW-UP

Follow-up is not required.

Theophylline Poisoning

Theophylline intoxication in children is usually iatrogenic although it may also be accidental or deliberate, particularly in older children. Convulsions and serious arrhythmias are more common after chronic over-medication than acute overdose (unless the plasma theophylline concentration is > 100 mg/l), whereas the reverse is true of hypokalaemia, metabolic acidosis and hypotension.

TREATMENT

1. Prevention of absorption

   a) Syrup of ipecacuanha is ineffective if more than 5 minutes have elapsed since overdose. Moreover, it will induce or potentiate vomiting and thus prevent the administration of activated charcoal.
   b) Activated charcoal 10–50 g depending on ingested dose is effective if administered 30 minutes after acute overdose; its efficacy thereafter is unknown.
   c) The value of gastric lavage has not been investigated formally.

2. Supportive measures

   a) Treat convulsions: these are usually short-lived but if persistent may be treated by diazepam 2.5–10 mg i.v. or phenytoin 50–250 mg i.v. In persistent cases the child should be paralysed and ventilated until fits have been adequately suppressed. Repeated convulsions may give rise to rhabdomyolysis and acute renal failure.
   b) Correct hypotension with volume expanders and inotropes, such as dobutamine 5–40 µg/kg/minute. Give low-dose dopamine 1–2.5 µg/kg/minute to dilate the renal vascular bed.

3. Correct metabolic abnormalities

   a) Infuse potassium 20–60 mmol/hour to correct hypokalaemia. Alternatively, if the hypokalaemia is severe and a supraventricular tachycardia is present, consider i.v. beta blockade, but remember that the child's asthma and obstructive airways disease may be exacerbated by this therapy.
   b) Correct severe metabolic acidosis by improving cardiac output, preventing convulsions and, if necessary, by infusing sodium bicarbonate i.v.

4. Methods to increase theophylline elimination

   a) Repeat doses of oral activated charcoal 25–50 g 4-hourly will increase theophylline elimination.
   b) If oral charcoal is impossible to administer due to theophylline-induced vomiting, consider charcoal haemoperfusion if the clinical condition warrants this.

PROGNOSIS

- As there is only a general relationship between the clinical features of poisoning and the plasma concentration, theophylline levels can only act as a general guide to the severity of intoxication. A single theophylline concentration on admission may be misleading particularly when a slow release preparation has been ingested. The plasma level should be re-estimated two hours later and subsequently if there is an initial rise in concentration.
- Most symptomatic patients have plasma theophylline concentrations > 25 mg/l and severe intoxication is uncommon at concentrations < 50 mg/l.
- Marked hypokalaemia, metabolic acidosis, repeated convulsions, coma and severe hypotension are poor prognostic factors.

FOLLOW-UP

Monitor compliance and plasma levels in those children who were iatrogenically intoxicated.

Tricyclic Antidepressant Poisoning

Tricyclic antidepressant poisoning remains a significant cause of childhood morbidity and mortality. Sometimes, the drug ingested has been prescribed for the child concerned or a sibling for the treatment of nocturnal enuresis.

TREATMENT

1. Methods to prevent absorption

   a) The value of syrup of ipecacuanha has not been formally evaluated but is contraindicated because of the hazard involved if the child subsequently becomes comatose.
   b) Gastric lavage and activated charcoal may be of value for up to 12 hours after overdose because of impaired gastric emptying due to the anticholinergic effects of tricyclic antidepressants.

2. Supportive measures

   a) In severe cases, intubation and/or mechanical ventilation will be required.
   b) Hypotension should be corrected by volume expanders and inotropes.
   c) If cardiac arrhythmias supervene sodium bicarbonate should be infused intravenously, even if metabolic acidosis is not present. If this fails, lignocaine may be given, although it may depress myocardial function further.
   d) Convulsions are usually short lived, but if they persist diazepam 2.5–10 mg may be given i.v.
   e) Metabolic acidosis should be corrected with sodium bicarbonate i.v.
   f) Confusion during the recovery period often requires sedation; diazepam is effective.
   g) Physostigmine mesylate cannot be recommended as its action is short lived and it may itself induce serious complications.

PROGNOSIS

- The severity of intoxication may be gauged from:

   a) The clinical features, particularly the degree of coma and cardiovascular impairment.
   b) Associated metabolic disturbances, e.g. metabolic acidosis.
   c) The width of the QRS complex on ECG. If > 0.11 s the patient is severely poisoned.
   d) The plasma tricyclic concentration. If $> 1000\ \mu g/l$ the child is severely poisoned.

FOLLOW-UP

No follow-up is required.

Iron Poisoning

Approximately 5% children admitted to hospital from suspected acute poisoning have taken iron. Between 1968 and 1983, iron accounted for 10 of 1558 deaths in England and Wales in children under the age of ten.

TREATMENT

1. Prevention of absorption

   a) Gastric lavage should be undertaken if > 10 mg/kg body weight of elemental iron has been ingested less than 4 hours previously.
   b) Although desferrioxamine (2 g in 1 litre of water) is customarily added to the lavage fluid or left in the stomach after lavage, its value is unproven although it is unlikely to be harmful.
   c) Syrup of ipecacuanha and activated charcoal have no role in prevention of absorption.

2. Supportive measures

   a) Measures to correct hypovolaemia, hypotension and hepatorenal impairment will be required in a few cases.
   b) Convulsions, if persistent, may be aborted by diazepam 2.5–10 mg i.v.
   c) Metabolic acidosis may be corrected by the infusion of i.v. sodium bicarbonate.

3. Desferrioxamine

   a) If the serum iron concentration is > 90 µmol/l (5 mg/l) and the patient is symptomatic, desferrioxamine should be considered. However, the value of desferrioxamine in acute iron poisoning has not been evaluated as part of any formal clinical trial.
   b) Desferrioxamine is administered in a dose of 15 mg/kg body weight/hour i.v. A maximum of 80 mg/kg body weight should be administered in any 24 hour period. Such a regimen should not lead to complications such as hypotension, although rashes and anaphylaxis have occasionally been reported.
   c) Desferrioxamine may be discontinued when the orange/red colour imparted to the urine by ferrioxamine disappears as this implies that iron is no longer available for chelation.
   d) Desferrioxamine appears to be safe in pregnancy and may save the life both of the mother and her child.

PROGNOSIS

- A child who does not develop one of the following clinical features within 6 hours of ingestion of iron is not at risk of serious toxicity: vomiting, diarrhoea, leucocytosis $> 15 \times 10^9/l$, blood glucose > 8.3 mmol/l or a positive abdominal x-ray for iron.
- Haematemesis, hypotension, metabolic acidosis, coma and shock are poor prognostic features.
- If the serum iron concentration is > 90 µmol/l (5 mg/l) less than 6 hours after overdose, clinical features are likely to be present and the child may need treatment with desferrioxamine.

FOLLOW-UP

Follow-up is not required.

Household Products

The ingestion of household products by children, usually aged less than five years, is a frequent cause for alarm among parents and doctors alike. Serious harm rarely ensues, with the exception of corrosive substance ingestion.

Household detergents

TREATMENT

1. Ingestion of anionic or non-ionic detergents does not require treatment.
2. If a substantial overdose of a cationic detergent has been ingested, expert advice should be sought from a poisoning treatment centre.

PROGNOSIS

- The toxicity of household detergents is determined by the nature of the surfactant used in their composition,.
- Anionic and non-ionic surfactant-containing detergents (carpet shampoo, dishwashing liquid, dishwashing rinse aid (for dishwashing machine), fabric rinse conditioners, fabric washing powder and flakes, general purpose household cleaning liquids and powders, household soaps, scouring liquids, creams and powders) are essentially harmless.
- Cationic detergents, e.g. cetrimide, are far more toxic than anionic and non-ionic detergents, but are rarely found in household cleaning materials and then only in low concentrations.

FOLLOW-UP

Follow-up is not required for anionic and non-ionic detergent ingestion. The complications of cationic detergent ingestion should be followed-up on merit.

Household bleach

Household bleach consists typically of a 3–6% solution of sodium hypochlorite.

TREATMENT

When, as is commonly the case, only small quantities have been ingested, no specific treatment is required, although demulcents may relieve any 'burning' sensation in the mouth and oesophagus.

PROGNOSIS

- As small children usually swallow only small quantities, recovery should be uneventful.
- Older children who deliberately swallow large quantities may develop mild pharyngeal and/or laryngeal oedema.

FOLLOW-UP

Follow-up after hospital discharge is not required.

Corrosive agents

It is rare in the UK for a large amount of a corrosive material such as in oven cleaners (sodium hydroxide), kettle descalers and bath stain removers (formic acid), dishwashing machine powders (silicates and metasilicates), drain cleaners (sodium hydroxide or sulphuric acid) to be ingested, and then it is usually the result of deliberate intent on the part of an older child. The widespread use of these materials in North America particularly, has been accompanied there by a greater number of serious poisoning incidents.

TREATMENT

1. General measures

   a) Pain from ulceration may be severe and opiates are often necessary to achieve satisfactory relief of pain.
   b) Gastric lavage and emesis are contraindicated but demulcents may be used to provide symptomatic relief.

c) Intravenous fluids and blood transfusion for shock and haematemesis.

d) Broad-spectrum antibiotics should be administered.

2. Specific measures

a) Alkali ingestion (including silicates and metasilicates)

i) Endoscopy should be performed within 12 hours of ingestion on all children at risk of serious oesophageal damage (suggested by the presence of visible lesions in the mouth, severe retrosternal or epigastric pain, or if the ingested agent has a pH > 12.

ii) The use of steroids should be considered, to reduce oedema and subsequent inflammation (although there is no good evidence for their value in full thickness lesions in man).

b) Corrosive acid ingestion

i) Correction of acid–base balance with i.v. bicarbonate.

ii) The use of steroids should be avoided unless aspiration has occurred since they may mask the development of abdominal signs and there is no evidence for their value in third-degree burns.

iii) Further management is surgically orientated because most children who ingest significant amounts of acid undergo surgery, if not because of immediate complications, then because of late development of antral or pyloric stenosis.

iv) Contrast radiography, using a water soluble agent, should be undertaken within one hour of ingestion of the acid, followed by endoscopy to the most proximal area of damage (to avoid perforation) within 12 hours.

v) If there is evidence of second or third degree oesophageal or gastric burns, and if signs of sepsis or peritonitis develop, then laparotomy should be undertaken to remove non-viable or marginally viable stomach. A 'second-look' procedure should be considered.

vi) If perforation has not occurred by the seventh day, experience suggests that a laparotomy should be undertaken with a view to antrectomy or pyloroplasty.

PROGNOSIS

- The prognosis and complications, both short- and long-term, are determined by whether the corrosive material is acid or alkaline.
- Oesophageal and gastric damage can occur in the absence of visible oral ulceration.
- In 80% cases, acids spare the oesophagus when ingested but cause coagulative necrosis of the stomach.
- Alkalis damage the oesophagus but spare the stomach (because of the protective effect of gastric acid).
- Immediate and life-threatening complications of corrosive substance ingestion include laryngeal and glottal oedema, and perforation of the oesophagus and stomach.
- Formic acid may also cause acute renal failure.
- Oesophageal stricture formation is a common long-term complication of alkali ingestion.
- Antral and pyloric stenosis are common long-term complications of corrosive acid ingestion. Achlorhydria and protein-losing gastroenteropathy may also occur as late complications. Oesophageal strictures develop in a few patients.

FOLLOW-UP

Follow-up for at least six months to a year is required to exclude the development of oesophageal, antral or pyloric stenosis.

Lavatory deodorants and sanitizers

Modern lavatory deodorant blocks and moth-repellent products contain paradichlorobenzene which possesses little intrinsic toxicity.

TREATMENT

Symptomatic treatment only is necessary.

PROGNOSIS

- Serious poisoning has not been reported in children.

FOLLOW-UP

Follow-up is not required.

Other cleaning products

The combination of cleaning agents may lead to the production of noxious fumes. Chlorine gas and oxides of sulphur are generated by the addition of household bleach to powder or granular lavatory cleaners containing bisulphite. Bleach mixed with ammonia generates chloramine gas, and sterilising tablets (which contain sodium dichloroisocyanurate) mixed with water cause evolution of chlorine gas.

TREATMENT

1. Nebulised salbutamol and humidified oxygen for cough and bronchospasm. If the response is poor, then the use of corticosteroids should be considered.
2. Diuretics and antibiotics have not been shown to produce any definite advantage.

PROGNOSIS

- Serious poisoning is unlikely to have occurred if the child is asymptomatic at the time of arrival at hospital.
- Serious poisoning is indicated by the presence of persistent cough, bronchospasm and pulmonary oedema. Ulceration and oedema of the oropharyngeal mucosa may also be seen in these circumstances.

FOLLOW-UP

Follow-up after hospital discharge is not normally required.

Paraffin oil (kerosene)

In addition to paraffin oil itself, petroleum products form a substantial part of other cleaning materials such as window and mirror cleaners, wax-based polishes and metal polishes.

TREATMENT

1. Gastric lavage and emesis should be avoided

because of the increased risk of chemical pneumonitis.
2. There is no evidence that steroids and antibiotics reduce mortality, respiratory complications, or radiological and pathological changes.

PROGNOSIS

- Pulmonary and neurological complications determine the outcome in children.
- Death in children is usually due to pulmonary toxicity as a result of aspiration and this may develop within one hour of ingestion.
- Serious poisoning is unlikely if respiratory symptoms or radiographic abnormalities (which can occur independently of each other) have not developed within 12 hours of ingestion.

FOLLOW-UP

Follow-up after discharge from hospital is not normally required unless there are persistent radiological changes on the chest x-ray. In these circumstances, the child should be followed-up until such changes have resolved.

Button battery ingestion

Small disc batteries are now frequently employed as energy sources for watches, hearing aids and cameras. They usually contain an alkaline electrolyte (potassium hydroxide or, less commonly, sodium hydroxide), a zinc anode and a cathode of either magnesium, silver or mercuric oxide.

TREATMENT

1. On admission to hospital, an x-ray should be taken to determine the site of the battery.
2. If the battery has lodged in the oesophagus, endoscopic removal should be attempted immediately.
3. It is both unnecessary and impracticable to remove a battery from the stomach or beyond; cathartics may hasten intestinal transit.
4. The use of syrup of ipecacuanha is neither indicated nor effective.

PROGNOSIS

- The outcome should be uneventful provided the battery does not lodge or disintegrate in the oesophagus (usually only when the diameter of the battery exceeds 15 mm).
- If a battery lodges in the oesophagus, pressure and liquefactive necrosis (due to electrolyte leakage) is likely to occur with fatal consequences.
- Leakage of mercuric oxide from a split battery is not usually a toxicological problem as mercuric oxide is converted to non-toxic elemental mercury in the presence of gastric acid and iron dissolved from the corroding steel container of the battery.
- The majority of ingested button batteries (90%) pass through the gut spontaneously, usually within 72 hours.
- Symptoms rarely develop, unless the battery lodges in the oesophagus when anorexia, fever, dysphagia and vomiting may occur. Unless treated promptly these children may die.

FOLLOW-UP

Follow-up after hospital discharge is not normally required.

Abbreviations

AATD	alpha-1-antitrypsin deficiency	**CGD**	chronic granulomatous disease
ACTH	adrenocorticotrophic hormone	**CH**	congenital hypothyroidism
ADA	adenosine deaminase	**Ch1VPP**	chlorambucil, vinblastine, procarbazine and prednisolone
ADH	antidiuretic hormone		
AH	acquired hypothyroidism		
AIDS	acquired immunodeficiency syndrome	**CLH**	chronic lobular hepatitis
		CLT	chronic lymphocytic thyroiditis
ALL	acute lymphoblastic leukaemia	**CM**	cardiomyopathy
		CMI	cell-mediated immune response
ALT	alanine aminotransferase		
ANA	antinuclear antibody	**C-MOPP**	cyclophosphamide, vincristine, procarbazine and prednisolone
ANF	antinuclear factor		
AML	acute myeloblastic leukaemia		
		CMV	cytomegalovirus
ARF	acute renal failure	**CNS**	central nervous system
ASD	atrial septal defect	**CoAo**	coarctation of the aorta
AST	aspartate aminotransferase	**CPAP**	continuous positive airways pressure
AV	atrioventricular		
AVS	aortic valve stenosis	**CPH**	chronic persistent hepatitis
		CREN	continuous rate enteral nutrition
BAS	balloon atrial septostomy	**CRF**	chronic renal failure
BCG	bacille Calmette–Guérin	**CSF**	cerebrospinal fluid
b.d.	*bis die* (two times per day)	**CVP**	central venous pressure
BMT	bone marrow transplant		
BPD	bronchopulmonary dysplasia	**DDAPV**	1-deamino-8-D-arginine vasopressin (desmopressin)
		DHF	dengue haemorrhagic fever
CAH	chronic active hepatitis/congenital adrenal hyperplasia	**DI**	diabetes insipidus
		DIC	disseminated intravascular coagulation
CALLA	common acute lymphoblastic leukaemia antigen	**DM**	diabetes mellitus
		DMSA	dimercaptosuccinic acid
CAPD	continuous ambulatory peritoneal dialysis	**DNA**	deoxyribonucleic acid
		DOCP	deoxycorticosterone pivalate
CCPD	continuous cycling peritoneal dialysis	**DPT**	diphtheria, pertussis, tetanus
CDH	congenital dislocation of the hip	**DSS**	dengue shock syndrome

DTPA	diethylene triamine pentacetate	**HIV**	human immunodeficiency virus
		HP	hyperphenylalaninaemia
EBV	Epstein–Barr virus	**HPV**	human papilloma virus
ECF	extracellular fluid	**HRIG**	human rabies immune
ECG	electrocardiogram		globulin
EDTA	European Dialysis and Transplant Association/ ethylene diamine tetracetic acid	**HTIG**	human tetanus immunoglobulin
		HV	height velocity
		HVA	homovanillic acid
EEG	electroencephalogram		
EHBA	extrahepatic biliary atresia	**ICP**	intracranial pressure
ELISA	enzyme-linked immunosorbent assay	**IDDM**	insulin dependent diabetes mellitus
ENL	erythema nodosum leprosum	**IDM**	infants of diabetic mothers
		IE	infective endocarditis
EPH	extrahepatic portal hypertension	**IFAT**	indirect fluorescent antibody test
ESR	erythrocyte sedimentation rate	**IHD**	ischaemic heart disease
		i.m.	intramuscular
ESRD	end–stage renal disease	**INAH**	isonicotinic acid hydrazide (isoniazid)
FH	familial hypercholesterolaemia	**IOL**	intraocular lens
		IPD	intermittent peritoneal dialysis
FHF	fulminant hepatic failure		
FNH	focal nodular hyperplasia	**IPH**	intrahepatic portal hypertension
FSGS	focal segmental glomerulosclerosis	**IPPV**	intermittent positive pressure ventilation
FSH	follicle stimulating hormone	**IPV**	inactivated poliomyelitis vaccine
GA	general anaesthetic	**IQ**	intelligence quotient
GAG	glycosaminoglycans	**ITP**	idiopathic thrombocytopenic purpura
GBM	glomerular basement membrane		
GFR	glomerular filtration rate	**IUGR**	intrauterine growth retardation
GH	growth hormone		
G6PD	glucose-6-phosphatase deficiency	**i.v.**	intravenous
		IVH	intraventricular haemorrhage
GSD	glycogen storage disease		
GVHD	graft versus host disease	**IVP**	intravenous pyelogram
		IVU	intravenous urography
HB	hepatoblastoma	**IWL**	insensible water loss
HBV	hepatitis B virus		
HCC	hepatocellular carcinoma	**JAS**	juvenile ankylosing spondylitis
HDCV	human diploid cell vaccine		
		JCA	juvenile chronic arthritis

LCT	long-chain triglycerides	**PKU**	phenylketonuria
LDL	low-density lipoproteins	**PN**	parenteral nutrition
LFT	liver function tests	**PNP**	purinucleoside
LRF	luteinising hormone		phosphorylase
	releasing factor	**PPD**	purified protein derivative
LVOTO	left ventricular outflow	**PPHP**	pseudopseudohypopara-
	tract obstruction		thyroidism
		PRA	plasma renin activity
MCN	minimal change	**PT**	prothrombin time
	nephropathy	**PTH**	parathormone
MCT	medium-chain	**PTU**	propylthiouracil
	triglycerides	**PUJ**	pelviureteric junction
MEN	multiple endocrine	**PVD**	pulmonary vascular
	neoplasia		disease
MODY	maturity onset diabetes of	**PVR**	pulmonary vascular
	the young		resistance
MOPP	mustine, vincristine	**PVS**	pulmonary valve stenosis
	(Oncovin), procarbazine		
	and prednisolone	**q.d.s.**	*quarter in die sumendum*
MPS	mucopolysaccharidosis		(four times per day)
MSUD	maple syrup urine disease		
MTC	medullary thyroid	**RDS**	respiratory distress
	carcinoma		syndrome
MVPP	mustine, vinblastine,	**RF**	rheumatic fever
	procarbazine and	**RHD**	rheumatic heart disease
	prednisolone	**ROP**	retinopathy of
			prematurity
NDI	nephrogenic diabetes	**RSV**	respiratory syncytial virus
	insipidus	**RVOT**	right ventricular outflow
NEC	necrotising enterocolitis		tract
NHL	non-Hodgkin's lymphoma		
NT	nasotracheal	**SAS**	subaortic stenosis
		s.c.	subcutaneous
ON	ophthalmia neonatorum	**SCID**	severe combined
OPV	oral poliomyelitis vaccine		immunodeficiency
ORS	oral rehydration salts	**SGA**	small for gestational age
	(solution)	**SLE**	systemic lupus
OTCD	ornithine transcarbamylase		erythematosus
	deficiency	**SMA**	spinal muscular atrophy
		SSPE	subacute sclerosing
PDA	patent ductus arteriosus		panencephalitis
PEEP	positive end expiratory		
	pressure	**TAPVC**	total anomalous
PHP	pseudohypoparathyroidism		pulmonary venous
PIE	pulmonary interstitial		connection
	emphysema	**TB**	tuberculosis
PK	pyruvate kinase	**t.d.s.**	*ter die sumendum* (three
			times per day)

TFT	thyroid function test	**VLDL**	very low density lipoproteins
THAM	tromethamine		
TGA	transposition of the great arteries	**VMA**	vanillylmandelic acid
		VSD	ventricular septal defect
TPN	total parenteral nutrition	**VUJ**	vesicoureteric junction
TRH	thyrotrophic releaser factor	**VUR**	vesicoureteric reflux
		VZ	varicella–zoster virus
TSH	thyroid stimulating hormone		
TSI	thyroid stimulating immunoglobulin	**WBC**	white blood corpuscle
		WD	Wilson's disease
		WHO	World Health Organisation
UCD	urea cycle defects	**WMS**	Wilson Mikity syndrome
UTI	urinary tract infection		
		YAG	yttrium aluminium garnet (laser)
VDRL	venereal disease reference laboratory		
VLBW	very low birthweight	**ZIG**	zoster immune globulin

Index

HEINEMANN
MEDICAL DICTIONARY

Bernard and Mary Lennox

"Excellent short (611 pages) medical dictionary which avoids the obvious and obscure, so concentrating on what is likely to be useful to the average working doctor."

Doctor

Over 20,000 entries
Up-to-date and easy to use
Concise and clinically relevant
Lists generic and proprietary drug names
Explains common abbreviations
Essential for the practising doctor

A new kind of dictionary!

Today's clinician needs a new kind of dictionary. One which is up-to-date, includes only useful information and excludes obsolete and self-evident terms.

Based on a six-year word search of newly published medical journals and textbooks, and updated a year after its first publication, this is just such a dictionary. It is an essential companion for hospital doctors and clinical students.

0 433 19154 6
611 pp, limp, 198 x 129 mm

Further volumes . . . .

This is one of four volumes in the
Treatment and Prognosis series. Other titles
will appear in the near future. The series includes
titles on:

Medicine
Surgery
Obstetrics and Gynaecology

Updated editions will also be published from time
to time. If you are interested in receiving details
of these volumes together with special subscription rates
for the entire series, please write to:

Department TP
Freepost EM17
Heinemann Medical Books
22 Bedford Square
London
WC1B 3BR